Monographien aus dem Gesamtgebiete der Psychiatrie

22

Psychiatry Series

Herausgegeben von
H. Hippius, München · W. Janzarik, Heidelberg
C. Müller, Prilly-Lausanne

G. Guntern

Social Change, Stress and Mental Health in the Pearl of the Alps

A Systemic Study of a Village Process

With 45 Figures

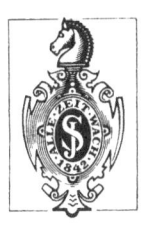

Springer-Verlag
Berlin Heidelberg New York 1979

Dr. GOTTLIEB GUNTERN
Psychiatrie Oberwallis und Psychosomatische Abteilung,
Oberwalliser Kreisspital,
CH-9900 Brig-Glis

ISBN 978-3-642-88193-0   ISBN 978-3-642-88191-6 (eBook)
DOI 10.1007/978-3-642-88191-6

Library of Congress Cataloging in Publication Data. Guntern, G. 1939-. Social change,
stress, and mental health in the Pearl of the Alps. (Monographien aus dem Gesamtgebiete
der Psychiatrie- Psychiatrie series ; 22) Bibliography: p. Includes index. 1. Social psychiatry--
Switzerland--Saas-Fee. 2. Saas-Fee, Switzerland--Social conditions. 3. Saas-Fee, Switzer-
land--Statistics, Medical. 4. Psychology, Pathological--Social aspects. 5. Social change--
Psychological aspects. I. Title. II. Series: Monographien aus dem Gesamtgebiete der
Psychiatrie ; 22. RC455.G86. 301.29'494'7. 79-19790

2125/3130-543210

I dedicate this book to the village of Saas-Fee, also called "The Pearl of the Alps". Its history provoked my keen interest, and its structure, past and present, taught me more about life and human fate than I could have anticipated.

Foreword

I first became acquainted with Dr. Gottlieb Guntern's work at several scientific symposia and was impressed by the way he combined originality and imagination with the proper use of careful, multidisciplinary epidemiologic approaches.

Dr. Guntern has attacked some of the cardinal aspects of the consequences, in terms of health, well-being, and social function, of rapid social change in an originally isolated rural community — a phenomenon that is occurring at an accelerating rate in developing, as well as in developed, countries.

This worldwide problem is approached by Dr. Guntern in a holistic manner. Health and social function are seen as integrated elements of human existence and are studied accordingly. His analysis of social events and their consequences for health and well-being in a small Alpine village can serve as a paradigm for the study of the process of social change and its various consequences elsewhere.

In view of the problem's importance and being impressed by the thoroughness and ingenuity of Dr. Guntern's multifaceted approach, I encouraged him to make the study available to an international readership. Dr. Guntern's book is warmly recommended not only to epidemiologists, sociologists, anthropologists, and psychiatrists, but also to all those interested in psychosocial and psychosocially induced problems in today's and tomorrow's environments.

Stockholm, July 1979

Lennard Levi, M.D.
Director
Laboratory for Clinical
Stress Research

It is wonderful the way a little town keeps track of itself and of all its units. If every single man and woman, child and baby, acts and conducts itself in a known pattern and breaks no walls and differs with no one and experiments in no way and is not sick and does not endanger the ease and peace of mind ot steady unbrocken flow of the town, then that unit can disappear and never be heard of. But let one man step out of the regular thought or the known and trusted pattern, and the nerves of the townspeople ring with nervousness and communication travels over the nerve lines of the town. Then every unit communicates to the whole.

The Pearl
John Steinbeck

Preface

This study attempts to shed some light on one of the dark spots on the descriptive-explanatory map of the contemporary social science. In general, political power, money, decisionmaking, information processing, and cultural events are concentrated in the big cities. City life seems to be *the* life form of our centrury. The question is whether or not this is really the case.

Today more than two-thirds of the world's population live in rural areas. Only few conceptual maps are available describing this territory. There is no coherent systems of coordinates to be spread over the rural areas. This seems to be a conceptual lag of the social sciences.

Comparatively little is known about the life-styles of rural populations and their existential problems. These gaps of knowledge are easily filled with projections. Rural areas are often perceived as scattered fragments of an Arcadian paradise or as the back-yard of society. Both assumptions constitute the end of continuum. They indicate inadequate information. Better information would yield a picture which places rural areas more adequately. In my opinion, the social sciences should try to build bridges over the gulf which separates rural minorities from big cities. This is a difficult endeavor because we deal with a process and not with an immovable object.

Life, one aspect of the great cosmic dance, means change and evolution. Life is a never-ending spiralic process. There are stages in the process when recalibration is needed, when readjustment of all the subsystems and the system as a whole seem to be of vital importance for a given population. A rapidly increasing speed of social change constitutes one of the possible stages of this process. Not every human system is capable of finding an adequate readjustment within the necessary time span. A system lacking the capacity for adequate recalibration is a system in crisis. The crisis is apparent to the observer who tries to look behind the folkloristic make up of the presupposed Garden of Eden or behind the fence of the pressupposed backyard.

Since World War II, more and more rural areas have become industrialized and urbanized. The advent of tourism is one of the many socioeconomic processes affecting villages, towns, and whole rural areas in many parts of the world. In my view, the impact of tourism on the mental and physical health of given populations during the phase of disequilibration should be one of the important fields of social research.

Saas-Fee is a village in the Swiss Alps with a native population of less than 800. Following the construction of a road in 1951, it opened the doors for mass tourism which increased the population considerably at times. 1951 was the time marker of the rapidly increasing speed of social change which had started at a slower speed before. This social change created major problems of a psychosocial and psychosomatic nature.

X

The Saas-Fee study is a follow-up study aimed at the investigation of social change, stress, and mental and physical health in a circumscribed human system — a mountain village. A full and concrete description of these changes is the central goal of my investigation. The methodological goal of my investigation is to demonstrate the systemic or, as I prefer to call it, the syngenetic approach; an approach which aims at the elucidation of the relationships between the subprocesses of social change in the different supra-systems and subsystems of the village. The guidelines of my approach are threefold — I will try to avoid reductionism, which often explains complex social phenomena by reducing them to the features of one element; I will try to show the manifold roots of the social phenomena and their determinants within the web of relations between the innummerable interconnected processes; and, finally, I hope to avoid the role of Procrustes, who adapted a changing and complex reality to the dimensions of his cognitive bedstead which rigidly withstood accommodation to the reality it was supposed to encompass.

This book describes the village process from the prehistoric time, when the first settlers arrived, until 1970. From a purely psychiatric point of view, it is a cross-sectional study analyzing the mental health of the population in 1970. The next cross-sectional study will be made in 1980, followed by another cross-sectional study every decade.

Acknowledgments

In one way or another, there were many individuals involved in the present study. It is virtually impossible to mention, or even to remember, everybody who has offered advice, criticism, or some kind of feedback since I started the investigation in 1968. Thus, I will mention only a few persons whose contributions were especially helpful for the realization of this book.

Professor Christian Mueller, M.D. director of the *Clinique Psychiatrique Universitaire* of Lausanne gave me much support, guidance, and directions; he offered suggestions and criticisms which shaped this study in many aspects; he organized two leaves of absence without which I could not have written this book.

Werner Fischer, Ph. D., sociologist of the *Centre Psychosocial Universitaire* of Geneva gave practical advice concerning methodological problems; he organized the codification, processing, and elaboration of the data of the questionnaire. Mrs. Brooke, Hopital Sandoz, University of Lausanne, was a part-time consultant for statistical questions. Professor Raymond Battegay, M.D., director of the *Psychiatrische Universitäts-Poliklinik* of Basel reviewed the original formulation of the questionnaire. Mrs. Wyss, librarian of the *Clinique Psychiatrique Universitaire* of Lausanne was very helpful in the organization of the bibliographic material.

To all these persons I express my gratitude for their help and cooperation.

I am also indebted to Dr. rer. pol. Anton Bellwald, Brig, an economist whose information was crucial for the understanding of the economic process in Saas-Fee. I am grateful to Beat Mutter, director of the *Schweizerische Kreditanstalt* of Zurich, for his information concerning banking policies of Switzerland.

I wish to express my gratitude to Paul Parin, M.D., Zurich, an ethnopsychoanalyst, for suggestions and advice.

Professor Lennart Levi, M.D., director of the WHO-Laboratory for Clinical Stress Research, *Karolinska Institue* of Stockholm, read the manuscript and suggesting modifications and theoretical clarifications. I am extremely grateful for his critical help.

Part of this study was made possible by a research grant from the Swiss National Foundation for Research; I express my gratitude for this financial contribution which enabled me to work 6 months exclusively at the elaboration of the data gathered during the different field observations.

I should also like ot thank to Mrs. Marcia Vitiello, Philadelphia, who read the first draft of the English manuscript which I had translated from its original German version and who suggested stylistic corrections. My special thanks go to Mrs. Mary Daniels, Ph. D., Philadelphia, who edited the book and whose critical mind proposed many a clarification.

Last, but not least, I wish to express my deep gratitude to the whole population of Saas-Fee. Without the friendly and openminded cooperation of the villagers of Saas-Fee, this study could not have been made.

San Francisco, July 1979   Gottlieb Guntern

Contents

Conceptual Framework and the Methods of Investigation

Development From an Isolated Mountain Village to an International Tourist Resort: Sociological and Socio-Psychological Aspects of the Village Process

Social Change and Stress

Stress Indicators Observed in 1970: Physical and Mental Health Aspects of the Village Process

Conceptual Framework and the Methods of Investigation

1. General Introduction

1.1 Accelerated Social Change in Rural Areas

For centuries rural areas were a symbol of immobility, traditional life, unpretentious contentedness, robust health, and cultural retardation. The lifestyle of yesterday was the lifestyle of today and there was no reason to assume it would change. However, suddenly, to the utter amazement of the inhabitants of these areas, the lifestyle changed, and changed greatly.

Rural areas in the European Alps, following the rhythm of nature, smoothly adapted to the minor changes life generally imposed on human beings. As though in imitation of the gigantic immobility of the surrounding Alps, rural life was petrified in the *conditio humana* of the tradition-directed society with its rigidly maintained social structures. Suddenly, rapid social change, like an earthquake, jolted the rural populations out of their peace and flung them into the chaotic reality of modern life.

Essentially, this era started after World War II. It came in waves of varying intensity and it reached different areas with variable power and efficiency. Some areas were on shaky ground for a long period of time, being unnerved and disoriented — their world changed enormously. The economic infrastructure changed from agriculture and stock farming to the tourist industry, influencing and being influenced by the sociocultural suprastructure. This social change occurred within a few years. It affected all the subsystems of every involved human system and the qualitative and quantitative aspects of this unbalancing and rebalancing process are as yet unknown.

How did this change come about? What are the different threads of events making up the fabric of the social reality analyzed throughout this book? At this point, I will give a global overview of the process of social change. Later, I will analyze it in detail, using the Saas-Fee study as a paradigm for a worldwide process.

The rapid social change in the second half of our century embraced rural areas all over the world — especially in Europe. It has to be seen as a *Gestalt* arising out of the gloomy background of the first half of our century. World War I and its ensuing economic crisis and World War II brought Europe and parts of the western hemisphere to the brink of total catastrophe. Millions of people were killed and the survivors were threatened by famine. The general frustration level was incredibly high and so was the complementary need for relaxation and regression, recreation, and the restructuring of a world in ruins. Apart from the physiological famine, there was a general psychological starvation for joy, fun, and exuberance.

As soon as the economic situation recovered, as a result of the Marshall Plan instigated by the American President Truman, these latter demands became imperative. The society of conspicuous consumption was born. Vacations, formerly a social institution reserved for the upper class, became a democratic custom. Needs create institutions and institutions create demands and these demands need to be channeled and organized. Thus, in a spiralic dialectic process of supply and demand, the upcoming tourism provoked the construction of more and more tourist facilities and these, in turn, increased tourism.

The mountains and the seashores were the preferred sites of tourist institutions. In Europe, the Alps and the Mediterranean were overrun by mass tourism. In the United States, the Rocky Mountains and the Caribbean Sea, as well as the shores of the east and west coast, became fashionable. A similar process occurred, although on a different scale, in many other parts of the world.

Skiing became a sport for the masses, as did swimming, which formerly had been restricted to purely practical goals. Both became expressions of the new fun-oriented morality. A suntan became the status symbol of the new social elite that was widespread, cosmopolitan, and democratic and became a badge of physical and mental health — a symbol of toughness and achievement.

Suddenly, some villages in the Alps — formerly isolated for 6-8 winter months — were discovered and thrown into the vortex of rapid and turbulent social change. Roads were built, new lodging facilities destroyed the architectural homogeneity of the old villages, a web of cablecars and ski lifts began to spin over hills and mountains like spiderwebs, and slopes were cut through the forests, tearing deep wounds into groves of spruce and larch. These examples were only the most obvious indicators of a fundamental social change.

The speed and thrust of social change were often faster and stronger than the prudence of sober minds, and consequently, there was little planning. When the rush was over, villages and entire landscapes were damaged — often irreparably. It seems to be a natural law of modern tourism that it destroys the landscapes which engendered it — growing like a cancer with multiple autonomous centers and escaping control and invading and destroying the very life substance from which it is nourished. Thus, the inhospitability of the big cities, deplored and attacked by Mitscherlich (256), reached the villages of the Alps, often breeding in its midst bastards and monsters, at least from an esthetic point of view.

Nature and man are related elements within an ecological system; they influence each other. Thus, as the environment changed in Saas-Fee, the behavior of the villagers changed. This latter change was of a less obvious nature than the change in the landscape. In fact, it affected the deepest layers of the human (i.e., people) ecological system. The villagers changed in multiple ways — in behavior, roles, ideas, beliefs, attitudes, and values. Their somatic, psychological, and social identities altered. The profound social changes created stress. The inhabitants of this changing human system tried to cope with the stress using all the strategies available. Not every one was resourceful or successful. Some of the people developed a great number of pathological symptoms which are the observable indicators of a disturbed homeostasis.

Tourism introduced industrialization, urbanization, and the above outlined social change with all its consequences in different rural areas the world over. Such worldwide processes deserve the attention of social scientists — including psychiatrists. To my knowledge, the study of Saas-Fee is the first comprehensive contribution by a psychiatrist to this topic.

The village process in Saas-Fee can be seen as a paradigm of a more general process. Thus, the results of this study will help to understand corresponding processes of social change in other rural areas transformed by modern tourism or other forms of industrialization and urbanization.

1.2 Synergetic*Approach to the Study of Saas-Fee

The investigator of a process of social change faces a series of basic and interconnected questions. How do the people of a human system — in our case an isolated village in the Swiss Alps — react when it is transformed almost overnight into a famous tourist resort? What happens to people who give up agriculture and stock farming in order to manage a beautiful landscape — a scarce resource — or by renting and selling it to tourists? What are the social institutions and the roles and behaviors which change? How do these people cope with stress and the vast range of stressors which impinge upon their daily life? What is the role of acculturation (i.e., the taking over of new values, attitudes, and behaviors) in the process of social change? How does acculturation influence the process of socialization [i.e., of in-formation (cf. 151)] of the younger generations? How do the physical and mental health of the population change under the impact of stressors and stress? Is it possible to integrate into a program of preventive health care the preventive and/or curative procedures suggested by the results of this study?

The investigation of a social process requires special conceptual tools. In my syngenetic[1] approach, I use a holistic concept integrating, among others, theories of social change, stress, communication, cybernetics, structuralism, system theory, and general system theory. These conceptual tools will be discussed later.

What is the syngenetic viewpoint?

A village process, i.e., the change of village structures in time, cannot be described in isolation from the surrounding world. A village is only one thread within a social web that includes the whole world. The single thread can only be fully understood in terms of the whole web and within the context of all the relations of the eco-social network which constitutes the world.

I agree with Ribeiro (294, p. 149) that the world has become a symbiotic system since the Industrial Revolution. In this system, the big cities and the small villages are interconnected. There is a continuous flow of matter-energy and information which maintains the homeostasis of the whole world structure. A change at a given point will influence all other points, although to a varying extent. This means that we have to deal with a very complex reality. Whenever we face complexity, the pitfall of a simplifying reductionism is wide open and we are easily trapped. There are many fallacies in an easy, monocausal, reductionist explanation of the process of social change.

One could, for instance, try to reduce the complex process of social change to the dimension of economy. Marx (240) maintained that a social structure will never change unless all the forces of production are fully developed and that new forms of production never arise unless they have been hatched in the nest of the old society. To a certain extent, this holds true for the process of change affecting the Alps and their population.

---

* *syngeneia* = relatedness, relationship; syn = together; *gignomai* = become, grow, evolve.

Here, agriculture and the economy of subsistence for centuries formed the only important economic base. Technological rationalization and optimal use of the soil soon reached their natural frontier, determined by the geographic situation and especially by the long and hard winters. A growing population at the end of the last century bypassed the production capacity of this economic system. Recurrent famines were the result of an unbalanced ecological system. Emigration was the available strategy to restore the threatened homeostasis. This means that, at this point, economic reductionism has to be given up in favor of the two-dimensional syngenetic approach. The economic and the demographic process were obviously linked.

The Walsers (population of the Swiss Alps) emigrated at different periods to occupy the valleys around the southeast border of Switzerland. Emigration into the cities and – especially at the turn of the century – to North and South America followed. The situation, therefore, was ripe for a basic reconstruction of the economic subsystem. Here lies one, but only one, of the many roots of industrialization in the Alps. We will see later that there were many other reasons for social change – reasons which were interconnected and partly supporting and/or paralyzing each other.

At this point of the discussion, it is important to stress that the process of social change had many causes and many consequences or, more accurately, it produced innumerable phenomena which, depending on the vantage point of the observer, can be described as causes or consequences. Tourism brought bread and alienation simultaneously. Sometimes cultural critics point out only the aspects of alienation. They would prefer to keep the rural areas like a Walt Disney World to which the urban population can escape from their stressful living conditions in the cities.

Alienation is one aspect of the reality; the other is a new self-realization. Alienation, on the one hand, and self-realization and a new way to survive, on the other hand, are the contradictory aspects of reality for the mountain people. Later discussions will outline how the syngenetic approach integrates the different threads of the different structures and processes, weaving them into a rich tapestry – the tapestry of a village with its lights and shadows, lines and plains, hopes and distresses.

The syngenetic approach takes into account this interconnectedness between the different subsystemic processes, causes and consequences, and the apparently paradoxical complementarity of coexisting positive and negative aspects. The syngenetic approach aims at the description of *relations*. While the systemic approach often emphasizes hierarchy and boundaries, the syngenetic approach is directed toward the synapses which link systems and systems, subsystems and subsystems, and processes and processes. In this respect, it is relativistic because we will see again and again that the definition of, for instance, hierarchies depends on the vantage point of description, as does the structure of boundaries.

The syngenetic approach implies certain redundancies since the description of one subsystem or one process sometimes repeat what has already been said in the description of other subsystems or processes. Such redundancy cannot be avoided because it is due to an inherent contradiction between the structure of "outer" reality and the structure of our mind. Reality is a process and processes are of an analogous nature – relations are codified in an analogous manner. Our mind, however, breaks this analogous reality down into binary bits and pieces. Concepts are codified in a digital manner. A digit implies a conceptual relationship of the type "either or" while reality is of an analogous "and-and" or "maybe-maybe" type.

If we construct the whole out of the digits, we necessarily must be redundant to overcome the inherent insufficiency of conceptual tools. This is a restriction in principle which the syngenetic approach shares with many other contemporary concepts. This restriction seems to be unavoidable, at least at the present stage of the epistemological process.

Another feature of the syngenetic approach is that it sometimes leads to seemingly paradoxical and contradictory statements concerning the same fact. Reality, however, *is* paradoxical as the modern theory of quantum mechanics unmistakenly demonstrates. Seen from a certain vantage point, a village, family, or individual is unstable. Seen from another vantage point, the same entity is stable. Relativity theory taught us that reality changes depending upon the position of the observer. The syngenetic approach implies a constant shift of the position of the observer and thus unavoidably leads to contradictory statements which are only the complementary aspects of what we call "truth."

1.3 Rural Areas as a Scientific Problem

1.3.1 Historical Neglect

According to Levi and Anderson (218, p. 47), 72% of the world population lived in rural areas in 1970 (the year I gathered most of the field material). Given this quantitative situation, we should assume that the social sciences have been eager to study the life conditions of rural areas. A short overview of the current scientific literature shows that this has not been the case.

In 1887, Knapp (cf. 199, p. 5) postulated a sociopolitical history of the rural population – a postulate which seems not to have affected the urbanocentrism of social science.

What are the possible reasons for this historical neglect?

Universities are mostly situated in the big cities and, consequently, the scientific process is centered around urban life due to political, economic, and psychosocial factors. The rural areas have remained a *terra incognita* with an aura of provincialism – another word for backwardmindedness – at least in the semiofficial etymology of many city dwellers. The lack of adequate knowledge about the rural topos fostered projection processes that instrumentalized the rural areas and made them increasingly taboo for cognitive and scientific exploration. Berner (27), quoting Lamarche, outlines the following reasons for the univestigated conditions of rural life: the myth of the healthy and natural rural life; the wrong assumption of many economists of the future world as an urbanized agricultural society without rural milieu; and finally, the lack of communication between urban and rural populations due to the country folks inability for articulation.

Jaeggi (175), one of the rare exceptions, made an important sociological study in a region of rural Switzerland.

There has been, however, an astonishing interest in the exotic cultures of so-called primitive rural societies, as illustrated by the works of many ethnologists [e.g., Bateson (16), Benedict (25), Levi-Strauss (219, 220, 223), Malinowski (235, 236) and Mead (246-248)]. The cult of the exotic was a catalytic antithesis to the urbanocentric thinking.

Epistemologically, the strange object of investigation and the cultural distance between observers and investigated objects facilitated the scientific investigation and, as a byproduct, it fostered interdisciplinary research. Anthropology and psychoanalysis, for instance, are combined in the works of Freud (105, 108), Morgenthaler and Parin (259-260).

Levi-Strauss (219, p. 344) explains that ethnologists often hate their own culture and, therefore, have a fascination for exotic cultures. This may or may not be the case. In my view, love of adventure, romanticism, and the search for the perfect *bel objet* are equally important reasons for seeking the exotic. In short, the quest might be one for the lost paradise.

In 1949, Murdock (cf. 196, p. 187) proposed to compare modern social behavior with its prototypes in order to determine some basic universals. As fruitful as this may be, such a comparison has inherent pitfalls. Freud (105, p. 445), despite his own occasional indulgence in oversimplifications, warned against such shortcuts because they blur the cognitive field. Nevertheless, our cultures have been explained with conceptual tools developed in primitive societies and simple analogies often crystallize to structural homologies. The postindustrial society is explained in terms of neolithic microsocieties of the South Pacific.

In order to better understand our own culture, we should investigate its own prototypes, which are still existing, right in front of us. We ought to grasp them before they vanish in the process of an all-engulfing social change. These prototypes have survived in rural areas where the slower speed of social change has preserved the forerunners of our civilization. Their investigation, however, creates important problems. Since Einstein and Infeld (89) and Heisenberg (150), we know that the observer influences and changes the object observed. This is especially the case when the cultural distance between observer and object observed is small. This is a general epistemological problem (cf. 129).

Since World War II, this formerly stagnating topic has slightly moved. An increasing number of studies are published although they do not achieve the quantitative importance of the urban investigations. Wylie (373) described a village in the French Vaucluse and Myrdal (262) wrote a fascinating report about the village Liu-Ling in Central China in the process of social change introduced by the communist revolution. Both authors painted a vivid and colorful picture. Myrdal (262) avoided a theoretical analysis in order to preserve the authenticity of his report while Wylie (373) made some theoretical attempts to penetrate his topic.

Jaeggi (195), Koetter (198-200), and Wurzbacher and Pflaum (376) have advanced the theoretical grasp of rural populations. Strotzka (346) did an unusual mental health study of rural populations in Europe. My own attempt is to link the sociological aspects of a village with stress and mental health problems in a holistic manner. It is a comprehensive study dedicated to the life conditions of rural areas. Partial results have already been published (cf. 124-128, 132), although without the broad theoretical approach of the present study. Here, I link the different aspects in a syngenetic way to the underlying and/or concommitant changes in the different subsystems of the ecosystem Saas-Fee.

1.3.2 Myth of the Healthy Country Life

Where appropriate knowledge is lacking, myths flourish like mushrooms. Cassirer (52, p. 5) wrote that myths are the forerunners of history. History, however, presupposes written accounts which, due to the historical neglect of rural areas, are lacking.

The average city dweller who visits the countryside on weekends tends to perceive it as a peaceful homogeneous Arcadia devoid of quarrels and stress. He perceives what he wants to perceive. He walks or drives through the villages and projects the innocence and peaceful slumber of Sleeping Beauty onto them (199, p. 10). – "There is no sin on the alp." This verse in an old song aptly translates the stereotypical belief of the city dwellers. The countryside is the apple that conceals no worm. The sturdy sensuality of the villagers is nature personified. This easy anthropology is reinforced by the traditional architecture fitting organically into the landscape like in Frank Lloyd Wright's dream of the integrated ecological system.

But times move on, the projected colors are fading, and, as Oswald (266, p. 36) observed, the picture of the Arcadian village grows dim. Simultaneously, its negative aspects, denied for so long, become apparent and, for many observers, preponderant. Hacker (134, p. 16) emphasizes that the systemic denial of aggression tends to provoke its opposite. The alarmed citizen is full of indignation. He points his finger at the new picture which breaks through the brittle canvas. He sees a rural population either vegetating in apathy or shaken by rapidly changing times. All at once he sees the villagers unbalanced like himself – indulging in aggressions, drinking heavily, and sometimes showing signs of an incipient anomie.

The negative aspects are but one side of the coin. It may be helpful to remember what Mendel (250, p. 79) observed: the search for the absolute is undertaken by people governed by the archaic mother (i.e., the irrational fantasies). Relativity, however, is a feature of the scientific father (i.e., the principle of rationality). Although I disagree with this terminology, I accept its basic message. The process of relativism and the complementary description of both sides of the coin, according to the Chinese T'ai-Chi T'u, has to be guided by rational analysis. We only then will find the Yin and the Yang, the negative and the positive, which are the indispensable and complementary constituents of all reality.

1.4 Antithesis of Rural Versus Urban Areas

Thus far, the two terms "rural" and "urban" have been used in an antithetical way which simplifies and, consequently, distorts reality.

Niehaus (cf. 199, p. 9) conceptualized urban and rural areas as integrative phenomena of the same socioeconomic and sociocultural process. The philosopher Bloch (33) assumes that rural and urban areas are to be found at different positions on the diachronic axis – rural areas preserve cultural petrefacts and fossilia which cannot be found any more in urban areas. Koetter (199, p. 15) places rural areas in the position between yesterday and tomorrow. Old behaviors and new technological devices challenge each other and create the so-called cultural lag (Ogburn). Cultural lag refers to the difference in the developmental speed of economic infrastructure and sociocultural superstructure, the latter being retarded. Ultimately, this terminology refers to the thinking of Marx, as Dahrendorf (69) rightly points out.

For more practical purposes, it is important to note that rural areas actually experience two cultural lags — one inherent to their structure and the other in relation to the cities.

The rural-versus-urban antithesis is a dichotomy of historical value which has to give way to a concept of complementarity. In this sense, Koetter (199, p. 28 ff.) speaks of a rural-urban continuum whose corresponding process has been labelled as "rurbanization" (Galpin), a two-way processing of information leading to mutual interactions and adaptations. Rurbanization, although functioning in both ways, has a preferred direction: the flow from the cities to the countryside is more important than vice versa, i.e., the countryside is more influenced than the cities. The rural areas produce holiday resorts and new roles, but no longer cheap labor and agricultural products for the cities. The rural areas manage their old resources in a new way — they rent and sell nature with its sun, water, snow, and mountains. Nature, made accessible by modern technology, has become a merchandise to be traded to the urban guest.

Koetter (199, p. 158) ascribes four roles to rural areas: the production of agricultural goods, the organization of trade and industry, permanent habitation for its population, and recreational areas for the urban population. The three latter functions are particular to tourist resorts in all parts of the world.

Koetter (200, p. 604 ff.) formulates some operational criteria to allow for a differentiation between rural and urban areas. Rural areas are characterized by small communities with a low density of population, dominance of agriculture, natural environment, homogeneity of population, low stratification, and low mobility. Relationships are mainly of a personal and informal nature. Urban areas, by contrast, are characterized by large communities, high density of population, almost exclusively nonagricultural occupations, locations far from nature, heterogeneous population, extreme stratification, and extreme mobility. Secondary formal relationships are predominant.

Although such a differentiation can be helpful in certain cases, it is not adequate in the case of Saas-Fee. The tourist resorts show a reality for which an interconnected patchwork of the above criteria holds true.

When tourism affects the mountain villages in the Alps, the old relationships between rural and urban areas change. In the pretouristic periods, urban areas exploited rural resources, as Bellmann et al. (21, p. 119) made clear. Today, part of the urban surplus flows back to the tourist resorts where it is sacrificed on the altar of conspicuous consumption, according to the new philosophy that one is what one consumes. The villagers, of course, are interested in exploiting these rituals of self-realization.

Summarizing this chapter, we can say that there are differences between rural and urban areas. They are, however, dynamically changing in the industrialized and partly urbanized tourist resorts. Careful analysis reveals the chatacter of these differences.

1.5 Social Change in Rural Areas

The economic development of the postwar era has led to the phenomenon of mass tourism. The transfer of people and money to rural areas has been substantial. Scheuch (316, p. 802) indicates that in 1964 international tourism accounted for an expenditure of 30 million German Marks. In 1967, West German holiday makers spent approximately 6.4 billion German Marks in foreign countries. According to a Swiss study in 1974, 67 million Europeans spent their vacations in foreign countries.

The over-organized industrial man, accustomed to a well-defined time budget and clearly prescibed roles and functions, was unable to spend his vacations in a nonorganized way. The eager rush into freedom often ended quickly in boredom and irritation. A well-organized tourist infrastructure became increasingly attractive. Rural areas, fighting for their own survival, met the challenge and within a few years all the major tourist resorts in Europe were built. The people of Saas-Fee abandoned agriculture quickly and without much regret. They changed their economic basis, moved into new occupational roles, and made easy cash, an experience they had rarely had before. Their world changed rapidly and for the better. Gradually, they adopted a new identity and were no longer the pariah from the backyard of society − they were now right in the center. Geography, previously a handicap, was now an advantage. They could sell what they had in abundance − nonpolluted nature. The "retarded" mountain dweller was catapulted into the glamorous roles of the suntanned ski instructor or the adventurous mountain guide. He became the genuine prototype of the healthy life − the primal man of nature − roaming freely in the wide spaces between the mountain peaks and the valleys of the much admired Alps. His social clumsiness, ridiculed before, was now perceived as a symbol of authenticity.

This transition, however, was not as smooth as it might appear. In fact, it was stressful. The tourist facilities caused an important economic burden for community, families, and individuals. Their economy now unexpectedly depended upon the political and economic situation of Europe and the world to a degree they had never known before. The villagers made unilinear extrapolations from their actual situation and forgot the wisdom of their forefathers that the world process is spiralic, with recurring ups and downs. Soon, the whole population increasingly suffered from strain. They tried to cope with it and prayed to their Lord, worked harder, developed psychosomatic disorders, and increased their alcohol and drug consumption. Progress, obviously, had its price.

The new tourist resorts in the Alps developed a new sociocultural formation, a term coined by Ribeiro (294). Their economic basis had changed and the ideological superstructure, with its values and norms started to change as well. The formerly tradition-directed society (297) became increasingly achievement-oriented and inner-directed. The intergenerational gap widened and created additional stressors. The widening cultural gap between the development of the superstructure and the development of the infrastructure constituted, as Riesman (297, p. 57) pointed out, a dynamic factor pushing social change even further. Each stage of development had to be paid for with money, energy, and stress.

The specific features of this process in Saas-Fee will be discussed later.

1.6 Rural Areas in Crisis?

The question is: are the above-mentioned features of the village process indicators of a crisis or are they "normal" symptoms of social change?

According to Habermas (135, p. 39), a social cirisis is a situation in which the economic basis and the sociocultural superstructure threaten the identity of the individuals. Saas-Fee and many tourist resorts in the Alps, show certain signs and symptoms of such a crisis. The perplexity and helplessness of many natives, leading to heavy alcohol consumption and psychosomatic symptoms, are indicators of systems in which control by clearly formulated norms is insufficient. To paraphrase Fromm (111, p. 56), the villagers sometimes seem to be the helpless appendix of forces which are the rigidified expression of their world and of alien forces which they no longer understand. A man in a situation he is unable to control or direct is a man in crisis.

Different people deal with crisis in different ways. Fathers pay for what they believe will be a better future for their sons. This produces loyalties with either positive or negative characteristics. Progress has a Janus face — an adequate rebalance can only be achieved over generations. The partial separation from traditional Catholicism and traditional values leaves the individual in a vacuum which produces anxiety. According to Marx and Engels (cf. 110, p. 30), the mind is the matter translated into the head of a human being. This matter has yet to be translated to shed light into the *camera oscura* of the new reality of many villages. Anxiety and insecurity accompany this crisis which, at first sight, is not obvious to a visitor. To perceive it, we have to look for indicators which translate the system's crisis into observable units of interpersonal transactions.

The stress indicators in Saas-Fee will be discussed later.

1.7 The Village as a Habitat of Regeneration

The development of tourism ascribed a new role to formerly isolated villages. They were now expected to be quiet oases for the hustled urban population. Thus, the villages received a mandate to be what politicians and city dwellers wanted them to be — a habitat for regeneration. Koetter (199, p. 169) observed that attractive landscapes are a resource with pitfalls. The villagers who had freed themselves from the former fetters imposed by natural forces were now faced with the new fetters of urban fantasies and demands.

There was a basic misunderstanding because the villagers conceived the relationship with the urban populations differently. They focused on the syngenetic structure of a dyadic system of interaction in which both giving and taking have to be negotiated, but not prescribed. They refused to play the pawn in a game where money was at risk. They refused to accept the occasional city dweller's mentality of a bargain haberdasher and his claims of a czaristic duke. The villagers were, moreover, overburdened with the new roles of hotel managers for which they had not been prepared. Consequently, criticism by the guests were perceived as criticism *ad personam* or aimed at their role identity.

This basic misunderstanding is rarely perceived by the guests who want their "psychotop" (Neutra) to be free of central paraphernalia of normal human interactions. The villagers felt and partly understood the city dwellers' expectations. Because they wanted the guests to be happy and come again, they swallowed the occasional bitterness and tried to keep the urban people in good spirits.

Thus, the new role of the village constituted a considerable source of stressors, at least for one constituent of the interactional system (i.e., the villagers).

1.8 The Village as an Object of Research

The study of the process of social change requires adequate entities of observation which can be a single transaction, an individual, a communication system (including at least a sender, receiver, and communication channel), a family, a village, or the society as a whole. Each of these units is a legitimate entity of observation and yields a certain set of results. I chose the village. It is a microcosm and a well-defined human system which permits the integration of several conceptual approaches. Our century has witnessed the investigatory shift from the individual to the family and, therefore, my choice constituted a logical further step in the general scientific process.

Several authors stress the value of the village as an object of research. Redfield (291) shows that the village was at all times the predominant form of human organization. Koenig (195, p. 334) made clear that the small community articulates the image of the larger society in each of its inhabitants, thus shaping identity and fostering social integration. Bernard (26) writes that a community has to be seen in a systemic view and that it contains a hierarchy of subsystems and suprasystems whose interactions have to be carefully studied and analyzed.

It seems that this way of thinking is winning an increasing number of disciples. According to Ahrensberg (7, p. 498 ff.), the study of the community is gaining growing importance in the field of social sciences and, if it is studied with a systemic ecological approach, it will help to explain how almost identical environments create different cultures with different norms and behaviors and different styles of transactions. Knoetig (190) and Wein (365, p. 727) stress that this is a scientific problem of general importance.

The systemic ecological approach raises the question of the *oikos* — the environment of a human system. Human environment is, to a great extent, composed of history and ideas. How can we study ideas? Questionaires only provide information about rationalizations, but not about the implicit norms which govern human transactions. Direct field observation, however, yields valuable information about ideas and their governing rules and, thus, about the ecology of human systems.

Since the Saas-Fee study is a paradigm, the question arises whether or not similar research in other tourist resorts will lead to comparable results. If the principle of equifinality, formulated by von Bertalanffy (28, 29), holds true, we should be able to predict that human systems with identical organizations produce identical structures independently of their historical background. All tourist resorts have, for functional reasons, the same set of organizing principles and, therefore, comparable social organizations. This and many other questions can better be answered when future research sheds more light on the situation of small communities in rural areas raised to the status of international tourist resorts.

To readers who are not interested in purely theoretical and methodological considerations, I suggest to pass over the following chapter and to continue with part II (4 f.f.). Part II deals with the many aspects of the development of Saas-Fee from ancient times to 1970, when the village had become an extraordinary holiday resort.

2. Theoretical Problems of Social Change

The theory of social change developed by sociology is of crucial importance for the Saas-Fee study. It is, however, far from being comprehensive or sufficient (cf. 124-127). In the following section, the actual state of sociological concepts of social change will be briefly discussed in order to outline some aspects of the theoretical framework of this study.

2.1 Concept of Social Change

Social change is a term introduced by Ogburn (cf. 299). It has been used in an inflationary manner, a fate it shares with many other scientific constructs (378, p. 18). The notion of social change has, according to Bendix (23, p. 178), Eisenstadt (90, p. 76), and Zapf (378, p. 11), subsumed other notions such as development, modernization, social dynamics, transformation, revolution, evolution, differentiation, circulation, fall, specialization, and complexity. Obviously, this phagocytosis changed the character of the notion itself, making it increasingly vague.

Life without change is impossible. The world, as long ago stated by Lao Tsu and Heraclitus, is an ever-changing process. Change is synonymous with life, evolution, and process. Given all these definitions, it is understandable that the term of social change was overstretched or became meaningless. Tjaden (356, p. 131), for instance, mentions a definition by Gillette and Reinhardt: "whatever changes in society is social change". This definition embraces everything and, therefore, it is not a definition. We should at least differentiate between a simple social event (e.g., the construction of a church) and the historic process of evolution itself. Since the expansion of knowledge depends upon adequate cognitive tools, an increase of knowledge is impossible when terminology is suspended in a fog of nondifferentiation.

Fromm (110, p. 28) outlines that a competent definition of social change has to consider the view of historical materialism and, therefore, describe the processes of active and passive adaptation of man to his environment. These processes of adaptation (cf. 199) are increasing in rural areas where industrialization and urbanization are changing social structures and institutions at a high rate of speed.

2.2 Definitions of Social Change

When the basic terminology is vague, the definitions are also vague. The definitions presented in the literature are clearly insufficient. They are heterogeneous (i.e., based on different concepts) and usually reductionist in one way or another – a complex reality is reduced to or explained in terms of a one-dimensional factor. They are, moreover, difficult to operationalize and, therefore, useless in empiric social research.

For instance, Moore (258) defines social change as "the significant change of social structures, i.e., of the pattern of social action and interaction, of values, of cultural products and symbols." However, what are the criteria for "significant"? Don Martindales (cf. 378, p. 13) states that social change "refers to the formation and resolution of interpersonal relations," a definition encompassing everything and nothing. Heintz (149) writes that "social change is the totality of all the structural transformations of a society in a given time span." Again, this definition encompasses everything. Parsons (273, p. 43) identifies social change with the change of normative culture. This definition does not take into account the fact that social change often starts in the economic basis which creates, in an interactional process, with the ideological superstructure, the change in the normative rules. Nevertheless, Parsons's definition is important insofar as it considers the hierarchy of a social system in a quasi-quantitative approach. He speaks only of social change when the highest hierarchical level – the level of norms – is affected. However, a cybernetic model of explanation should not forget the feedback processes between the top and the bottom of a hierarchical system.

Boskoff (cf. 356, p. 151), obviously influenced by Parsons, writes that the social change is "the collective deviation of established patterns," a definition including simple social events as well as the historic process itself. Almond (9, p. 217) defines the change of a system as "the achievement of new capacities which change the whole structure." This definition aims at a specific form of social change in a political system. Deutsch (74, p. 330) gives a more comprehensive definition. He uses the term "social mobilization," defining it as a process in which major parts of old social, economic, and psychological ties are disrupted and people are prepared for new forms of social structures and behaviors. Bendix (24, p. 510) specifies that the above definition is only applicable to a particular case of social change, starting in the eighteenth century, consisting of the progress of a few pioneer societies and triggering the social change of their followers. This same notion is refined by the term "partial modernization," used by Ruesche-Meyer (307, p. 382) who defines it as "a process of social change leading to the institutionalization of relatively modern social forms side by side with less modern structures in the same society."

Jaeggi (175) gives a more operational definition – change can be measured indirectly by the change of patterns of behavior and interactions, by the transformation of institutions, and by the transformation of needs and expectations. Although this definition is certainly useful, it does not contain quantitative criteria to allow statements of emergent qualitative modifications. These criteria have yet to be developed.

All these definitions are often contradictory, always insufficient, and, at least partially, mutually exclusive. Yet, there is a growing consensus (cf. 378, p. 11) that "the transformation of social structures must be the central feature of the phenomenon of social change." Lockwood's (226, p. 124) definition is an indicator of this new consensus, "the notion of social change describes a transformation of the institutional structure of a social system and, more exactly, a restructuring of the predominant institutional order of a society, so that we can speak of a change in the type of a society." It remains to be defined what a social structure is.

The notion of social change is interconnected with the notion of "system crisis," especially when social change occurs at a high rate of speed. It is, however, difficult to define the boundaries and content of social systems which are supposed to be in crisis 135 p. 11) in a systemic language, because social systems change not only their elements, but also their target values, in order to resolve control problems. Watzlawick et al. (363, p. 136 ff.) stress that human systems have metarules which enable them to change their calibration as soon as the process of social change demands new forms of behavior and new value patterns. In this area, the terms "social change," "transformation of structures," and "systemic crisis" are sometimes overlapping.

Summarizing this discussion, we can say that none of the above-mentioned definitions is generally accepted. More detailed reasons will be discussed later. Here, two major causes for the wide range of definitions are mentioned:

1. The difinitions are based upon different conceptual frameworks (e.g., general or normative functionalism, old or the new theories of evolution, cybernetics, systems theory, conflict theories).
2. Different authors have different units of observation (e.g., international or national systems, complex or primitive societies, political subsystems, sociocultural subsystems.).

Since my unit of observation is a mountain village in the process of rapid social change and since this study is based on a syngenetic (e.g., systemic, cybernetic, holistic, ecologic) conceptual framework, I propose a special definition for my own purposes — *social change is the measurable transformation of system structures occurring in the different subsystems* (e.g., demographic, economic, technological, political, religious, sociocultural) *which have a specific social organization* (e.g., nuclear families, kinship systems, generations, interest groups) *and different roles for the individuals involved. Social change affects all the subsystems and all the suprasystems of the village, although in varying order and at varying speed, intensity, and direction.* This definition enables me to describe and analyze, step by step, how and to what extent social change occurred. As we will see later, the question of quantification of the different elements in this definition is still often unresolved.

2.3 Theories of Social Change

Since the definitions of social change are insufficient, it is likely that the theories of social change are insufficient too. This has been outlined by Jaeggi (175) and Dahrendorf (69), with the latter criticizing the theory of social change as "the underdeveloped nucleus of sociological theory." Similarly, Don Martindale (cf. 356, p. 121) holds that the theory of social change is "the weakest branch of sociological theory."

Parsons (270), p. 486) assumes that it is too early for the formulation of a comprehensive theory since we do not know enough about the process itself. This seems to be a convincing argument. On the other hand, Dahrendorf (69, p. 108) writes that Parsons is partly responsible for this lack of basic knowledge because his static view has fostered the neglect of the phenomena of change. In 1937, Parsons put the question of "what holds society together" before the question of "what makes it advance." Thus, problems of integration and maintenance of stability became preponderant. This development in scientific theory is historically explicable. In 1937, the world had experienced a world war, an economic crisis, and was heading for a second world war. Thus, stability — the nature of stability and the search for stability — was manifestly important.

However insufficient the attempts at a theory of social change are, some of them are outlined here for two reasons; first, for the sake of a brief structured overview of the state of theory which is essentially the available instrumentarium for describing the process of social change in Saas-Fee; and second, the later discussion of the conceptual insufficiencies will make clear why the description of social change in Saas-Fee shows some gaps, overlappings, or even contradictions.

2.3.1 Functions of a Theory of Social Change

A theory of social change for rigorous scientific research should provide, as Zapf (378, p. 14) and Homans (157, p. 97) make clear, a deductive system of propositions which does three things — formulates general assertions (i.e., laws of social change); defines the necessary starting and marginal conditions, and it deduces falsifiable hypotheses (i.e., the prediction of events). This deductive system of propositions should not only articulate a model of social change and translate it into a system of symbols using a functionalistic, conflict-theoretical, cybernetic, or related language, it should also explain the process. According to Dahrendorf (69, p. 110), such an explanation should reduce the observed complexity of phenomena to a few structural dimensions of the social system without falling into the trap of a psychological reductionism as do, for instance, Hagen (138), Homans (156) and Tjaden (356).

Dahrendorf's (70) criticism seems justified, but, from a syngenetic viewpoint, it has to be modified. Explanations in a cybernetic model should not reduce phenomena to one structural dimension. Rather, they should be put into *relations* with each other. Reductionism of a psychological or systemic-structural character has to be avoided. Social structures influence human beings and are, in turn, influenced by human beings. History is made by man (cf. 32) who is woven into a web of relationships in the space-time continuum of ecological systems.

2.3.2 Sufficient Conditions for a Theory of Social Change

In my opinion, an adequate theory of social change should fulfill three basic conditions — it should provide an exact description and explanation of systemic structures and of systemic processes, permit quantification of the variables of structures and processes and allow the prediction of future events in terms of probability.

In order to define the Gestalt of social change, we need to describe the matrix of the background — the boundaries of systems, subsystems, and suprasystems; the horizontal and vertical structures of subsystems and suprasystems; the hierarchical organisation of roles and transactions; and the basic functions of systems, subsystems, and supra-systems. According to Parsons (273, p. 35 ff.), the basic functions of a stable social system are pattern maintenance, integration, goal-attainment, and adaptation. The description of systemic processes should involve processes of maintenance and processes of change. The balance of both subprocesses indicates whether or not social change has occurred in a system or whether or not there was only a postcritical restabilization.

Models based upon system theory [e.g., Cadwallader's (49), Etzioni's (94), Parsons' (270-273)] allow for quantification of the described processes, although such quantifications cause considerable practical problems. I agree with Zapf (378, p. 26) that the above-mentioned models are able to outline interesting developments which, in turn, influence the structure of future theories. Models formulated in a cybernetic-systemic language which take into account probabilistic and stochastic processes allow for the later creation of "situational models," as postulated by Deutsch (73, p. 200). A preliminary condition (cf. 181, p. 500) for the formulation of such models is a grammar of transformation which describes the set of rules which govern intrasystemic transactions. These rules of transformation should indicate what kind of transformation occurs in a system whenever its homeostasis is disturbed by an interfering factor.

2.3.3 Actual State of the Theories of Social Change

As Rocher (299, p. 58) points out, the first theory of social change was formulated by Marx. According to Marx (240), the unequal distribution of property and control of the means of production leads inevitably to class conflict (i.e., a social revolution – the most extreme form of social change). It starts when the development of the material forces of society's production gets into an antithetical position with the current form of production (*Produktionsverhältnisse*). The inherent contradiction becomes the force which provokes the transformation of the economic infrastructure which, in turn, is followed by a transformation of the ideological superstructure. The cultural lag between the two partial processes is caused, as From (110, p. 59) claims, mainly by the inertia of the "libidinous" structures which need time for a learning process. The learning process – through socialization and acculturation – changes the character formation of the individuals involved in an economic change.

Many of Marx' predictions have been proved wrong by history. His position has been criticised by Koenig (196, p. 215) and Pflanz (274). Hacker (134, p. 147) stressed, moreover, that there is a loss of boundaries between infrastructure and suprastructure. I disagree with the one-directional model of explanation by Marx (240) and some of his orthodox followers. The observation of human systems and, in our case, the process of social change in Saas-Fee shows that economic infrastructure and sociocultural superstructure are changing together and are interacting on many levels. Nevertheless, it is interesting to note that Dahrendorf (69) has amplified the concept of Marx by explaining social change as unequal distribution of power in different social positions – it is the asymmetry of power, not the property, that leads to social change.

Newer theories of social change are found in the works of Cadwallader (49), Etzioni (94), Hagen (138), Kaplan (181), and Parsons (270-272). According to Cadwallader (51) and Kaplan (181) ultrastable systems (i.e., open systems maintaining homeostasis transformation which enables them to maintain homeostasis in the phase of change. As Kaplan (181, p. 502) points out, ultrastable systems "search" actively for new behaviors which restore the disturbed balance of the system. This, however, is not an explanation. The explicanda are already prefabricated and hidden in the definition of ultrastability. Kaplan (181) concedes this theoretical deficit. It seems that cybernetic models are more apt for the formal analysis of processes than for their explanation.

Parsons (270-273) views the social system as a rigidly structured hierarchical system. The level of values, the level of specific norms, the level of organized groups and roles are the constituents of the hierarchical ladder. The upper subsystem controls the lower subsystems. Each subsystem is in a steady state and governed by homeostatic processes and processes of transformation. Social change occurs only when a subsystem is no longer able to neutralize the exogenous and/or endogenous factors of transformation. In this way, the level of norms undergoes structural changes.

The major criticism of Parsons' theory is aimed at the preponderantly unidirectionally conceived model of thinking and its explicative insufficiency. Lockwood (226, p. 136) points out that the normative functionalism in sociology unilaterally underlines the moral aspects of social integration, thus neglecting the question of system integration. These theories also have a tendency to overlook the circular character of systemic hierarchies (cf. 129, 131) and, therewith, the fact that norms are governed by transactions, roles, and the socioeconomic situation as a whole.

Homans (157, p. 97 ff) argues that functionalism overlooks the fact that the carriers of roles — the lowest level in the hierarchy of Parsons — ultimately determine social change and, therefore, explanations have to be of a psychological order. Although I agree partly with this criticism, I am opposed to a psychological reductionism which operates with an either or dichotomy of monocausal models of thinking. Norms determine individuals and individuals determine norms; this is a fact which can be described clearly within a cybernetic model of thinking.

Etzioni (94) proposed a comprehensive theory for the description of macrosociological processes. He (96, p. 147 ff.) differentiates between ongoing and guided change. A theory has to explain the interaction of these two processes and in doing so, it has to avoid two pitfalls; first, reductionism to universal global laws which are too general and, second, reductionism to microsocial laws (e.g., explaining society in terms of individual psychology or of a theory of family systems). Etzioni (94) integrates the voluntaristic approach which stresses the importance of guided change and the collectivistic approach which further stresses the importance of ongoing change. He points out that society is not a monolithic and highly integrated system in which the problem of power can be neglected. Capacity for control (i.e.) power and cybernetic capacities and leadership (i.e., capacity to organize consensus) are central notions in an explanation of social change. Etzioni (94) is especially interested in the processing of information within macrosystems and the problem of decisionmaking. The latter is linked to the members of an elite. Elites decide if and how social change should be accelerated, retarded, or modified in its direction. The process of decisionmaking is also influenced by the actual level of activity (i.e., by the relation between available and potential social resources within a social system). It depends upon the level of activation whether or not mobilization or retardation of social change occur. The theory of Etzioni (94) combines functional, cybernetic, and conflict-theoretical viewpoints. He does not treat society as a perfect supercomputer; rather, he emphasizes that subsystems sometimes possess a high degree of autonomy and control. With all its advantages, Etzioni does not provide an explanatory theory.

One of the newest theoretical approaches to the problem of social change has been formulated by Hagen (138). He investigated social change in agrarian societies and his concepts, therefore, are potentially helpful for my purposes. According to Hagen (138), the loss of status in certain groups leads to insecurity and uncertainty about adequate behavior in the parental generation. The intergenerational conflict leads to a rejection of the norms officially held by the elder generation. In a complex process of interaction among all the constituents of the social web, social change finally occurs leading to innovative-creative behavior in the younger generation. According to Boskoff (cf. 356, p. 151), innovative behavior leads to a collective deviation from the esthablished value patterns. Problems are resolved in a new way and the interaction with the environment reaches a new level. Loss of status is certainly an aspect which produces the potential for change. Again, however, we are dealing with a monocausal reductionism — a simplifying concept — and not at all with a comprehensive theory.

This is, then, the chain of approaches leading from Marx and Ogburn to Hagen. There is no comprehensive satisfactory theory. There is only — in the words of Zapf (378, p. 15) — a collection of different methodological approaches, with different levels of abstraction and varying patterns of logical propositions. We will see later to what extent these theories are useful for this study.

2.4 Factors Responsible for Social Change

The first models of theory for social change were based upon monicausal and unidirectional models of thinking (cf. 123) which logically led to a theory of predominant factors responsible for social change. As discussed previously for Marx, the responsible factor was to be found in the material forces of production and, for Ogburn, in technology. Eisenstadt (92, p. 75) criticises that these authors perceive existing tendencies, overemphasize them, and lift them to the status of central factors and causes.

Today, cybernetic models of thinking have replaced the monocausal and unidirectional models of thinking (378, p. 17). Parsons (270, p. 493) holds that the principle of interdependence of several factors is the central organizing principle in the formation of theories. In a cybernetic system where the different subsystems are controlled by feedback processes, each change in a subsystem constitutes both a cause and a consequence for change in other subsystems. It is difficult to define where a process starts and where it ends. In reality, the beginning and end of the process are defined by the way an observer, at a particular moment, decides to cut into this circle and "flattening" it out to a straight line or "punctuating" it. In a dynamic process, cause and consequence form an interlinked whole (74, p. 329). Again, the same factor can be defined as cause or consequence. In the same sense, economic, political, and social changes occur interdependently and not in a linear sequence (138, p. 352).

Adopting this point of view, Bendix (23, p. 507) emphasizes that factors may be exogeneous and/or endogeneous. Some factors stressed so far by different authors are discussed in the next chapter, partly following a scheme developed by Rocher (299).

2.4.1 Structural-Material Factors

2.4.1.1 Demography

According to Durkheim (cf. 299, p. 38), an increase in the population necessarily leads to an increase in the number of interactions. This interdependence is clearly formalized by Bossard (cf. 196, p. 244):

$$x - \frac{y^2 - y}{2}$$

Where x stands for number of interactions and y for the number of persons involved in an interaction. The increase in interactions leads to a *densité morale* (Durkheim) in which the constituents of the interactional system stimulate each other, introduce a distribution of work, and create a better form of organization raising the society to a higher level of complexity and efficiency.

Observations do not always confirm this theory. In India, for example, the increase of population has not led to a higher form of social organization. On the contrary, increasing population may lead, as Koetter (200, p. 609) emphasizes, to increasing social control which inhibits social change.

2.4.1.2 Technology

For Ogburn (cf. 149), the technological factor is responsible for social change. In fact, the introduction of the steam engine, electricity, electronics, and the systems of telecommunication have changed the world, decreased distances, and increased intersystemic interactions. Rostow (303, p. 305) pointed out that the railroad system was the most important factor in the economic development of the United States, Russia, Canada, Germany, and France. Radio, television, and newspapers connect remote places to the centers and increase the speed of acculturation.

Gehlen (114, p. 13) emphasized that modern technology, natural sciences, and capitalist forms of production stimulate each other and, therefore, the technological factor cannot be separated from the economic factor. In accordance with this view, Ribeiro (249, p. 201) describes the spiralic process in which the speed of transformation continually increases.

Such views are contradicted by Marcuse (237, p. 14), although his arguments are not sustained by facts. Marcuse (237) outlines that the central feature of the technocratic era inhibits the process of social change. This is a prescriptive statement based upon preexisting concepts more than observation. The epidemiologic data prove (cf. 199, p. 156) that the technological factor is, in fact, of crucial importance, especially for social change in rural areas.

2.4.1.3 Economy

Marx (240, p. 15) was the first to emphasize the importance of the economic factor. He stated that "the form of production of the material life shapes the social, political, and spiritual life process." As discussed earlier, this statement is of partial value. It can be considered only in the framework of a comprehensive syngenetic theory. Nevertheless, the structure of the economic base is very important. As Rostow (303) made clear, its influence is crucial in the phase of the economic "take off" where investments in new economic sectors have to be made quickly and the incipient economic growth has to be maintained in such a way that a thorough transformation of the economic subsystem is possible.

2.4.2 Cultural Factors

2.4.2.1 Values

The influence of values upon history has been stressed by Weber (cf. 299, p. 70 ff.) who holds that Calvin's doctrine of predestination and the resulting Protestant ethic were necessary conditions for the modern capitalistic system. The uncertainty about life after death fostered an attitude of rigorous asceticism in which hard work seemed to be the most promising way to salvation.

Empirical studies have offered partial proof of Weber's assumptions. Knapp and Goodrich (cf. 299, p. 82 ff.) were able to show that Protestant institutes and universities in the United States produce significantly more scientists than catholic universities do. Furthermore, Rosen (c.f. 299) observed that American Catholics tend to fatalism, as compared to Protestants. The Catholics less frequently try to reach long-term goals via careful planning. Wendt's study in Germany came to similar conclusions (c.f. 299).

Other studies show that the sex-specific differencies in values might influence social change. Hoselitz and Merrill (164, p. 585) suggest that women are more bound to traditional values than men and, therefore, have a retarding influence on social change. Modern theoreticians, especially Hagen (138, p. 352), stress the influence of values upon social chance. Hagen states that economic growth is possible only when innovative-creative behavior is directed towards production rather than war, philosophy, or art. Lerner (212, p. 364) holding a similar position that describes the personality feature of "mobile sensiblity" is important for social change.

Many authors pay special attention to the transformation of values which occur especially in the process of acculturation as emphasized by Ruesche-Meyer (307, p. 383) and Zapf (378, p. 37 ff.). Acculturation occurs whenever two different cultural systems come into contact. Acculturation, therefore, influences the process of socialization and, with it, social chage.

2.4.2.2 Ideologies

Ideologies are coherent systems of values, ideas, and judgments primarily used by privileged groups to explain and justify their attitudes and behaviors. Conservative ideologies inhibit social change while revolutionary ideologies accelerate social change.

2.4.2.3 Conflicts and Contradictions

Conflicts play a central role in Parsons' concept of strain (270, p. 493). Dahrendorf (69) stresses that conflicts are due to an asymmetry in the distribution of authority. Since authority, unlike power, depends on the social role, the dichotomy between roles endowed with authority and roles without authority generates the conflict which produces social change. In accordance with these views, Riesman (297, p. 252) sees social contradictions as the source of change. He (297) stresses the contradictions between the social character of adults and their social roles as accelerators of social change. Habermas (133, p. 11) holds that social change occurs whenever structural imperatives within a social system contradict one another. Systemic contradictions produce control problems. These, in turn, influence the speed and direction of social change. Finally, Parsons (273, p. 39 ff.) and Hagen (138, p. 358 ff.) hold that loss of prestige and status create social conflicts leading to social change.

Tantler and Midlarsky (350, p. 426) and Davies (70, p. 400 ff.) propose the interesting hypothesis that social change occurs whenever a slowly developing social progress is suddenly interrupted. The resultant discrepancy or "revolutionary gap" between demands or expectations and reality mobilizes the population for social change. In order to make the discrepancy between yesterday and today virulent, the society should have an "active" organization. "Active," according to Etzioni (94, p. 168), means effective control and high consensus steering the process of change. When consensus is high and control ineffective, a drifting social change throws a society into a lower form of organization or chaos.

2.5 Agents of Social Change

The above enumerated factors do not function by themselves. They are mediated and organized by people. History is made by man, although not by every man to the same extent. To paraphrase George Orwell, all men are equal, but some are more equal. There are certain persons with charismatic qualities and there are groups who organize transactional fields. They are able to display leadership, organize the masses, and articulate what others only vaguely feel.

Three specific groups bring about social change — elites, pressure groups, and social movements.

2.5.1 Carriers of Role

2.5.1.1 Elites

The notion of elite was introduced in sociology by Pareto (cf. 299, p. 30 ff.). It was modified by Mosca (cf. 299) who saw in the elite the carriers of power of a class character. In a study made in the United States, Mills (cf. 299) showed that an elite is a group of people who are organized to gain power and dominate society (i.e., a group with special interests, but not bound to any class). Parsons (273, p. 40) explains the efficiency of elites in a topological way — elites are on top of the pyramid of the personality system and, therefore, their influence is virtually unlimited.

2.5.1.2 Pressure Groups

A pressure group has a common political and/or economic goal. It uses money and power (e.g., through strikes, threats and similar means) to reach its goals. It directly influences the political power structure of its country.

2.5.1.3 Social Movements

Social movements are hierarchically organized human systems, formed ad hoc for the pursuit of specific goals (e.g., the protection of civil rights, the protection of the environment). When they are able to spread their ideas, reach consensus, and mobilize the masses, they succed in bringing about social change. They usually influence the political power indirectly via mass media.

2.5.2 Psychological Qualities of the Role Carriers

Elites, pressure groups, and social movements are made up of individuals with particular characteristics. Gandhi, Hitler, Mussolini, and Churchill had special psychological features which, as we know, enabled them to mobilize the masses and, thus, accelerate social change.

Weber (cf. 299, p. 166) claims that the spirit of enterprise was crucial for the rise of early capitalism. McClelland (243) stresses the importance of "achievement motivation" to bring about the industrial era. Parsons (272, p. 114) makes clear that achievement motivation has its functional equivalent on the level of values. For him, achievement is a characteristic value of our time.

Achievement motivation, like other character features, is learned in the process of socialization. McClelland (243) proved that there is a correlation between achievement ideology (i.e., as measured in school tests) and achievement levels of different countries. Toynbee (cf. 299, p. 172) pointed out that achievement motivation depends upon the structure of the goal. If the goal is within realistic limits, it prods the energy and initiative of people; if the goal is too high, it discourages people. Hagen (138, p. 354) describes the psychological features of what he calls the "lower elites, "whose display of creative-innovative behavior is extreme achievement motivation, organization, and a well-defined sense of the lawful structure of their environment. These features enable the lower elites to overcome resignation and apathy and initiate social change.

The appearance of charismatic personalities is, for Eisenstadt (90, p. 86), a social analogy to the notion of mutation in the biologic theory of evolution. Social mutation produces social change. This hypothesis seems to me like an explanatory *deus ex machina* which has a knot of impenetrable intricacies. An adequate theory of elites must explain why and how elites appear at a given point in a process, how and why they are charismatic, and how and why they are able to mobilize the masses. For the time being, we are far from answering these questions.

2.6 Factors Retarding Social Change

According to Parsons (270, p. 496), the direction of social change depends upon two factors – gratification and the possibilities for realization of goals and values. If ongoing social change threatens such gratification or the possibilities for realization, social change becomes retarded. Retardation is also influenced by the requirements of a given system (90, p. 76). Davis (71, p. 486) posits that these systemic requirements are, in themselves, the sufficient conditions of change and, therefore, determine wheter or not social change is accelerated or retarded.

Ogburn (cf. 274, p. 47) describes the following kinds of resistance to social change: the utility of the old culture, vested interests, the power of habituation, forgetting the disadvantages of the old social organization, social pressure, and, finally, the difficulties of innovation. Parsons (270, 271) stresses the retarding function of vested interests which are especially strong in totalitarian systems (i.e., political or religious systems). As times go on, these systems tend to stagnate and to rigidify their structures. Thinking becomes canonized and the developmental process stops or degenerates (cf. 131). Rueschemeyer (307, p. 383) points out that totalitarian systems tend to inhibit any form of social change. From this point of view, we better understand Parsons' (273, p. 40) claim that we can speak of social change only when the level of norms is changing its structure. In totalitarian systems, norms are rigidly fixed, the systemic processes stagnate, and social change only occurs when a revolutionary group imposes other norms.

2.7 Consequences and Manifestations of Social Change

The consequences and manifestations become especially apparent in the phase of the cultural lag which, in itself, is a consequence of the time lag between economic change and sociocultural change. These consequences are especially manifest when change occurs rapidly. If it occurs rapidly, the cultural lag widens and, suddenly, man lives in the economic world of today, although he still maintains the values, ideas, and attitudes of yesterday. As a consequence, there is now a human system in which the control subsystem (i.e., sociocultural subsystem) is partly disconnected from the other functional subsystems (i.e., mainly economic subsystems).

According to Parsons (273, p. 41 ff.), the characteristics of social change depend upon five variables: the quantitative aspects of inductors of change, the number of involved subsystems, the structure of the involved subsystems, the functional importance of the involved subsystems, and, finally, the degree of resistance of the different subsystems. The specific configuration of these variables determines the nature of change, its speed, and its consequences. The most extreme consequence is the dissolution of the system. Eisenstadt (92, p. 79 ff.) and other authors offer similar concepts.

Before we discuss the consequences of social change, a basic methodological problem has to be pointed out. How can we differentiate between consequences of social change and consequences of adaptations to this social change? The observer sees a conglomerate of phenomena whose genetic and structural positions are difficult to define. An example may illustrate this problem. Various authors describe the changes in the family structure of our century as the result of industrialization and urbanization. Koenig (196, p. 215) proved, however, that these changes were preexistent or coexistent to industrialization. This means that changes in the organization of social subsystems and changes in the organization of the economic subsystem mutually determine one another. There is a process of active adaptation which aims at a better fit of the two subsystems. In this perspective, the question as to cause and effect and consequences and adaptations to consequences cannot be strictly answered. Ultimately, such questions are rooted in a one-dimensional and unidirectional cause-effect framework which has to be given up in favor of an interactional framework which is circular and describes reality in terms of cybernetic loops.

2.7.1 Transformation of the Instrumental Complex

Social change abolishes old roles, creates new roles, and threatens vested interests. Organizations change first and the involved individuals change later. For example, the division of labor creates changes in the occupational roles which, in turn, influence the identity of the individual involved.

2.7.2 Change of Adaptive Structures

Institutions change and, later, the power structure of individuals and groups change. The United States, up to World War I, was characterized by a business era in which capital and the spirit of enterprise played a major role. Later, technology and management occupied the strategic positions because organizations became very complex. Such is Parsons's (270, p. 500 ff.) view. In my opinion, institutions and individuals change simultaneously and their transformation is governed by feedback processes and realized by multifold interactions.

As Parsons (270) points out, once the instrumental complex has changed, the family structures also change. Koenig (196), however, holds that the changes in the family structures are preexistent or coexistent. In Saas-Fee, the extended family of the preindustrial era has shrunken to the nuclear family. The women increasingly work outside the home, a fact which changes the roles of men and women and, with it, certain aspects of the family organization. Together with the changing roles, the process of socialization changes and, thus, the character of the younger generations.

Increasing mobility, caused by urbanization and industrialization, changes the structure of the community and, thus, the subsystems of values, attitudes, and customs. Class barriers become more permeable and decisionmaking more decentralized. The desecurized social climbers reach for more and more status symbols to gain respect and inner security. Usually the status symbols are those of the class they enter. They tend more to large quantity than to exquisite quality. The styles of verbal and nonverbal communications of the upper class are copied. The social climbers rigidify the boundaries between their former class and the new one.

When social change is accomplished, the society demands affective neutrality to allow its competitive members to function optimally within the new technological and bureaucratic system. The expression of emotions is now rejected, but nature finds a way out. In fact, history illustrates that after rapid social change a new passive hedonism is born. Television football games, and parties provide outlets for repressed emotions in the village.

The gratification system changes. Technological professions, in Saas-Fee, are highly rewarded while philosophers or artists are little esteemed. Science accelerates technological progress and, therefore, assumes a position of power. As the belief in science increases, religious and other beliefs decrease. The transcendental god is often replaced by a technological utopia.

Adaptation to social change can lead to tensions. According to Pflanz (274, p. 47), these tensions take the form of magical practices, personal conflicts, economic disturbances, and health disorders. The notion of the diseases of civilization is, however, often overstated and today it is generally discarded as obsolete.

The tensions especially occur in the family — the smallest social unit of the human system in which all the social forces are focalized. As Hoselitz and Merrill (164, p. 586) point out, the dissolution of kinship structures may liberate constructive economic actions, on the one hand, and lead to social conflicts, or even anomie, on the other hand. In both cases, the family process is influenced.

I agree with Ribeiro (294, p. 181) that one of the big challenges of our society is to cope successfully with the consequences of social change. The question is: are we able to dominate the forces we have freed or, in the words of Fromm (110, p. 172), are we able to find new modes of production and existence without irreparably damaging mankind?

The positive consequences of social change are, for instance, economic take off, abolishment of rigid hierarchies, permeability of boundaries between social classes, new possibilities of self-realization, better school systems, and better lodging facilities.

In Saas-Fee, the new mode of production stopped emigration. Rationalism and utilitarianism pushed aside older principles which had mainly helped the few privileged people, as Wurzbacher and Pflaum (376, p. 283) observed. Nevertheless, progress has a Janus face, bringing about advantages and disadvantages. Both dimensions demand a qualitative and quantitative analysis before we can evaluate the balance between advantage and disadvantage.

After this discussion of the theoretical problems of social change, it seems to be clear that international literature provides bits and pieces of concepts, but no coherent theory of social change to describe the process in Saas-Fee.

3. Problems of Methodology

3.1 From the First Field to the Formulation of an Adequate Conceptual Framework

Although Koenig (197, p. 1278) warns against an inflation of methodological discussions which can lead to the point of forgetting their object, the indication of some of the methodological problems I was faced with seems to be useful.

In 1968, I worked in Saas-Fee for several months. As the general practitioner of the village replacing the chronically ill village doctor, I soon became acquainted with many individuals and families and the general situation of Saas-Fee. The practice served the village with its population of about 800 persons; the 600 employees of varying nationality; and the tourists whose number varied between 6,000 and 12,000, depending on whether or not the daily visitors from nearby areas were included.

The medical practice dealt with bone fractures, wounds, infections, and the whole spectrum of health disorders of a given population. Through my frequent home visits, I got to know the general and the specific problems of the village population. My first impression was that Saas-Fee did not fit into the picture of the current mythology of a healthy mountain village. The population was, on the contrary, under considerable stress, as indicated through heavy alcohol and tranquillizer consumption and frequent psychosomatic symptoms (e.g., chronic "nervousness", irritability, and insomnia).

How did this surprising situation come about?

The villagers referred to the construction of the road in 1951 and the subsequent mass tourism overwhelming the formerly isolated mountain village with its unprepared population. Tourists, in great numbers, now rushed in. They brought money, new values, beliefs, and customs and threw the villagers into a vacuum between the old and new world. The rapid social change was perceived as a battery of stressors and they coped with it as well as they could. Alcohol and drug consumption increased in proportion to the stress experienced. The construction of the tourist facilities had swallowed large amounts of money, loaned from the banks, and the success of the tourist resort depended upon the unpredictable international and economic situation.

This was the picture of the informally interviewed villagers which shaped my first impression. Painted with rough strokes of the brush, it doubtlessly contained oversimplifications. People under stress tend to glorify the "good old times," which are rarely more than an agreeable myth replacing a mediocre past. Nevertheless, the village had experienced a rapid social change whose structure and history increasingly intrigued me. Could a theoretical and practical study of Saas-Fee provide a paradigm for social change occurring in rural areas all over the world?

The two major problems consisted of the choice of the unit of observation and the conceptual framework. A few selected individuals could be described as ideal types, as Parin has personally suggested to me. A few selected households (346), or families (196) could be described. I chose the village as a whole. A village is a model of society in which the "diffuse whole" is concentrated (199). It bundles all the forces of society into a comprehensible structure. It is a special type of human system whose investigation has been neglected by social sciences and, especially, by psychiatrists.

What was the adequate conceptual framework?

I did not fulfill the ideal requirements of social science as postulated by Myrdal (cf. 197, p. 1280) because I had no polished theory in advance. Rather, theory and practice interacted in a spiralic process leading to a theoretical framework. Observation of facts provoked theoretical questions and new theoretical insight provoked more search for new facts. Piaget (277) describes this process in his theory of the equilibration of cognitive structures.

There was no readymade theory for a systemic description of a village. I developed an approach which I call *syngenetic*. The syngenetic viewpoint is comparable to the ecological, holistic, cybernetic, and systemic viewpoints, but the term is more general. It does not evoke distorted, often mechanistic and sometimes discipline-bound, associations. It focuses upon relationships between systems (i.e., physical, social, and cognitive) or between structures and processes. It became increasingly clear that none of the entities or parts of social structures and processes were important in themselves. The whole web of the relational network which defined the identity and functional importance of each part within the whole had to be investigated. Neither was there a readymade syngenetic theory nor a theory of relationships. An interdisciplinary approach had to be developed, integrating intradisciplinary and interdisciplinary theories and concepts.

Such an approach has inherent dangers. What is true in one framework (e.g., theories of learning, psychoanalysis, cybernetics, theory of communication, system theory, ecology, sociology, psychiatry) does not necessarily hold true in another. The assumptions and hypotheses which are the results of one framework are often only the starting point for the thinking within another framework. What is given in one framework is questioned in another. Hummel (165, p. 1169) outlines the further danger that certain notions, taken out of their conceptual context, lose their meaning or suggest structural homology and identify where only superficial analogies exist.

I agree with Popper (cf. 40, p. 157) that science is the result of the free concurrence of thinking. Therefore, it seemed necessary to integrate critically the different concepts despite the inherent pitfalls. Today, the boundaries between the different disciplines are breaking down, a necessary development if we want to grasp the complexity of reality. Von Bertalanffy (28, 29) and Gehlen (114, p. 48) emphasized that the advantage of interdisciplinary or transdisciplinary concepts is that an object viewed from different vantage points adopts new aspects and is not cut down to meaninglessness by a simplifying, unilateral, monocausal, or reductionist approach.

In the following chapter, no comprehensive discussion of the different frameworks is attempted. Only certain aspects, important in the context of this study, are emphasized.

3.2 Problems of Methodic Pluralism

3.2.1 Problems of Empiric Social Science

A village has a social organization which, like in every human system, is responsible for its structure and function. The social organization is composed of an ever-changing pattern of transactions.

According to Firth (cf. 291, p. 42), a social organization is an arrangement of elements which determine what has to be done and when and how. It is both the programmed schedule and its realization; therefore, it is important to describe this social organization. However, such a description is difficult in a human system with rapid changes. Koetter (199, p. 155) holds that structures, the documents of the dynamic historic process, are not crystallized into easily recognizable forms whenever ideas, rules, behaviors, and institutions are pulled into the stream of rapid transformations. This was in fact the case in Saas-Fee. Agriculture was replaced by tourism within a few years. The new occupational and social roles were often diametrically opposed to the roles of yesterday. The values and the norms were floating freely and nobody seemed to be sure about what was right and what was wrong. The new distribution of work led to asymmetries between sexes, seasons, and social classes. The process of acculturation, in which attitudes and beliefs of several cultures were melting, did not yet have a definitive shape. In short, the social organization of Saas-Fee was in a turbulent flux. It was like burning magma not yet cooled to hard lava.

In a village, the social organization has a horizontal structure and composed of elements which are the subsystems — kinship system, families, couples, and individuals; institutions, administrative organizations, schools, professional groups, and interest groups; the church, tourist facilities (e.g., lodgings, shops, discos, transportation systems); and many other elements of a social organization. Because the overall structure of the social organization is difficult to study, I attempted to describe it element by element or subsystem by subsystem. Such a procedure, however, risks losing sight of the whole which is composed of elements and relations between the elements.

Among the subsystems of a social organization, the family has a central position. It is the basic unit of society and a whole social organization discloses its unsharp features within the family in a focused way. The analysis of the family requires an integration of the structural-functional approach and the analysis of interaction, as postulated by Koenig (196, p. 206). Moreover, since World War II, psychiatry has developed a new theory of the family system, as seen in the works of Bateson (17), Jackson (171, 172), Bowen (37), Haley (140, 141), Minuchin (253), Minuchin et al. (254, 255), Wynne et al. (374), and many others. Its basic concepts, which are used for the description of the village, are outlined elsewhere (cf. 130, 131).

In addition to its horizontal structure, a social organization has a vertical structure. The hierarchy can be analyzed within the conceptual approach of Parsons (270-273), who differentiates between a cultural system and a social system. The cultural system includes the norms and values which govern the social system. The social system has the following hierarchical level: norms, collectives, roles, and status. Within this network, individuals transact. Each of the different actions is governed by rules and goals whose hierarchical structure is analysed in the concept of transactional topology (cf. 129).

The vertical and horizontal subsystems of the social organization are integrated in a web of relations and are governed by feedback processes in such a way that a change in one subsystem affects to a varying extent all the other subsystems. Since the social organism is not a mechanistic device, it has many degrees of freedom, resonance, and coping capacities. This principle of social interdependence as a main feature was stressed by Mayntz and Ziegler (242, p. 451). Since the pure formalism of cybernetic thinking tends to overlook the question of power, as critizised by Habermas (133), we have to describe the living social reality and not an abstract computer model of society.

Social organization is maintained by the life of the human system. A village is an open system processing information and matter-energy. The process of in-formation, described by Thayer (351), needs special attention. In-formation occurs in the process of socialization and acculturation. Here, we touch upon the problem of how "the exterior conditions are reflected in the brain," to use Marx's famous phrase. How does character formation within an ever-changing environment occur? Can we discern the three historical types described by Riesman (297) — the tradition-directed, the inner-directed and the other-directed character? Are they characteristic for a specific social organization with a specific demographic, economic, and cultural subsystem?

As Linton (cf. 356, p. 87) points out, character is the result of a compromise between the needs of an individual and the needs of its context. In a changing context, needs change and so does the character of a population. Character and personality structure depend, to a large extent, upon the economic structure — a fact often stressed by Fromm (110) and Reich (292). Moreover, different personality structures react differently to social control — one complies and another resists. The concept of the hierarchy of control, outlined by Parsons (270-273), tends to treat human beings like norm-guided robots as Schwanenberg (321, p. 203) criticizes. In order to describe the social organization of the village in an adequate way, we need to take into account the specific personality structure of the villagers. We have to focus upon the interactions between characters, institutions, and norms.

These are but a few of the problems empirical social science faces within a concrete research project.

3.2.2 Psychoanalytic-Socioanalytic Approach

The problem of character formation leads to the problem of personality theories. Today, we have a basic lack of knowledge in the field of personality theories (cf. 130). We have the theory of affectivity based on Freud and, therefore, upon the scientific paradigm of the last century, on the one hand, and the cognitive theories of Bruner (45) and Piaget (275, 276) who are to some extent nonsystemic and atomistic, on the other hand. Moreover, their theories derive from different conceptual frameworks. Therefore, the two parts can probably never be integrated, although Haynal (147) for instance, attempts to do so. Bateson (17) and Grinker (120), however, made clear that no possible bridge exists between psychoanalysis, based upon an outdated energy concept, and modern behavioral science.

Since there is no general personality theory available, we have to use the psychoanalytic and the socioanalytic concepts developed by Fromm (110, 111), Horn (160),

Mendel (250), Morgenthaler and Parin (259, 260), and Schwanenberg (321). To combine the sociological with the psychoanalytic approach is questionable, though it yields some interesting results. There is an important conceptual gap between individuals and society at large. This gap (92, p. 12) and the fusion of the two topics (i.e., individual and society), criticized by Spiegel (337), are often overlooked and lead to psychoanalytic reductionism which often oversimplifies reality instead of introducing more differentiation. It increases entropy where structures should be differentiated. Benedict's view (cf. 291, p. 64) is a good example of the conceptual confusion as critizices by Spiegel (337). She views culture as a kind of individual superpsychology where intrapsychic contents are "thrown large upon the screen, given gigantic proportions, and a long time span."

With these problems in mind, some aspects of the socioanalytic approach are outlined. According to Fromm (110, p. 16 ff), it is the goal of analytic sociopsychology "to understand the libidinous drive structure *(Triebstruktur)*, the mostly unconscious attitude in terms of its socioeconomic structure upon which it is based." This approach combines views of historic materialism with psychoanalytic concepts − the "drive structure" is supposed to be rooted in biology, but it can be modified by economic conditions; sociocultural phenomena are understood as results of a passive and/or active adaptation to the economic structure of an ecological system; culture, norms, and values are influenced by the "drive structure" and, thus, by the economic basis; character is a product of adaptation; and certain character traits (e.g., ruthlessness) are the results of adaptation to the economic structure of capitalism.

3.2.3 Approach of Historical Materialism

Historical materialism explains social structures, values, ideas, and rules which govern behavior as mere epiphenomena of the economic basis of a society.

For Marx (240), material existence determines consciousness. Interactional styles depend upon the modes of production and a thorough analysis of the economic structures explaines, *eo ipso*, all the other features of society. This is an oversimplification of reality. According to Wyss (375, p. 31), Marx deserves credit for introducing a new anthropology which explains society with system-immanent criteria and without being based upon the abstract philosophic or theological categories obscuring the thinking of his time. Still, as Schaff rightly criticized (cf. 250, p. 112), Marxist thinking had not led to the development of an adequate psychology.

For my purpose, it is interesting to confront Freudian psychology with the psychology of historical materialism. The apparent antithesis between the two concepts often turns out to be complementary as soon as we apply the concepts to concrete phenomena. For instance, the drive for possession, according to Marx (cf. 375, p. 61), is determined by the economic basis of capitalism. For Freud (117, p. 105 ff), it is a biologic reality, necessary to produce capitalism. From a syngenetic viewpoint, there is an interaction between both of them and it is difficult and meaningless to determine which is the chicken and which the egg (i.e., which is cause and which is effect). Moreover, since biologic traits are hard-programmed, one wonders why all societies have not developed capitalism, as suggested by Freud's theory.

3.2.4 Ecological Approach

As previously pointed out (cf. 123), social science increasingly understands the importance of the environment. The holistic ecological approach is used by a growing number of researchers to describe complex systems. Some go so far as to reduce phenomena to the impact of the environment only. Skinner (329, p. 196) states that "a scientific analysis of behavior dispossesses autonomous man and turns the control he has been said to exert, over to the environment." Again, this is an oversimplification of reality. In order to see clear, we need to study the theoretical premises of such statements.

Haeckel (cf. 190, p. 26) introduced the term "ecology" in 1866 and gave it the following definition: "ecology means the comprehensive science of the relations of an organism to its surrounding environment, which consists ultimately of all the conditions of existence." This is an all-encompassing view of the environment, but since ecology is born as a branch of biology, we tend to forget that most of the human environment consists of the history and actual structure of ideas, beliefs, values, and norms. This is one of the reasons why Redfield (291, p. 30) thinks that the value of the ecological approach is limited for the description of small communities.

However, human ecology has modified some of its basic concepts. For Tietze-Weight (cf. 190, p. 28), human ecology is the theory of life cycles *(Lebenszyklen)* of man in relation to the physical environment. The physical environment *(Umwelt)* is defined by Uexkull (cf. 190, p. 103) as the sum of all the stimuli perceived by the animal according to the structure of its receptors. This idea of environment is too limited for our purpose. Recent developments try to overcome these limitations. Odum (cf. 190, p. 33) introduced problems of human interaction, values, and ideas. But, as Hawley (cf. 190, p. 38) points out, human ecology still does not have any explanation for interactions and conflicts in human systems; it only describes the context in which interactions and conflicts occur.

Also, Knoetig's goals (190, p. 11) are too limited for the description of Saas-Fee. He writes that "ecology has to study the relations between ecological potence (total pattern of genetic reaction patterns) of living organisms and the ecological valence (pattern of all the environmental structures." This approach neglects the syngenetic program (discussed later) which is composed of all the determinants of behavior due to multiple learning processes in different contexts. The genetic program has to be taken into account when we describe the ecological structure of the man-nature system in Saas-Fee. The ecology of a tourist resort is shaped by a specific relationship between man who exploits nature and nature which lends itself to exploitation. In other words, the ecological approach is helpful when the above described modification is included.

3.2.5 Cybernetic-Systemic Approach

Cybernetics, the theory of control and communication, has been developed mainly by Wiener (367, 368). It is very valuable for the formal analysis of system processes. I have outlined the basic tenets of cybernetics and its application in technology and science (cf. 130). The cybernetic model of explanation allows for more flexibility than its predecessors. Cybernetic thinking often finds a way out of the theoretical deadlock in which monodimensional-unilinear models, binary models, or the dialectic model have led us. In cybernetic thinking, the feedback of the result to the input and the modification of the input are given facts. Therefore, I consider it the best model for describing processes of interaction and overcoming dichotomies [e.g., the antithesis between the position of Marx (240) that existence determines consciousness and the position of Schelsky (cf. 274) that consciousness determines existence]. Both positions are partly correct; they are complementary and their individual development is controlled by feedback.

The cybernetic approach is linked to systemic thinking, even though the latter has different historical roots. Systemic thinking (cf. 130, 131) has been developed in our century; first in the field of quantum physics, later in biology, and finally it reached psychiatry in the 1950s. It should not be mistaken for general system theory as developed by von Bertalanffy (28, 29), Boulding (35), and Rapaport (290) who studied structural isomorphisms in different physical and conceptual systems. System theory is a theory of the structures and functions of a whole composed of parts and existing in the matrix of one or more contexts. Ackoff and Emery (1) and Miller (251, 252) excellently formulated the following theory of human systems: human systems are open systems which maintain their homeostasis by means of constant transformation and by exchanging matter-energy and information with their environment. The exchange of information is explicitly analyzed in the theories of communication as developed by Shannon and Weaver (324), Ruesch and Bateson (306), Bateson (17), Jacobs et al. (174), Jaeggi (175), and Thayer (351). The basic unit of a communication system consists of a sender, a communication channel, and a receiver. The theories of communication have to be modified for the description of human interaction (cf. 129).

A combination of these three approaches (i.e., cybernetics, system theory, and the theory of communication) is used throughout this study for describing the social change in the village. It can be described as a human system with step-functions and metarules which allow for new calibrations (i.e., for adaptive changes) whenever the homeostasis of one or several subsystems has to be restored or a special goal has to be attained.

One of the concepts of general systems theory is pertinent to the present study. Von Bertalanffy (28, 29) described the principle of equivalence which holds that different systems with a different history can reach the same terminal state if their organization is the same. Since tourist resorts all over the world have essentially the same social organization, the results of this study can be important for rural areas under the influence of mass tourism.

3.3 Methods of Information Gathering

I used three different methods for gathering information — direct field observation, interview of key persons, and interview of a representative sample of the population by means of a questionnaire. The data thus obtained sustain, modify, or invalidate one another in varying ways. The data concerning the state of mental health were gathered in 1970 and those concerning the village process between 1968 and 1975 during different periods of my field work.

3.3.1 Direct Field Observation

3.3.1.1 Function of Direct Field Observation

The investigation of a representative sample of a population has a wider operational range and the direct field observation has a higher degree of penetration, as mentioned by Katz (182).

Direct field observation is aimed at the study of institutions, roles, and transactions. I studied the behavior of villagers in families and in public places (e.g., on the streets, in the church, in restaurants). I studied the organization of families, kinship systems, schools, associations, customs, myths, and legends. I observed the demographic, economic, political, religious, and sociocultural structures of the village. I analyzed the distribution of work, worktimes, workrhythms, and the resulting battery of stressors and stress indicators.

A village has not only a structure, but also an evolving process. The past processes constitute its history. In order to study its history, I used old chronicles and newspapers, community reports, and reports of jointstock companies and associations. I discussed with old and young and the redundant observations and information gave hints for hidden structures and relations.

Direct field observation led to the formulation of hypotheses which could be falsified or supported later by comparing them to the results of the questionnaire. At the same time, it was valuable for checking distorted information in the questionnaire.

3.3.1.2 The Type of Direct Field Observation

In 1968, I was the general practitioner of the village for several months and was making, at the same time, preliminary observations. In 1970, 1971, and 1975 I returned to the village for a total of approximately 18 months, mainly in the function of the village doctor. During this time I made contact with most of the villagers and all the families and established a relationship of mutual trust to create the necessary conditions for a successful investigation.

To avoid disrupting the smooth process of direct field observation, the representative sample was investigated only at the end of 1970. A participant observer always changes the field of observation, especially when the observer is the village doctor. Therefore, I did not reveal the intended investigation before it was necessary.

The fact that I spoke the dialect of the natives was certainly helpful in the contact with the generally rather suspicious people.

3.3.1.3 Process of Direct Field Observation

In 1968, first impressions and information were gathered and contacts with key persons established to develop the questionnaire and my conceptual approach in 1969.

In 1970, the direct field observation continued until the end of the year when the sample was interviewed. Key persons in important hierarchical positions provided me with very valuable information.

In the following years, I occasionally went back to the village to fill in informational gaps which had become apparent while screening the material and writing the first manuscript.

In 1977, the village council of Saas-Fee, after reading the manuscript in a German version decided to have the name of the village mentioned. Notwithstanding, the data of the investigation are disguised; the individuals cannot be identified. The anonymity is further protected by the salient fact that this book is a history of the village and its present and former population and not a story about a few individuals.

3.3.2 Interviewing Key Persons

I interviewed the old priest, the old doctor, the director of tourism, the president, the school teacher, and other key persons holding positions which gave them access to important information.

The key persons were interviewed individually, in an informal setting, by means of a semistructured interviewing process. I had discussions with several key persons at later times, complementing and modifying earlier information. This method of information gathering is especially helpful to understand the historic development of behaviors, roles, customs, and values.

3.3.3 Interviewing the Representative Sample

3.3.3.1 Selection of the Sample

In 1970, at the time of the interview, the village had a population of 895. I excluded foreigners who had been living in the village for less than 5 years. This procedure left a sample of approximately 800 inhabitants. I selected 120 individuals (i.e. 15% of the population). I tried to avoid the investigation of several members of the same family or household to guarantee a higher degree of anonymity. Family-bound pathology could have been easily identified. Due to the method of selection, however, several members of the same family occasionally were interviewed.

The selection of the individuals was made according to a certain key which I cannot disclose for reasons of anonymity. The sample can be regarded as random. Two women refused to cooperate, therefore, I selected, in alphabetical order, the next persons in the same age group.

3.3.3.2 Stratification of the Sample

I interviewed 60 men and 60 women. They were members of six age groups, each group composed of 10 men and 10 women:

Group I: born between 1895 and 1905
Group II: born between 1905 and 1915
Group III: born between 1915 and 1925
Group IV: born between 1925 and 1935
Group V: born between 1935 and 1945
Group VI: born between 1945 and 1955

At the time of the interview, the oldest probands were 75 and the youngest 15 years old. This distribution of age groups facilitated studying the process of social change with its changing attitudes, beliefs, and values.

3.3.3.3 Information Given to the Sample

In accordance with Cannel and Kahn's (51, p. 13) argument that optimal information only motivates individuals to participate adequately in an investigation, I gave the probands preliminary information about the goal of the interview: they were partcipating in a "health study" investigating the correlation between their life style and their health problems.

The questionnaire was composed of clearly formulated questions allowing different types of answers. The subjects were instructed to ask for clarification whenever it was needed.

3.3.3.4 Design of the Questionnaire

The questionnaire contained 76 items with a total of 829 subitems. The sample was informed to add personal items or additional observations and statements at the end of the questionnaire if they wished to do so.

The general section was composed of questions concerning age, sex, marital status, and many other general questions taken from the sociopsychiatric questionnaire developed by Blaser and Poeldinger (30). I developed the special part of the questionnaire basing it on the findings of the direct field observations.

There were open and closed questions following the funnel approach, suggested by Cannel and Kahn (51), beginning with general questions and ending with more personal ones.

3.3.3.5 Content of the Questionnaire

The sample was asked about personal data; their occupational roles; distribution and rhythm of their work; their economic situation; their attitudes; judgments, beliefs, values, and behaviors; a description of their family life; their health disorders; their consumption of alcohol, drugs, and tobacco; and so forth. Usually the sample could choose between different, though not necessarily mutually exclusive, alternatives.

3.3.3.6 Place and Time of the Interview

The participants were mainly interviewed individually in their home. Some were interviewed in small groups of two-five individuals in a large room of the village hall. Here, they were placed in such a way that everyone could write undisturbed.

All the interviews were made in the fall of 1970 and each lasted 2-3 hours.

3.3.3.7 The Interviewer

All the interviews were conducted by the author.

3.3.3.8 Methods of Statistical Analysis

This chapter is a literal translation from German of the notes of statistical analysis and elaboration of the data of the questionnaire formulated by Dr. W. Fischer, a Swiss sociologist and director of the *Unité d'investigation clinique et sociologique* at the University of Geneva. He was willing and interested to participate in this study and took over the complex procedures discussed below.

(1) Elaboration of a Computer Code. Based on the 76 questions of the questionnaire, Dr. Fischer formulated a code for all the items. The proposed working hypotheses determined the variables of elaboration, determining the structure of parameters for the different indicators and the comprehensive indices. There were 316 indicators (i.e., variables of elaboration); secondary variables were sometimes added.

In a first phase, the code was tested and some corrections made.

(2) Codification. The codified information was transferred on code sheets which served as both a document for programming and for primary elaboration (i.e. for an elaboration without the help of the computer).

Codification and programming were performed according to standard procedures and with the necessary controls.

(3) Statistical Elaboration. The different phases of statistical elaboration essentially followed the subsequent sequence:

Global Counting. The first phase of elaboration yielded a global overview of the preliminary results. The global counting yielded the frequences of distribution which served to control the pertinence of the different variables. Extreme unilateral distributions on one or two categories in a continuum were discarded.

Elaboration of Sequences. According to the individual hypotheses and the groups of hypotheses combined on the basis of their content, the groups of hypotheses were elaborated in sequences. This procedure aimed at establishing the relations between the different parameters according to the correlations postulated in the working hypotheses. Tests of significance were completed.

This phase of elaboration provided the following:

– Specific results concerning the different aspects and dimensions of the problems investigated were now known.
– Pertinent and nonpertinent variables were discriminated.
– The global validity of hypotheses and a preliminary selection of significant correlations were established.

Variants Analysis. The variants analysis was aimed at the explicative variables with respect to clearly pertinent parameters which belong to the dimensions to be explained. This procedure yielded the following results:

– The validation of the determining part of the structure of variables
– The determination of tertiary parameters influencing the correlations
– The stratification of the explicative aspects of different variables or indices

Control and Specific Elaboration. The above described operations (3.2), aimed at the explication of the preliminary formulated correlations, were controlled and elaborated specifically.

The above mentioned procedure (3.3) made it possible to investigate and illustrate empirically the correlations between the hypotheses necessary in this phase of elaboration.

Application of Special Techniques. Special techniques were applied for certain central aspects of the study. These special techniques were the configuration-frequency analysis and the sectorial controls of correlations and interconnections which were especially important for the analysis of the material and the interpretation of the results.

3.3.4 Collective of Comparison and the Follow-Up Study

It would have been interesting to compare these results with a comparative study of another tourist resort. However, there was no nearby village who had experienced rapid social change following an event similar to the construction of the road. Even given such a village, it would have exceeded my available time and finances.

It would also have been interesting to make a before-after study, as recommended by Campbell and Katona (50). This was impossible since I arrived in the village only in 1968, 17 years after the event which led to the dramatic social change. Given this situation, a follow-up study of the village every 10 years and a comparison of the results of each cross-sectional study seemed to be a valuable alternative. This procedure will test the reliability and sensitivity of my methods of investigation and allow me to describe the social change in a diachronic perspective.

In addition, I hope that this study will serve as a catalyst for comparable studies in other parts of the world to compare results and map out the vastly unknown reality of social life in rural areas.

The future follow-up studies will be done with an interdisciplinary team; an imperative conclusion resulting from the high complexity of the syngenetic approach of a human system.

Development From an Isolated Mountain Village to an
International Tourist Resort:
Sociological and Socio-Psychological Aspects
of the Village Process

4. Time Before the Construction of the Road

4.1 The Geographic Situation

4.1.1 Function and Meaning of Nature and Geographic Environment

Man and nature are constituents of an interactional network, an ecosystem, shaping and modifying each other. The fight with nature and its immanent dangers mold the character of a population which is responsible for the way nature is related to and/or transformed.

According to Jusatz (cf. 190, p. 28), geography has the function of describing and defining the space in which geofactors impinge upon man. History begins with geography, as postulated by Marx (cf. 110, p. 29) (i.e. with the natural foundations of a process and with its modifications through time).

In the case of the village of Saas-Fee, geography set a natural frame defining in advance the resources and the possibilities of socioeconomic development and shaping the character of the inhabitants throughout the centuries. Tocqueville (cf. 297, p. 123) observed that in the state Michigan in the USA the settlers were completely imprinted by the fight with a harsh nature and, thus, they seemed "not to be interested in man." The same holds true for Saas-Fee. Here, nature was so dangerous and unpredictable that after centuries of exposure to the severe winters, the avalanches, and other threatening phenomena the character of the villagers was marked by some suspicion and self-reliance. This influence might be difficult to understand in 1970 when nature has become controlled by technology. Grassi (119, p. 9) gives an eloquent expression to the potential of nature for terrifying man. When exposed to the mountainous landscapes of Chile, he wrote that nature, unmediated by technology, is "absolutely sinister."

Nature, dominated by technology and combined with a beautiful esthetic configuration, is an attraction mobilizing man and money. Financial investments in a technically controlled nature, as Ribeiro (294, p. 20) points out, become the basis determining the life condition of its inhabitants.

4.1.2 Geographic Structure of the Environment

Saas-Fee is one of the five villages of the Saastal. The Saastal is a narrow valley, branching off to the south at Visp near the Simplon pass. The Saastal is part of the larger and longer valley of the Rhone river in the Canton Wallis.

In the following chapters the Saastal will be called "the valley."

Near the west end of the valley, on a high rocky terrace, there is the village of Sass-Fee. It is surrounded on three sides by the Alps with their snowcapped peaks more than 4000 meters high. The geologic configuration forms a shell. At the base of this shell lies the village, like a pearl, at an altitude of 1800 meters. Saas-Fee is also called the Pearl of the Alps. See Fig.1.

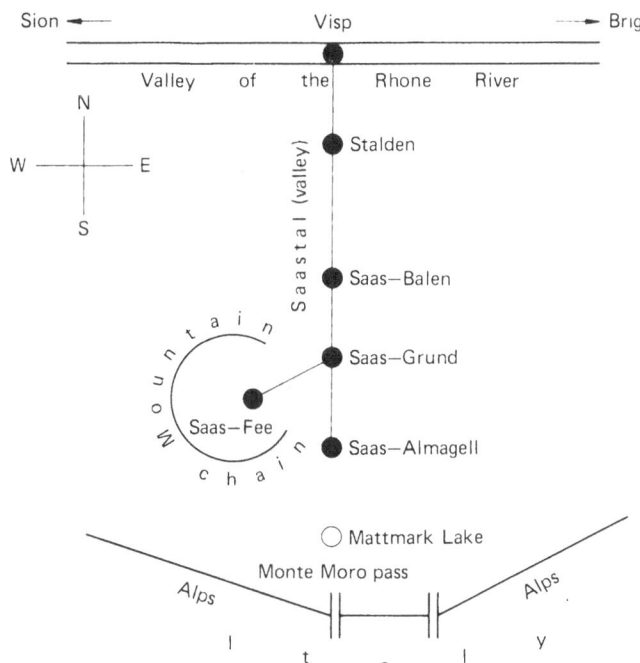

Fig. 1. The geographic situation of Saas-Fee.

The mountains are covered with snow and ice throughout the year. Glacier tongues hang from the mountains and reach towards the village. Many streams and rivelets flow in meandering ribbons down to the bottom of the shell. The landscape, thus structured, is beautiful and strange, for behind the beauty lies a hidden menace whose sensation increases the beauty of the landscape. Rilke's line, "the landscape is a verse in the psalter, it's gravity and weight and eternity," seems to be formulated especially for this area. The German writer Zuckmayer (381, p. 569), visiting the village at the end of World War II, wrote "you stand at the end of the world and at the same time at its origin, at its beginning and in its middle. Mighty, silver frame, closed in a semicircle, formed towards the south by snowcaps in an arrangement of inexplicable harmony, towards the west by a chain of towers of a gothic cathedral. . . . the foam-white ribbons of the mountain rivers move downward and their murmur and ringing fills the air and deepens the silence."

4.1.3 Climate

Despite the alpine location amidst numerous glaciers, the village climate is not of an arctic nature, as Supersaxo (348, p. 9 ff) points out. Situated near Italy and at the bottom of a kettle formed by the high mountains which keep the warm air during the night, the village has a mild climate as compared to other tourist resorts of the same altitude. The snowline of Saas-Fee is 300 meters higher than the usual snowline in the Swiss Alps and the forest line is the highest in Switzerland.

The amount of annual precipitation is equal to that in central Switzerland. According to Imseng (168, p. 126), the average annual precipitation is 866 mm and the winter precipitation 374 mm. The winters have sufficient snow for skiing while the summers are hot and dry.

According to Imseng (168, p. 124), the average temperature from 1907 to 1940, measured at 1.30 P.M., was +1.8°C in November, −2.4°C in December, −2.9°C in January, −0.9°C in February, +1.8°C in March, and +4.7°C in April. These are ideal conditions for tourism which depends not only on the international political and economic scene, but also upon weather conditions. The southern position makes the winters relatively warm.

Today, the glaciers are a tourist attraction. Between 1790 and 1840, they almost reached the village (166, p. 35 ff). Between 1915 and 1918, the villagers had to cut slopes into the woods in order to make space for the advancing glacier tongues. In the early tourist era they fetched ice for the hotels from the glaciers. They had to cover the hooves of their animals with sacks to walk them safely over unto the alps. Since 1918, however, because of decreasing precipitation, the glaciers have been receding.

Numerous rivelets create a constant sound which floats quietly over the village and produces a relaxing effect. The modern science of meteoropathology has demonstrated that exploding water droplets create a negative ionization of the air which has a psychotropic euphoric effect on people.

4.1.4 Forests and Flora

The village is surrounded by forests full of Spruce, Larch, Scotch Pine, and Mountain Pine. Dirt paths lead through the woods giving access to ecological niches for recreation and relaxation.

Over the centuries, these woods had gradually been destroyed by man until, finally, recurrent catastrophes — avalanches and landslides — brought about a new environmental policy. Bodenmueller (33) reports that the reforestation in this century was an expensive enterprise. Old trees are, therefore, rare in this area. It was a special event for the villagers when, in 1895, a Larch was felled which was estimated to be 700 years old (cf. 166, p. 9).

Imseng (169, p. 171) emphasizes that the flora is one of the richest in the Alps. In 1936, the State Council, in order to protect this flora, made it illegal to collect and/or sell more than ten plants at any one time.

4.1.5 Fauna

In addition to the unusual flora, mountain goats, capricorns, and marmots may be found in abundance. The region is situation within a national park where hunting is prohibited. The Marmots – described long ago by the Roman historian Plinius I, as the *mures alpini,* or mice of the Alps – have a long tradition in the region. They are tame and eat out of the hands of people. This presumptive contact with "wild" animals is highly appreciated by the tourist, as Bellwand's and Jaeger's (22) investigation showed.

4.1.6 The Village and Its Means of Transportation and Communication

Originally, the village consisted of several separate hamlets which were the settlements of different clans and ethnic groups. They were composed of a few houses, stables, barns, and granaries. They were the nuclei around which the village, over centuries, developed into an integrated whole.

The village is approximate 1500 meters long and 400 meters wide. It has an S-shaped ellipsoid form whose future development is strictly planned by the magistrate. It is the intention of the population to maintain the settlement's traditional character by keeping its growth within certain spatial limits.

A main road traverses the village. It splits into two lanes with many small branches and alleys within the village. Automobiles are prohibited in order to keep out pollution and noise. Transportation is done entirely by electrocars, whose number has increased with increasing economic prosperity. Today, they are a plague for the pedestrians. The development has far outgrown the original plan. The village intends to develop a special system of transportation leaving the central road free for pedestrians.

4.1.7 Ecological Function of the Geographic Situation

In Saas-Fee, nature has three potential resources – minerals, agriculture, and tourism. Minerals have not been seriously explored. Agriculture and stockfarming had been the prevalent economy for centuries. Tourism has replaced agriculture. Its potential has not yet been fully exploited.

Nature as a resource constitutes a physical component in the ecological system man-environment. It influences the character formation and the identity of man who, in turn, modifies the face of nature. The degree of modification depends upon the available technology.

4.2 History of the Village

4.2.1 Function of a Historical Perspective

The philosopher Dilthey (cf. 365, p. 736) stated that "man does not know who he is by self-reflection, he discovers it by studying his history."

In order to understand the structure of the village and its population in 1970, a brief outline of its history is required. Watzlawick et al. (363) pointed out that a chess game contains all the information at a given moment because it is a closed system. A village, however, is an open human system whose actual structure has been developed by a chain of transformations. We have to go back, therefore, and study the "metabolism of nature" (Marx) and the interactional process between man and nature to understand the actual pattern.

The following chapters are organized in a diachronic perspective. Social change is a process and human systems are the memory of this process. Problem resolution and human action is measured at parameters in the information pool of individual and collective memory which shapes present and future actions.

The diachronic perspective is also used to demonstrate that social change did not start after the construction of the road, as the villagers generally believe. In reality, social change started back in the obscure shadows of prehistoric times when the first people settled down in the area. It reached different speed at different times and accelerated tremendously after 1951.

For a long time, the valley and Saas-Fee formed a political and existential unit, sharing the same history for many centuries. Therefore, the history of Saas-Fee is the history of the ecological system Saas-Fee Valley. Although all four villages (i.e., Saas-Balen, Saas-Grund, Saas-Almagell, Saas-Fee) became autonomous political communities more than 200 years ago, tourism has forged them again into a unit.

4.2.2 Prehistoric Times

4.2.2.1 First Settlers

The first settlers in the valley were probably gatherers and hunters. The rare archeological sites and discoveries indicate (cf. 167, p. 21) that in primitive times glacial periods alternated with periods of abundant vegetation, a periodical process which must have influenced the settlers and the settlements. An old stone lamp is attributed to Neolithic man, but Duebi (82, p. 12) rightly points out that the production of stone lamps had an uninterrupted tradition up to recent centuries.

Thus, prehistoric times remain in the dark grottoes of oblivion. We do not know when man changed his life condition from a hunter to a stock farmer or a cattle breeder, to the sedentary condition of agriculture. This point in the village process, important for the history of every culture and, perhaps, the most important change in a culture (114, p. 71), cannot be exactly dated.

4.2.2.2 Ethnic Blend

The names of fields, woods, hills, and mountains give some clues about the ethnic nature of the first settlers. According to Imseng (167, p. 23), the valley was first settled by Sallassers, a tribe of Liguria, a region in northwestern Italy. Ligurians do not belong to the Indogerman race. According to various Roman historians, the Ligurians lived in the area of the Canton Wallis up to 400 B.C.

Names such as "Galen" (pastureland) and "Gand" (hillside boulders) were coined by the Celtic tribe. The Celts immigrated to Switzerland in the forth century B.C., founding, among others, the famous La-Tene culture at the lake of Neuchâtel. There is a rock near Saas-Fee which has certain patterns of inscriptions supposed to be a cult object of Celtic druids. I doubt, however, about Imseng's (167, p. 38 ff) interpretation. The rock might just as well have been formed by the forces of nature or served completely different purposes.

The Celts migrated over the passes toward the south. It is highly probable that they passed through the valley on their way to Rome, which they reached in 387 B.C. At the end of the third century B.C., Roman legions attacked the intruders and forced them back. At this point, the Roman politics of expansion began. In 58 B.C., Caesar defeated the Helvetians (i.e., the old name for the Swiss, a Celtic tribe, on Helvetia's territory). Thereafter, the Roman administration made major contributions to build and maintain the roads and passes leading over the Alps because an efficient system of communication along the south-north axis was vital for the Roman legions.

From time to time, the roads were cut off by the Sallassers who would lay siege to the passes. In 25 B.C., the commander of the Roman troops defeated them. In 69 A.D., following a decree of the emperor Vitellus, the population of the whole region became Roman citizens. According to Duebi (82, p. 13), Roman documents of that time prove that the valley was in contact with the Roman troops of occupation.

The first mountain path from the valley to Italy was built probably around this time. Roman names of mountains and slopes suggest their importance for the transport of troops and supplies. An old coin, found on top of one pass, had been stamped in the eastern Roman Empire between 324 and 333 A.D. (167, p. 67).

Although the name Saas-Fee has been given various origins — Celtic, Roman, and Arabian — it is probably derived from the Ligurian dialect: *sausa* meaning steep hillside with scarce vegetation, and *feya* female sheep. This name would fit the fact that the vegetation of the region was scarce and could, therefore, sustain only flocks of sheep in those times. Between the fifth and tenth century, the valley was invaded by Francs and Burgunds (167, p. 72 ff). The existence of an important wine culture in the Canton Wallis and certain family names (e.g., Burgener) in the village and the valley seem to sustain this fact.

The question of the immigration of Arabian Saracenes is still in dispute (cf. 33, 82, 166-169, 308, 348). In my opinion, there are more arguments for such an influence than against it. Some authors, among them Imseng (168), leap into an etymological *salto mortale* to deny any immigration of the "godless Moors." In fact, there are no documents proving their immigration, but there are several indirect indications for it:

— Meyer (cf. 33, p. 32) reports that the Saracens crossed the Western Alps in 906 A.D. They arrived in 913 in Piemonte and reached the Great Saint Bernard in 921, pillaging the abbey of Chur in 936 and the abbey of Saint Moritz in 940. They were defeated by the French king, Hugo of Arles, in 941. The king hired them as mercenaries putting them in charge of controlling the passes over the Alps. They had to protect him against his Italian enemy Berenger, Duke of Ivrea. The Saracens set up customs and demanded fees from the pilgrims who crossed the Alps to reach Rome and Jerusalem.

— According to Bodenmueller (33, p. 32), the Saracens were defeated in 942 on the "mountain of the Moors," today called Monte Moro, over which the Romans had built the first road. Evidence that the Saracens were probably in contact with Saas-Fee appears in a legend which, according to Duebi (82, p. 72), describes a troop of riders which was seen by the settlers.

— Hess (cf. 33, p. 31) claims that the previously mentioned deforestation and the vestiges of forest fires in the region were due to the influence of the Saracens. Such vestiges can be found in all the countries under the influence of Moslems because the Koran orders the burning of forests to create pasture land. Hess (cf. 33, p. 31) made studies in the Maroccan Atlas and found a situation comparable to Saas-Fee.

— Evidence for the historic presence of the Saracens is given by some of the contemporary practices of slaughtering sheep and in the absence of rearing pork. Duebi (82, p. 68) noted that the villagers still slaughter a sheep and prepare the meat in a way which is otherwise found only among the Berber tribes of North Africa. A killed sheep is scalded before the wool is shaven, the skin remains, and the meat is air dried without losing its fluids. For the Moslem Saracens, eating pork is prohibited by the Koran. To this day, there is very little pig-rearing in the valley, unlike nearby regions outside the valley (33).

— The names of mountains (e.g., Allalin, Balfrin, Mischabel), villages (e.g., Almagell), and mountain passes (e.g., Monte Moro) suggest an Arabian origin.

— It also seems that certain anthropological features (e.g., the structure of the human crane, the colors of the old costumes) suggest a middle eastern influence.

Between 800 and 1100 A.D., the Alemans immigrated to the valley. They spoke German, the actual idiom of the valley. They settled in all the high regions of the Alps and introduced cattle. Each kinship system had its settlement which was obviously responsible for the formation of the hamlets. Many names of pastures, mountains, and families (e.g., Antamatten = on the pasture, Bumann = construction man, Zurbriggen = to the bridge) are derived from the Alemans.

When the Alemans were settled, the ethnic melting pot became quiet. The same families intermarried over centuries and inbreeding was the consequence. This changed only in our century when modern tourism intruded upon the sleeping valley.

In summary, social change had been going on from the earliest history of Saas-Fee. It accelerated at times and slowed down to a quiet rhythm again. The early changes laid the foundation for the complex ethnic, demographic, and sociocultural structure of the village.

4.2.3 Historical Times

4.2.3.1 Era of Feudal Law

According to Duebi (82, p. 16), the actual name of the valley is mentioned for the first time in a document of August 1, 1256. Abbot Conrad of Arona invested Giudotto Visconti with five alps, one of them connected with the Saastal, mentioned as *vallis solze.*

At this time, the valley was property of the Count of Huebschburg who resided in Visp, the small market town at the entrance of the valley. Later, the Italian Count of Biandrate, by intermarriage, got sovereign rights over the valley. He was interested in a well-functioning system of communication and, therefore, restored the roads over the passes which obviously had not been used for a considerable time. This revival of the traffic must have been of some economic interest for the valley and the villagers.

A treaty signed Augst 2, 1267, between the Bishop of Novara and the Bishop of Sion (i.e., capital of the Canton Wallis), describes that two of the passes are open and used. Commerce seems to have improved the economic situation of the valley because Duebi (82, p. 21) reports that they were able to buy an alp from the Duke of Biandrate for a price of 40 pounds in October, 1300.

At the beginning of the fourteenth century, the valley consisted of four small villages — Saas-Fee, Saas-Almagell, Saas-Grund, and Saas-Balen. The chronicler Zurbriggen (cf. 308) reports that when the four quarters of the valley assembled, each village sent approximately 20 men. Shortly before this meeting, the valley had become partly independent from the market town Visp which constituted a parish of its own.

The name of Saas-Fee is officially mentioned for the first time in a document of August 24, 1456 (cf. 84, p. 30). It deals with the use of the pastureland ("Almenden") and the forests by the inhabitants of the valley who buy land within the territory of the village. The document contains a law prohibiting the construction of houses or stables on the pastureland.

A geographic map constructed by Sebastian Muenster in the 16th century mentions several names of mountains around the village, but not the village itself (169, p. 165).

It seems that the population lived in a tradition-directed society (297) making a living from cattle breeding, dairy farming, and agriculture and gradually developing their identity characteristic for the countryfolk. Duebi (82, p. 32) reports that a document of May 9, 1596, shows that during this period the four communities of the valley had elaborated a set of conditions for the acquisition or loss of citizenship. It specifies that a person loses citizenship if his real estate is worth less than 60 pounds. This law concerned all four villages which, at this time, were one single political unit.

William James (cf. 365, p. 737) calls habituation "the great fly-wheel of history," but history is also made by nonhabitual events which interrupt the habitual course of life. This is especially true when the contradictions within a human system increase, for then the expanding centrifugal forces become the pacemakers of social change. The centrifugal forces must have accumulated in the valley because the four villages separated on February 24, 1763. From then on, Saas-Fee had been politically independent.

4.2.3.2 Independence

As Duebi (82) points out, the separation of the four villages was the first and most important step toward an autonomous community and toward the development of the modern municipal community of the nineteenth century. Nevertheless, cooperation to some extent continued and, even today, some alps are managed cooperatively by the four villages.

The new autonomy was soon threatened. In 1798, Napoleon's troops entered the valley; marauding and pillaging. The chronicler Zurbriggen (cf. 82, p. 39) deplores the devastations of the Napoleonic troops in the valley and their request of large sums of money (i.e., "5400 crowns within 24 hours"). Between 1802 and 1810, Wallis and, with it, the valley and Saas-Fee were an independent republic under the protection of France, Italy, and the Helvetic Confederation of Switzerland. The valley perceived this "protection" mainly as the presence of custom's officers demanding high taxes for the import of Italian merchandise.

In 1810, Wallis and, with it, the valley became a department of the French Empire. Again, being part of the "Grande Nation" was marked by heavy taxes. For the first time in their long history, the villagers needed passports to cross the passes to Italy. Passports, of course, cost money. Furthermore, the young men had to do military service. If they refused to perform it, they had to pay large ransoms every 3 years, a procedure causing considerable impoverishment. The chronicler Zurbriggen (cf. 308) reports that the 2 years 1814 and 1815, until Napoleon was definitely banished to the island of St. Helena, cost the valley approximately 1200 crowns.

In 1815, Wallis became the 20th Canton of the Confederation of Switzerland. The period which followed was quiet from a political point of view. Economically, however, the indicators of an impinging social change were gradually developing.

4.2.3.3 Precursors of Tourism

For centuries, the valley had a subsistence economy based on agriculture and cattle breeding and, intermittently, supplemented by trade over the passes. Natural catastrophes (i.e., fires, avalanches, and repeated overflowings of Mattmark lake) temporarily destroyed the economic basis of the valley.

As Oswald (266, p. 41) holds, the local orientation creates a high degree of integration in the preindustrial village fostering the sociocultural development of the personality structure and enforcing the sense of identity.

When the economic basis is repeatedly destroyed, however, the feeling of identity is threatened, especially if famines lead to death and emigration, as in the village and the valley.

The villagers felt that something was wrong in their ecology and that the evolution of their economy was retarded, as compared to the rest of Switzerland. Ribeiro (294, p. 47) explains that economic retardation occurs because the adaptive system (i.e., the action system vis-à-vis nature and the production process) is based upon a technology with low production efficiency. Thus, Saas-Fee was prepared, at least unconsciously, for the transition to industrialization.

The first tourists in Saas-Fee and the valley were the precursors of this transition. They were scholars whose publications made the world aware of the existence of these small sattlements high up in the Alps. The map of Gabrielis Walteri, a copper plate engraving of 1768, mentions two mountains of the valley and Supersaxo (348, p. 165) assumes that the author must have known it personally. In 1788, Sigmund Gruner (cf. 82, p. 104) described the valley in his book called *Travels Through the Strangest Regions of Helvetia*. His experience must have been frightening for in his unflattering description he refers to the valley as "the Swiss Greenland," and "the most horrible wilderness of Switzerland." A few years later, Abraham Thomas, another scientist, wrote an enthusiastic report about the valley and, in 1825, William Brockedon, an Englishman and author of an illustrated travel guide, visited the valley. By the end of the nineteenth century, the traffic through the valley had slightly increased.

At the same time, courageous tourists, with the help of native guides, started to climb the lower mountains and to cross a few mountain passes. In 1835, Christian Moritz Engelhardt wrote two major publications about the valley and distributed them in

Germany and France. The first officially registered tourist in Saas-Fee was the English natural scientist James D. Forbes. All these visitors, some of them illustrious, made the village and the valley known to a larger public.

In the middle of the nineteenth century, the first tourists, on their way to Saas-Fee, often spent the night in Saas-Grund, the main village of the valley. Because there was no tourist infrastructure, the travelers stayed at the prist's house. It is, therefore, not astonishing that the idea of exploiting tourism started in this very house. The priest Imseng was an intelligent and somewhat charismatic man. He belonged to the elite, instigating social change. An old photograph shows a bearded man with large eyes, a sensual mouth, a bold nose, and a piercing look on his stern face. He looks like a man who not only knows what he wants, but is also bold enough to carry out his intentions.

The priest, or "Kilchherr" (i.e., master of the church), was an enthusiastic hiker who was also interested in the geographic and topographical problems of the region. He contacted various scientists, several of whom (i.e., Melchior Ulrich, Jakob Siegfried, Heinrich Schoch, and Gottlieb Studer) made first ascents on several mountains with him. The chronicler Ruppen (308), himself a priest, although a less successful one, reproachfully called his fellow clergyman *ein leidenschaftlicher Bergfex,* a passionate mountain climber.

In 1850, the priest Imseng organized the first "hotel," transforming an old barn into a dining room and an old stable into a cellar. Again, the chronicler Ruppen (308) exclaims in oblique admiration that it is "amazing what can be made out of nothing with some spirit of speculation." The hotel was obviously a success because in 1856 the priest built a second hotel and planned a third near Mattmark lake. The farmers angrily rejected this project, pointing out that the tourists would destroy the grass on their idle walks through the pastureland. This can be taken as a good example of the way that vested interests retard social change (270, 271). Apparently, the clergyman did move too fast because 3 years later, on July 15, 1869, his corpse was found at the bottom of Mattmark lake. Nobody seems to know whether or not he died of cardiac arrest and fell into the lake or was pushed into it by one of the jealous or angry parishioners. Gossip, however, names the person who pushed the priest into the lake.

By now, the tourist development was advanced by other pacemakers of social change. In the middle of the last century, Englishmen started the run unto the highest peaks of the Alps which up to then had been taboo. Legends reported terrible catastrophes killing any villagers who were bold enough to challenge the taboo. However, taboos have power only within the human system which creates them. Englishmen, at the zenith of their economic and political power, were not inclined to abide by local superstitions. In 1865, Whymper and his expedition climbed the Matterhorn, a mountain peak in a nearby area, the renowned symbol of the invincibility of the Alps. This was a widely publicized event, applauded by the whole world.

Several members of the expedition were killed in a tragic accident during the descent. This fact remobilized the old fears of many a mountain dweller. The taboo, however, had essentially lost its magic power. A new sport and economic activity for the villagers was officially initiated. The ascent of the Matterhorn was the definitive signal for the new era. From now on, the villagers worked as porters and guides for mountain expeditions.

4.2.3.4 Development Between 1850 and 1950

Many villages of the Alps underwent a gradual transformation. More and more tourist came. In Saas-Fee and Zermatt, primarily upper class Englishmen came to spend a few weeks making excursions and first ascents on yet unchallenged mountains.

In 1880, under the guidance of an energetic president, Saas-Fee built its first hotel in cooperation. It belonged to the whole community. According to the amount of taxes one paid, each citizen had to work a certain number of days on the construction plant. By the end of the nineteenth century, Saas-Fee had a modest summer tourism. The English tourists influenced, in a slowly developing process of acculturation, the life style of the villagers. For example, they introduced the custom of afternoon tea. The strictly Catholic villagers even agreed to build an Anglican chapel for the English people. Thus, the village entered the chain of liabilities which connects the development of rural areas to the development of metropoles, a process described by Bellman et al. (21, p. 11).

In the following years, more lodging facilites and hotels were built. During the summer months of 1894, a mule transport brought daily mail and merchandise to the village. Around the turn of the century, foreign investors built four hotels with a total number of 460 beds. The conditions for a rising capitalism, according to the criteria of Marcuse (237, p. 126), were given. There was a class of monied foreign investors and a class of poor villagers who sold their labor for low wages. The resulting distribution of work had never existed before. In the agricultural society, men and women had worked closely together. Now men worked as mountain guides and porters and women worked as servants, chambermaids, or kitchen aids in the hotels.

Adler (2, p. 42) points out that the distribution of work is a necessary institution for the solution of new problems and for creating new life conditions. The new distribution of work in the village was the consequence of the adaptation to a new economic situation.

Although tourism slowly increased, the only means of communication between Saas-Fee and the valley was a path used by men and mules alike. During the 6-8 winter months, the path was covered with several meters of snow and, thus, Saas-Fee was cut off from the rest of the world.

In 1905, when the nearby Simplon tunnel was opened, the chronicler Ruppen (308) wondered whether or not the general economic takeoff would be followed by a moral takeoff. He vaguely felt that the patriarchal system in Europe was on the brink of dissolution, as discussed by Fromm (110, p. 71).

In the first decade of our century, the village founded the first ski club. In 1910, the first racing competition was organized, challenging ambitious young men. Between 1911 and 1914, villagers won several international competitions in Europe. Achievement motivation and the triumph of success gradually fostered a new identity, reinforced by repeated victories. This was a major factor accelerating the pace of social change in the village.

At the same time, a new project promised, with a single stroke, to vastly change the economic basis of the village. Ruppen (308) reports that in 1910 the village gave a concession to an engineer who intended to build a railroad from the market town of Visp to Saas-Fee. The project was supposed to cost 50 million Swiss francs, a horrendous sum in those days. The railroad was planned to run mainly in covered tracks in order to protect it from avalanches and landslides. The project was never realized because the organization of the finances turned out to be too difficult for the ambitious engineer.

In 1914, World War I broke out. Imseng (166, p. 11) reports that the villagers were terrified for weeks to the point of "leaving the hay on the meadows." Tourism stopped. After the war an infrastructure was slowly built up. It prepared the conditions for modern tourism.

In 1923, the electric light was introduced. In 1930 an adequate water supply was provided. In 1925, the villagers founded a tourism association. In 1927, a club for mountain guides was founded.

The economic crisis of the 1930s stopped the incipient tourism again. In 1939 World War II broke out. However, the social change, which had begun, slowly moved on. During and shortly after World War II a nationalism on community level flourished (cf. 124, p. 298 ff), a collective consciousness with strongly narcissistic features arose. In the context of the military service, the villagers formed an elite of sportsmen, the ski champions who had won over forty victories in international competitions. Five times a villager was Swiss champion in the so-called Nordic Combination, i.e., cross-country skiing and ski jumping. In 1948, eight villagers of a population of less than 500 participated in the Olympic Winter Games of St. Moritz. The villagers won the gold medal in the military patrol. Suddenly, these men experienced themselves as the authors of history — no longer as its passive material. Their names and pictures were spread in newpapers and on radios. So was the name of the village. Saas-Fee had become known world-wide overnight.

Stimulated by their successes, the villagers planned the immediate construction of a road to connect the village with the outside world throughout the year. Originally planned in the 1930s, this road was finally built in 1951.

Its tremendous impact on Saas-Fee will be discussed later.

4.3 Development of the Demographic Subsystem

4.3.1 Sources of Information

The old sources and chronicles (33, 82, 166-169, 308, 348) disclose little information relevant for an adequate description of the demographic structure of the village. The same holds true for the statistical yearbook (342) which is not detailed enough before the construction of the road. Therefore, precise statements about the generative structure of the population (i.e., rates of birth and death) are possible only after 1951.

4.3.2 Ecological Control of the Demographic Subsystem

A community constitutes an ecological system in which different subsystems, (e.g., the economic, demographic, sociocultural) influence each other. The demographic subsystem of a community is controlled by the whole ecological system, as observed by Redfield (291, p. 21) in his study of a Maya community.

Changing conditions in Saas-Fee (e.g., the advance and retreat of the glaciers, overflowings of Mattmark Lake, political events) had always demanded an adaptation of the structure of population to the economic situation. Some villagers had to emigrate periodically or definitively. They often contributed to the proletariat of the big cities, at least until the cities also needed adaptation by sending parts of their population overseas (294, p. 149). Intrasystemic tensions and unbalances can be removed by exporting the disturbing factors. Saas-Fee and the valley exported their members to Italy, Austria, France, or Spain and, in mainly two waves, to the United States. After each emigration, the homeostasis of the ecological system was, at least for a while, restored. Later, the same mechanism repeated itself.

4.3.3 Demographic Development

According to the sources indicated by Duebi (82, p. 120), the growth of population in the village and in the valley had the structure shown in Table 1.

Table 1. *Increase in population from the Middle Ages to 1900*

Time	Saas-Fee	Valley
14th century	15 men	60 men
1421	20 men	80 men
1501	30 men	120 men
1816	180 inhabitants	741 inhabitants
1860	217 inhabitants	839 inhabitants
1900	280 inhabitants	1114 inhabitants

In the fifteenth and sixteenth centuries, we have information only on the number of men; evidence that the census occurred within a patriarchal society. The times for survival were rough and the men, who were mainly responsible for the economic situation, seemed to have been more important than women, at least for the chronicler.

The generally slow development of the population was probably due to the high infant mortality and to emigration. A greater population increase can be observed in the nineteenth century (see Fig. 2). The major world population growth around 1650, according to Riesman (297, p. 42), occurred later in Saas-Fee.

The figure indicates that the demographic development was almost stationary from 1850 to 1900. The population was in the phase of high turnover which is characterized by high mortality rates and high birth rates. This demographic situation is, according to Riesman (297), typical for the tradition-directed society of the preindustrial era.

After 1900, the population increased and the social organization changed in the direction of the inner-directed society, as we will discuss later. This was the phase of the new identity, the new ambitions, and a high achievement motivation. The village was preparing for the leap into industrialization and urbanization.

According to our information, the village at the turn of the century still had a patrilocal structure (302, p. 333). A young couple usually lived with the family of the husband. The family itself was an extended multigenerational group tied into a wider kinship system. The agricultural economy was based on this type of social organization.

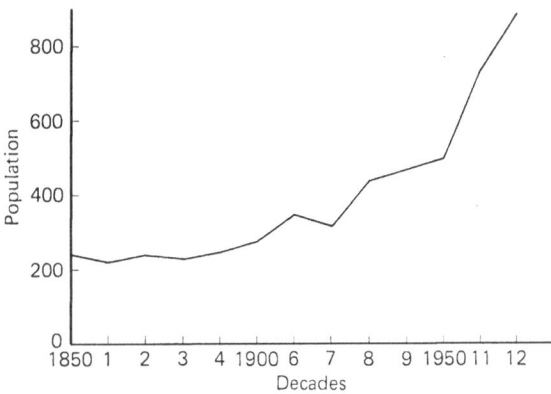

Fig. 2. Increase in population in
Saas-Fee from 1850 to 1950

Birth and death rates were high, especially the death rate of infants. In their reports on the frequent, and expensive, infant burials, old chroniclers use the term "child marriages." According to the Catholic ideology, "innocent" children who died were believed to have married the Lord. The ones who survived were, indeed, the fittest and had a fair chance in the struggle for life in the Alps. Little is known about health or hygienic procedures, except to say that they were based upon old wisdom and old superstition — in somewhat equal proportions. The village had no doctor until the twentieth century. The statistical yearbook gives exact data only after World War II, which make it possible to analyze the demographic structure of the village. See Table 2.

Table 2. *Demographic structure of the population in 1941 and 1950*

Statistical data	Inhabitants in 1941	in 1950
Population	475	504
Marital status		
Single	307	300
Married	156	163
Widowed	12	21
Divorced	-	-
Religion		
Protestant	9	8
Roman Catholic	466	496
Language		
German	473	503
French	1	1
Other	1	-
Employed		
Total	210	240
Self-employed	88	90
Households	108	130

56

There were no major changes in the population structure in the last two decades before the construction of the road. Some small changes become apparent when we compare the age groups separately.

The age groups in Fig. 3 differ from those usually given in demographic reports, therefore, a detailed analysis of the demographic structure in 1941 and 1950 is not possible.
Essentially, three changes can be deduced. In 1950, there are fewer children who are less
than 4 years old and fewer adolescents who are between 15 and 19 years old; there are
more adults between 20 and 39; and, the number of women over 65 increases relative
to the same age male group. The first two transformations can be explained by the natural vertical displacement of the population pyramid. The relative increase in the number
of aged women is due to the higher mortality of aged men. It is difficult to judge whether or not stress or more exposure to accidents is responsible for the increased mortality
of men.

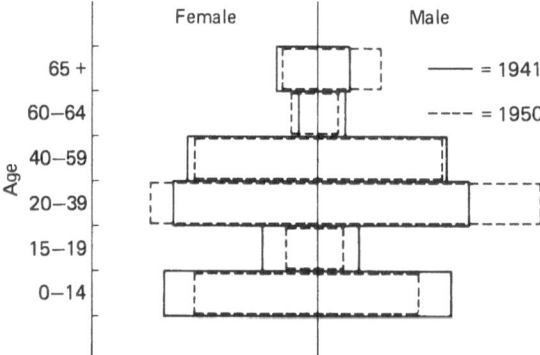

Fig. 3. The demographic comparison
of the age groups in 1941 and 1950

It is not possible to tell whether or not the figure indicates a bell-shaped structure
of population which is, according to Mackenroth (232a), typical for a stationary population or whether or not we have a pyramid-shaped population structure typical for an
increasing population. However, analyzing the development of the birth and death rates,
we find some indicators of a static population. See Fig. 4.

The birth rate remains stationary until 1950; so do the death rate and the rate of
marriage.

4.4 Development of the Economic Subsystem

This chapter deals with social change in the economic subsystem, due especially to the
influence of exogenous factors.

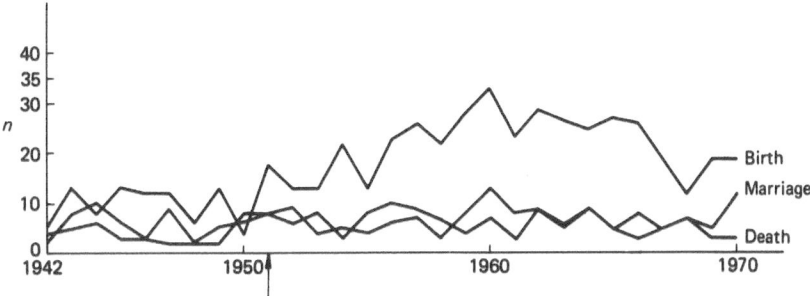

Fig. 4. The development of the population structure between 1940 and 1970

4.4.1 Determinants of Economic Development

The Economic subsystem of a human system is the indispensable basis of life. As Parsons (270, 271) rightly holds, it is the economic subsystem which has the function of adaptation (i.e., the function of organizing the means for the goal attainment of a given human system). The economic subsystem is interrelated to the other subsystems and suprasystems of a human system. Changes in one subsystem or in a suprasystem affect all the other subsystems.

In order to simplify a complex situation, it is important to emphasize that the economic basis of Saas-Fee has been governed by four basic types of determinants – by nature (i.e., the geographic situation and the climate), the means of communication connecting the village to the outside world, quantitative and qualitative characteristics of the population, and the economic and political situation outside the village. Every modification in one of the four determinants changes the direction and speed of the economic development. Moreover, this development is influenced by microdeterminants (242, p. 456), such as economic rationality (e.g., in the organization of a shop), maximal efficiency (e.g., the type of work distribution), and individual contentedness and self-realization (e.g., in the selection of occupation). Such normative elements influence the way in which a population, governed by macrodeterminants, organizes economic development.

4.4.1.1 Influence of Nature

Over centuries, a changing climate led to periodical significant retreat of the glaciers. Legends mention wineyards above the village. It is known that at particular times the overall surface of the fertile land increased.

At other times, it decreased because the protruding glacier tongues blocked the outflow of the lake leading to flooding and devastations of the valley and because the growing glaciers covered more fertile soil.

Since the village formed an economic and political unit with the valley, the village was directly concerned. According to Duebi (82, p. 42), there were more than 20 overflowings between 1589 and 1800. In 1663, for instance, the whole valley was covered with deep layers of mud and boulders. Half the population had to emigrate because the economic basis was almost destroyed. The other half, not discouraged by the mud which, according to the chronicler, "reached the middle line of the chamber stove" in many houses, started to reconstruct their houses and roads and to clean the pastureland. These devastations were definitely stopped in 1925 and 1926 when a tunnel was built to evacuate the backwaters stowed by the glacier tongue.

The precipitation and, especially, the snowfall were factors influencing the economy. Duebi (82, p. 45) reports that the "wild snow," a finely granulated snow without cohesion falling when no wind blows, was especially feared because it produced heavy avalanches. In 1741, 1849, 1917, 1918, 1931, 1945, and 1955 the avalanches did enormous damage to cattle, houses, and stables. Nineteen persons were killed on one occasion and a mother with her six children on another. To fight against "the white death" and further devastation, the people built vaults into the hillsides. Later, as technology improved, they also improved their preventive strategies. They erected wooden fences high up in the mountains.

The important economic losses due to these devastations retarded development. The avalanches were caused by economic policies of earlier times which had, at first, advanced economy — the forests were burnt to create pastureland. In the middle of the nineteenth century, the trees of entire forests were cut to produce ties for the Loetschberg-Simplon railroad or poles for the wineyards of the Canton Wallis. Moreover, wood was continuously used for the construction of houses and stables or for fuel. Short term advantages have a tendency to lead to long term disadvantages. Systems have a built-in "memory" which interferes with the balancing maneuvres whenever homeostasis is to be restored. Thus, systems can punish. The population of the village and the valley had been punished repeatedly, but it is the sons who pay for the sins of the fathers.

4.4.1.2 Influence of the Means of Communication

Systems are interconnected by a special means of communication which carries matter-energy and information and is, therefore, responsible for the development of the elements and units it connects. Saas-Fee and the valley were connected to the north and the south to two different ecological systems which influenced the economic system of the village.

(1) Passes Over the Alps. Three passes connect the valley with Italy; two of them, the Monte Moro and the Antrona pass, have always been especially important. Over centuries, the three passes were open or closed depending upon the ice formation or the political situation. The Roman troops used these passes to reach and conquer the north of the Alps. The historian Aegidius Tschudi (cf. 82, p. 19) reports that the Roman historiographer Livius called the Monte Moro pass the *jugum cremonis.*

In the fifteenth century, the count of Biandrate encouraged the restoration of the pass in collaboration with the valley. Five men of the valley and 29 men from Italy agreed in a document of May 20, 1403, upon the restoration. A document of 1440 (cf. 82, p. 89) mentions the pass as a *"becchia strada,"* an old road. The same document indicates that travelers and pilgrims bound for Rome and Jerusalem traversed the pass, a fact which must have had some repercussions upon the economy of the valley. In the sixteenth century, traffic increased and the Monte Moro pass was mentioned in several books. In the seventeenth century, traffic decreased, partly for climatic reasons and partly because the Simplon pass had become important for the north-south traffic. In 1642, a market in an Italian village which depended on the traffic over the Monte Moro closed down "for lack of interest." From the end of the seventeenth to the end of the eighteenth century, due primarily to the trade of salt, traffic revived. Duebi (82, p. 94) reports that in 1719 the Antrona pass was restored with much work and money.

However, political turbulences prevented an optimal use of the pass. The magistrate of Sion, the capital of the Canton Wallis, wrote a letter to the king of Sardinia on December 7, 1724, complaining about difficulties and asking the king for an opening of the pass on the Italian side. The king did not answer and, after some waiting time, the villagers repeatedly started to remove the obstacles by themselves. In a letter dated July 26, 1788, the royal government of Turin protested the action of the villagers. Nevertheless, a few months later an agreement was reached and the villagers were allowed to transport 1055 sacks of salt over the passes. This treaty seemed so promising that 4 years later the villagers built a salt shelter on the Monte Moro. This investment, however, was of brief advantage. The construction of a paved road over the nearby Simplon pass, organized by Napoleon between 1801 and 1805, created a more efficient means of transportation for the international traffic.

During the two world wars, the border to Italy was closed. The old Monte Moro road, built at enormous expenses, withered. Today, all the passes have returned to their conditions of ancient times. Hunters and hikers walk over the old stones which once bore the feet of Roman soldiers. From an economic point of view, the passes are now meaningless. A few smugglers occasionally carry cigarettes and other contraband over the mountains.

(1) Communication With the Market Town Visp. The path connecting the valley to the market town Visp had to be maintained throughout the centuries. It led through a steep ravine and was often destroyed by rain, landslides, falling rocks, avalanches, or the overflowings of Mattmark Lake.

According to Duebi (82, p. 27), a document dated December 10, 1522, mentions this path first. It indicates that the valley and the market town were bound to pay ten pounds each for the maintenance of three bridges. This path became economically important only in the nineteenth century when tourism started. Prior to this, the valley had traded almost exclusively with Italy.

With the incipient tourism, a better infrastructure was needed. In 1929, a road was built leading from Stalden for several miles into the valley, but without reaching the next village. This piece of road had an immediate reinforcing effect upon tourism, as Supersaxo (348) reports. In 1931, four more lodging facilities were built in Saas-Fee. This event confirms the observation of Wurzbacher and Pflaum (376, p. 17) that increasing means of communication accelerate industrialization in rural areas.

The small piece of road attracted more tourists. It shortened the walk to Saas-Fee and decreased the hardship of the trail. In 1938, the road reached Saas-Grund and, again, the number of lodging facilities increased. According to Supersaxo (348), the village tourism reached a total of 1,300 lodging nights the same year. From 1939 to 1951, due to World War II, the economic development stagnated.

4.4.1.3 Quantitative and Qualitative Characteristics of the Population

Growth of population increases the number of interactions between individuals and creates a *densité morale,* according to Durkheim. This leads to a general stimulation which accelerates social change. An increase in population occurred especially in the nineteenth century. It unbalanced the homeostasis between the demographic and the economic subsystems of the valley. People were forced either to emigrate or to change the economic base. Thus, the quantitative characteristics of the population stimulated a qualitative change in the economic system.

The economic basis influences the "drive structure" *(Triebstruktur)* and the process of socialization and character formation, as observed by Fromm (110, 111). On the other hand, character, specifically cognitive operations, control the "drive structure." As Max Weber (cf. 176, p. 97) holds, the drive or the need to make a living does not by itself foster enterprise and capitalistic development. It needs a rational organization of the economic subsystem which depends upon the character of the people involved. Therefore, a brief discussion about how character features influence the economic subsystem seems to be adequate.

The only sources of information about the character traits of the villagers are the old chronicles. The chroniclers were priests originating in the same area and members of certain family clans. Since their value judgements must have influenced their evaluation of the villagers' character, they have to be taken as relative statements. These informations combined with constructions deduced from general psychological knowledge have given a picture, however partial, of the character of the villagers.

Character is formed in the interaction process between man and man or man and nature. Nature in Saas-Fee was wild and, therefore, the fight for survival must have been hard. Natural selection and adaptation led to character features such as taciturnity, tenacity, suspicion, need for control, capacity to renounce, self-sufficiency, self-reliance, parsimony, high tolerance for stress and frustration, courage, capacity for planning, solidarity, and mutuality.

The southern position and, perhaps, the genetic pool fostered a choleric temperament, a constitutive element of character which the villagers still have today.

The contact with travelers and trade with Italy fostered character traits such as flexibility, cunning, capacity for quick adaptation, self-control and, perhaps, suspicion.

The overall picture shows two fundamental traits important for economic development — creative aggressiveness and the belief in a better world which was, however, present only intermittently, especially at the turn of the century when the tradition-directed society changed into the inner-directed society, which tried to go *per aspera ad astra* (297, p. 126). This transition fostered the achievement motivation (243), the basic condition for the development of a new economic basis. This achievement motivation of the villagers is illustrated as follows: shortly after the construction of the road, a mountain guide climbed nine mountains, all over 4000 meters high, within 24 hours. He gave up climbing the tenth mountain because his companion was exhausted.

This overall character enabled the villagers to build up a tourist industry. Other villages in the Alps with a similar potential for tourism never "made it." Tourist industry, however, required new traits of character. It was not easy for the mountain people to develop kindness, warmth, extreme flexibility, and cautious respect.

Three men, the members of the elite, especially well displayed the typical character features — the priest Imseng who built the first hotel in the valley in 1850, the first man who realized the economic potential of the landscape; the president of Saas-Fee who, in 1880, initiated the construction of the first hotel in Saas-Fee; and the young president of Saas-Fee who stimulated the construction of the modern tourist resort between 1948 and 1968. The priest belonged to the charismatic elite and the two presidents to the technocratic elite whose importance is discussed by Rocher (299, p. 136). These men articulated the hidden potential of the population. Their leadership was vital on the way from agriculture and cattle breeding to industrialization and urbanization.

4.4.1.4 Economic and Political Situation Outside the Valley

We have seen how the economic and political situation in Italy and Europe interfered with traffic and commerce in the valley.

An incipient tourism started to change the economic basis in Saas-Fee. The specific character structure of the villagers fostered the specific development of industry which, in the nineteenth century, was created by noble Englishmen whose Empire was at the zenith of power. This illustrates the interdependence of many factors leading to an event. Here, we focus on the economic and political factors only and, therefore, on the economic and political situation of England of the nineteenth century.

In 1800, the British conquered Malta and, during the following century, it expanded its colonial territory all over the world. In 1920, at the zenith of its power, the British Empire covered 37.8 million square kilometers. Their economic takeoff and considerable political power fostered an identity of strength and power. There was no task in the world which could not be resolved by English genius and enterprise.

The rise of the British Empire is an example of the way in which economic growth is based on social violence and exploitation, as discussed by Habermas (133, p. 46). Imperialism pressed money and goods out of the conquered countries, and in turn, some of this wealth was transferred to where the English took their vacations. Thus, to a certain degree, the economic growth in Saas-Fee was indirectly based upon exploitation. The British elite, looking for adventures, invaded the Alps to conquer the mountains, the last unmet challenge in Europe. Whymper, the first conqueror of the Matterhorn, was typical of the spirit of these early tourists.

After the initial economic change in the village, the process slowed down and stopped completely with World War I, the economic crisis of the 1930s, and World War II. An impoverished Europe, at the brink of famine after World War II, was rescued by President Truman and the Marshall Plan which was designed to restore the economic and political situation in Europe and, thus, keep communism under control. It led to the so-called economic miracle *(Wirtschaftswunder)* in Germany and other central European countries. In the meantime, the British Empire had shrunk and the British tourists stayed away. Instead, the Germans came and revived tourism in Saas-Fee.

This outlines the extent to which a human system is bound to the processes of its context and ecological suprasystem. It demonstrates the vulnerability and dependence of tourism upon the international situation. Thus, although the village had escaped from the uncertainties of a wild and untamed nature, it found itself prey to a new kind of uncertainty — the threat that one day, for whatever reason, no tourists would come.

4.4.2 Economic Structure of the Village

The economic structure of the village — its architecture, the shape and the organization of its economic units, the distribution of work, the rhythm of work, the number of workhours, and the number and pattern of occupations — have changed throughout the centuries.

4.4.2.1 Architecture

Architecture is the materialized spirit of an epoch and, as archeology proves, we can deduce many important things from its structure, even when a culture and its inhabitants have vanished.

The traditional house in Saas-Fee, built up to the construction of the road in 1951, was a simple block house planned according to rigorous and functional rules. The building timber was originally larch, resisting the weathering process for several hundred years. Later, for economic reasons, the less costly spruce was used. See Fig. 5.

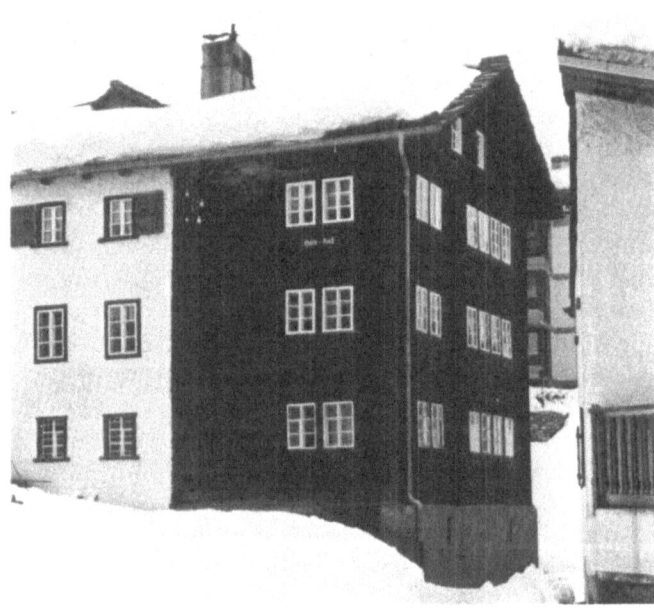

Fig. 5. A dwelling house
(photo: G. Guntern-Gallati)

The entrance, called port, (derived from the Latin *porta* = door) was situated at the long side of the house. A short stone stair led into a small room or directly into the kitchen. The kitchen was in the masonry part on the mountain side of the house or, less often, in the wooden part of the house. It was very small with a tiny window which scarcely gave light. In the corner of the kitchen was a *Trächa,* a stonework construction with a chimney flue. On the *Trächa* a fire was banked day and night. The women cooked in iron pans on an iron tripod. Water had to be fetched at a fountain outside the house and sanitary installations were lacking. People went to the stable to perform necessities. In later centuries, a wooden partition contained a latrine.

The classic house was two- or three-storied, each level with three rooms – a kitchen, living room and chamber. The same stone stove heated the kitchen and the living room while the chamber often was without heat.

The family ate in the kitchen. The parents slept in the living room which was always very tidy and the place where family festivities or official events were celebrated. It was also the place where the children were born, the sick were cared for and, in case of death, the corpse was laid out and the wake was held. The ceiling of this room had a *Binnu*, a wooden beam with inscriptions of the names of the couple who built the house and often a pious sentence asking the Lord for protection and imploring his benediction.

As a rule, all the windows were very small in order to keep the house warm in winter and cool in summer. In the very old houses, there was sometimes a *Seelenglotz*, little hole for the souls – a small square outlet for the souls of the dead to escape, a relic of pagan thinking.

The children slept in the chamber. Often, one berth was placed above the other. The chamber also contained the working devices for the housewife – a spinning wheel and the weaver's loom. Since there was little space in the house, each room served several functions.

The gabled roof was covered with stone plates to sustain the weight of the large amounts of snow in winter. The old houses sometimes had a stone cellar which served as a storeroom. The barn and the *Spycher* were special store roomes (Fig. 6).

The *Spycher* was near the house. It stored dried meat, cheese, butter, tools, and sometimes clothes and costumes. It was erected on four poles, each covered with a stone disc look-ing like a mushroom. The stone disc kept mice out. The same device was used for barns and granaries.

The stable, barn, and granary were usually situated at some distance from the dwellings (Fig. 7). The stable was in the stone work part beneath the timber construction of the barn. The barn stored the hay collected during summer. The granary stored corn and wheat. Sometimes the barn was divided into many tiny compartments, a result of the "real division" of inheritance, dividing the property into as many parts as there were children. Stable and granary were divided in the same way. The real division often atom-ized a barn with the dimension of six by six meters into twelve parts with each a different owner. This required a complicated scheme of rotation which was especially energy and time consuming in winter. Each owner moved for a period of time, equivalent to his share, into the stable; then, he moved into another stable where he owned another part.

This situation was a constant source of litigations because space was a precious re-source and its occupation and use governed by the transactional Querencia Principle (cf. 129). If its antiprinciple, the Apertura Principle, is not effective enough, conflicts arise triggering mutual and never-ending hostility.

The local architecture, unchanged over centuries, created an image of homogeneous harmony. The chalets, burnt black by the hot southern sun, were the expression of an amazing congruence between structure and function. With tourism, the function of the buildings changed and with it the architecture.

The four granite and concrete hotels of the end of the last century were clumsy mon-uments of a new era. Their imperialistic aspect suggests their function of giving residence

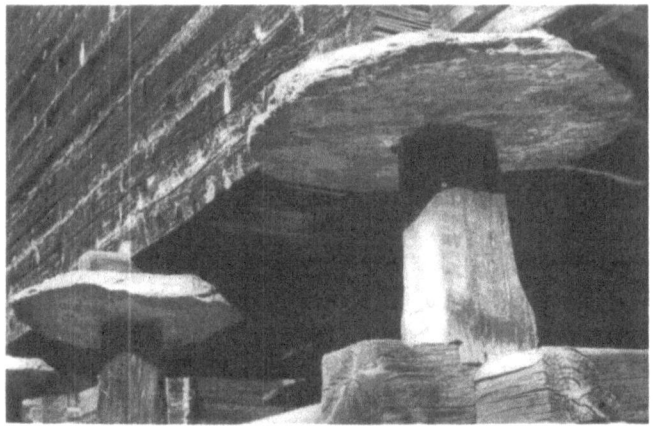

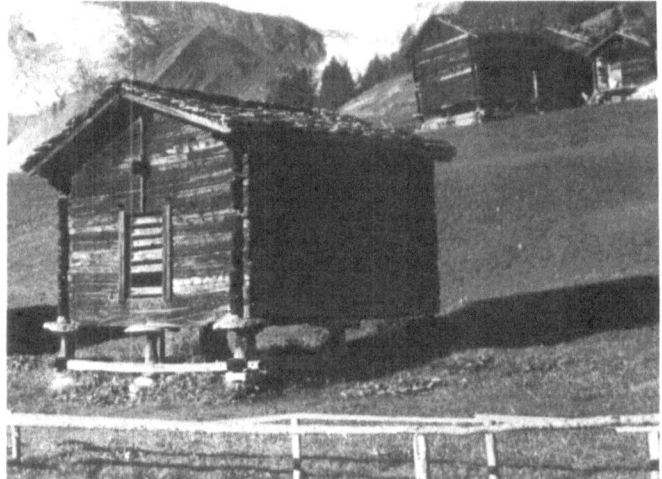

Fig. 6. The *Spycher*
(photo: G. Supersaxo)

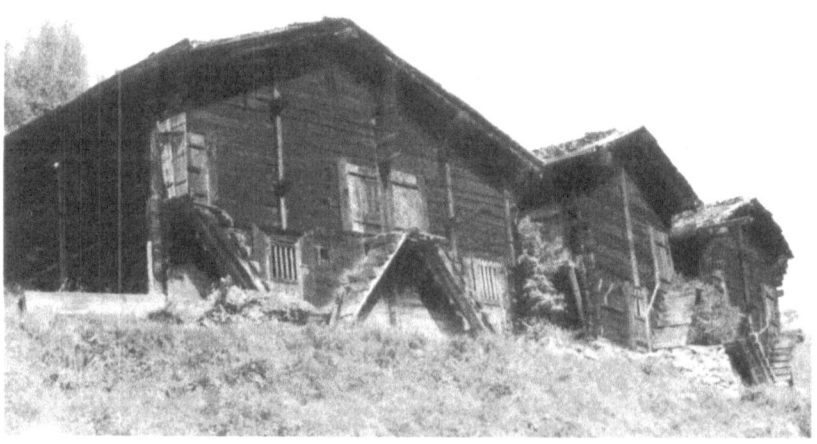

Fig. 7. The stable, barn, and granary (photo: G. Guntern-Gallati

to the upper class of that time. These hotels, with their rusty tin roofs and the ginger-bread architecture of the Côte d'Azure of the same time, have a kind of hideous pomp-ousness.

Thus, the new economic thinking, combined with modern functionalism, destroyed part of the ecological balance and architectural unity of the village.

4.4.2.2 Economic Sectors and Units

Clark (cf. 297, p. 25) differentiates three economic sectors – sector I, or the primary sector (e.g., agriculture, hunting, fishing, mining); sector II, or the secondary sector (e.g., manufacture, construction); and sector III, or the tertiary sector (e.g., trade, traffic, serv-ices).

The economic change in the village moved essentially from sector I to sector III. Sec-tor II had a major importance only during the construction period of the modern tourist facilities. Before, sector II had never been of big importance.

(1) Agriculture and Stock Farming. For centuries, the geographic situation of Saas-Fee provided the basis for an economy of subsistence. Its production nourished the few native families. The name Saas-Fee means mountain of the sheep; sheep raising and stock farming were the basis of the early economy.

The territory of Saas-Fee was divided into five functional zones – the highest zone consisted of the mountains, populated by eagles, marmots, mountain goats, capricorn, and sheep; the next lower zone consisted of the alps, grazed by the cattle during the few summer months; the third zone, called *Almend,* the pastureland, was owned by the com-munity and used by all the citizens; the fourth zone was private pasture and arable land; and the fifth zone was the zone of the dwellings or for construction.

The zones of the alps and "Almends" were worked by all the citizens, according to the number of cattle of each, measured by so-called *Tessel* units. They constructed and maintained paths and fences, felled trees, mended water channels, and cleared the pas-tureland of stones, mud, and branches. The first document describing the organization of these alps and *Almends* was written August 24, 1456. A second document of July 7, 1495, concerns a verdict of the magistrate of Sion which decreed that emigrated citizens who lived less than two-thirds of the year in the valley were excluded from the use of alps and *Almends.*

The marmots, described by the chronicler Zurbriggen (cf. 82, p. 34) as "a miraculous gift of the divine generosity," seemed to play quite an important role in the pretourist world. The villagers, as long ago as September 12, 1559, made a contract with their Ital-ian neighbors not to catch, dig, shoot, or kill by other means any marmots outside of their own communal territory. These rights, existing over centuries, were confirmed as late as 1944 by the State Council of the Canton Wallis.

As indicated earlier, the raising of goats and pigs was insignificant. Sheep and cattle raising was, however, of central importance for the economy of the village and the val-ley. Around the middle of the last century, the chronicler Ruppen (308) wrote that sheep trade was a major source of income and that each springtime the people of the whole valley bought approximately 1500 young sheep. They were fattened and sold in autumn. Goat trade was prohibited for fear of contagious diseases.

There are little exact data available indicating the number of domestic animals, but the valuable enumeration shown in Table 3, reported by Duebi (82, p. 124), gives a basic idea.

The number of cattle has a general tendency to decrease while the number of small animals varies. Apparently, pig, sheep, goat, and chicken raising increased as a result of a governmental policy during World War II. The number of mules, a means of transportation, increased during the construction of the infrastructure and before they were replaced by cars.

Table 3. *The number of domestic animals in Saas-Fee between 1866 and 1951*

1866	1936	1943	1951	Animals
1	-	-	2	Horses
1	12	3	1	Mules
148	122	97	100	Horned cattle
116	96	81	?	Cows
28	24	49	17	Pigs
133	138	235	222	Sheep
61	31	47	51	Goats
-	22	196	109	Chicken
-	12	10	18	Bees hives

The increase of sheep is an example of an interesting process, observed by Parsons (270, p. 512) in another context. Objects with an instrumental value in one context attain a different value in another context, where they may function as status symbols or cherished items in a new hierarchy of values. Today, there is a kind of sheep cult in the village comparable to the horse cult in the United States after the car had replaced the horse. In Saas-Fee, the sheep, although economically useful, are objects of nostalgia for "the good old times." They are symbols of archaic times, a kind of perennial totem of Saas-Fee.

Cattle breeding was a relatively easy enterprise because there had always been enough pastureland, especially during the centuries of low population. The meadows were watered by innumerable channels *(Suonen)* forming a tight network of irrigation. The use of the water was regulated in an elaborate system of rotation – each citizen had the right to "use the water" for a few hours per week. An optimal use of land, however, was disrupted by the legal process of the previously mentioned "real division," leading to an atomization of the parcels.

The farmers had to work on many different tiny pieces of land, a process which took a great deal of time and energy away from the work itself. Duebi (82, p. 85) reports that the average parcel in the village covered 400-600 m², an area half as big as the average parcel in the Canton Wallis.

In 1939, the structure of agriculture had already changed by a budding tourism (cf. 82, p. 122). There were 75 agricultural units; 33 of them were worked by a full-time farmer, 29 had a surface of 1-5 hectares, and 46 had a surface of less than 1 hectare. The average surface of a unit was 9600 m² and in each unit there were twenty parcels, each with an average of 480 m². The total irrigated surface in the village was 359,500 m².

The units were worked by the extended multigenerational family which, as Scherhorn (315, p. 844) stresses, made the family autonomous and independent of markets, since the production only covered its own needs. According to Rosenmayer (302, p. 333), this is the major reason why the extended family has persisted for centuries.

(2) Trade and Traffic. Sheep trade was the most important activity. Duebi (82, p. 100 ff) reports that in 1591 the village had to pay the enormous sum of 105 crowns because it did not abide by the then existing prohibition of sheep trade over the Alps. It also indicates that the wool was woven and "some years, over 900 pieces of fabric" were sold to Italy. The fabric trade started in 1630 and lasted until the nineteenth century when the Italian government stopped it by increasing taxes.

Milk was used for the production of cheese and butter. Before the tourists consumed a surplus of cheese and butter, these goods were traded with outside villages. Corn was never sold because the production was barely sufficient to cover the needs of the village. The increase in population, due to tourism, finally stopped all trade of agricultural products. The demand for food exceeded the production capacities of the decreasing agriculture.

The salt trade was important for a long period of time. According to Duebi (82, p. 95), the villagers made a treaty with the Kind of Sardinia, dated November 22, 1788, which allowed them to carry 1055 sacks of salt back to Saas-Fee. They paid 33 crowns for the royal permission and were obliged to intervene "against possible smuggling."

Other merchandise was traded over the passes, although this kind of trade was never really important. Ruppen (308) lists the items of the trade brought to the village in the last century; salt, tobacco, coffee, spices, copper, and gold rings. With the exception of salt, most of the merchandise was smuggled. The chronicler mentions that each transport brought considerable money to the valley [i.e., 80-100 crowns per transport (1 crown = 3.53 Swiss francs in the currency of 1850)]. Significant evidence for the extensiveness of the trade exists in the fact that the German speaking population of the valley spoke some Italian.

When the basic needs were covered, there was time for fun. Imseng (166, p. 6) mentions that wine was smuggled in milk vessels and saccharin "hidden in the bandages" around the men's legs used as a protection against snow.

There was some labor trade. Imseng (166, p. 5) indicates that between 1850 and 1880, several men worked in the gold mines of Italy or they collected hay in exchange for 15-20 kilograms of rice.

All traffic and trade with Italy was stopped officially by the beginning of the nineteenth century. The new road over the Simplon pass was now more efficient for trade. Only smuggling of coffee and cigarettes continued for a while. After 1920, the fabric and wool trade increased again in Saas-Fee because tourists now bought these products.

Trade with the market town Visp had always been insignificant. Imseng (166, p. 6) reports that two villagers traded butter. Other sources tell that the blacksmiths of the valley bought iron bars each autumn to make the nails they sold in Visp in spring.

Production of other goods was modest. Tailors and Shoemakers went on *Ster,* i.e., they worked at the customer's house for minimal wages. At the beginning of our century, a new branch of trade started. Imseng (166, p. 26) reports that between 1905 and 1907 a lady from Geneva taught twelve apprentices the technique of woodcarving during the winters. This trade survived for a short period, but as soon as new and better possibilities arose, the villagers abaondoned it.

(3) Tourism. Koetter (199, p. 122) points out that an economic potential can be optimally exploited by three means:

1. The modification in intensity of exploitation. In Saas-Fee, the intensity had always been high and could not be increased.
2. The transformation of the economic units. In Saas-Fee, a new law of inheritance would have been needed to avoid the atomization of the parcels and, thus, ameliorate the use of land. This law had never been changed.
3. The transformation of the capacity for work. In Saas-Fee, the work capacity had always been fully exploited.

Based on these factors, it is clear that the economic potential of agriculture could not be exploited further. The same holds true for trade. When the passes closed, it was time to create a new economic base, especially since there was an increase in population and emigration was an undesirable solution. Thus, the village was ready for the social change from sectors I and II to sector III. The farmers were ready because the forces pushing out of the old economy were strong and the forces pulling into the new economy even stronger. This fits with comparable observations in developing countries (164, p. 502). The human system Saas-Fee needed to be calibrated on a higher level of efficiency in order to feed its constutuents. Tourism was the organizing mechnism of this calibration.

The first small summer tourism started in the nineteenth century. It only slightly varied during the following 100 years. The village remained isolated during the long winters. These hundred years were the period of transition leading to the gradual development of the tourist infrastructure and the adaptation of the population to the new phenomena. It gradually prepared the village, however insufficiently, for the change into a new era which was retarted by two World Wars and the economic crisis of the 1930s.

4.4.2.3 Work Time, Work Rhythm, and Work Distribution

During the agricultural era, the time and rhythm of work depended upon the season and the daily weather. Winter was a time of general relaxation. During the short summer, production increased as did the workhours and intensity. The work schedule showed the features of the preindustrial era, i.e., work was distributed over the whole day with a slightly varying intensity (316, p. 777).

According to Mayntz and Ziegler (242, p. 475), the distribution of work is *la raison d'être* of an organization. The distribution of work in a given human system is the expression of the functions necessary for a certain economic structure and, for the human needs, this structure has to fulfill. Either a change in the economic base or in the needs will change the distribution of work. Theoretically, we can assume that the distribution of work, which is only one subsubsystem of the subsystem economy, changes whenever the whole system (i.e., the village) changes in its overall character.

In the agricultural era of Saas-Fee, the distribution of work was not very differentiated. Most of the jobs could be done by men or women. Since partial emigration of men was necessary — they were seasonal workers in various parts of Switzerland or Italy — women took on the vacated jobs. Already in the nineteenth century, many women had the double function of running the household and the economic units (i.e., agricultural), a feature typical for industrialized societies (196, p. 198). The distribution of work was introduced in the eighteenth century and, especially, in the nineteenth century. It led to the socioeconomic organization which I call the hidden matriarchy.

The worktimes in trade and manufacturing were very long, especially during summer. The worktimes in manufacturing even increased in winter, but trade stopped completely. Imseng (166, p. 7) reports that shoemakers and tailors on *Ster* in the customer's house spent from 7 A.M. to 9 P.M. at their tasks.

The work distribution in trade and production was such that men carried on trade, but both men and women were involved in manufacturing and construction. Women, clearly disadvantaged, earned lower wages than men. Imseng (166, p. 7) indicates that women tailors earned 0.50 Swiss Francs an hour while male shoemakers earned 1.90. Women were disadvantaged by the patriarchal society in which men were the official wage earners.

Tourism before 1951 increased the summer worktimes, but the rhythm of the long winter was not modified. The distribution of work led to an increasing sex-specific differentiation. Women took on a growing number of roles and functions while men were restricted to essentially two occupations — mountain guides and porters.

4.4.2.4 Occupational Role Pattern

As Koetter (199, p. 71 ff) points out, an increasing distribution of work creates new occupational roles. The very first roles in the valley were that of hunter, gatherer, and shepherd. Later, agriculture created the role of farmer. Trade did not differentiate the occupations; it was carried on as an additional activity. As Hoselitz and Merill (164, p. 570) show, developing countries have diffuse and nonspecified role patterns. In Saas-Fee, the same person had different occupations because specialization was practically nonexistent.

The chroniclers provide us with few, but more quantified, information about the agricultural era only in the twentieth century. In 1936, the village numbered 73 farmers and, in 1943, 87; an increase obviously due to the increasing population and the changing economic policy during the war.

The chroniclers tell us more about the role patterns in the valley's economic sector II. In the middle of the nineteenth century, there were 20 nailsmiths, 20 masons, 18 shoemakers, 16 carpenters, 16 furnacemakers, 15 tailors, 10 cellarmen, 8 blacksmiths, 8 wooldyers, 6 joiners, 4 turners, and 3 glaziers. The village provided approximately one-quarter of these craftsmen. The crafts were handed down from generation to generation. They were part-time jobs because there was never enough demand. Obviously, there were too many part-time specialists in the valley with a population of 839 in 1850.

Given this precarious economic situation, many men emigrated for seasonal work in the construction of water systems and roads, agriculture, the forests, and, in the nineteenth century, several road and railroad projects of the Canton Wallis. According to Horstmann (162, p. 49), this type of horizontal mobility has the function of making the size of the population congruent with the economic basis.

Tourism brought new occupations and stopped part-time emigration. Porters, mountain guides, and ski instructors were now needed in Saas-Fee. In 1902, the village had 14 mountain guides and, in 1952, their number had increased to 65. For each expedition, one mountain guide and several porters were needed because the English upper class preferred to travel unburdened. Later, the demand for hoteliers, innkeepers, and shopkeepers increased.

In 1902, the first skis were introduced in the village. In 1907, a few villagers climbed the over 4000 meters high Allalinhorn on skis for the first time. In 1908, a ski club was founded, the first in the Canton Wallis. Winter tourism, however, remained insignificant until 1951. The villagers started to work in other tourist resorts as ski instructors. Some villagers were icecarriers — they fetched ice from the glaciers for the hotels and restaurants of Saas-Fee until their job was eliminated by the introduction of the icebox.

Women worked as chambermaids, servants, and kitchen aids in the hotels where they worked hard for low wages. They were an example of the status schism that social change introduced in the former homogeneous social structure of the village. They were employees of the foreign investors. Later, these investors went bankrupt because of bad times and bad management. The hotels became property of the banks and, later, the villagers bought them back.

In summary, we can say that, during the 100 years before 1951, the first constituents of a new occupational structure were introduced in Saas-Fee. Although they were mainly part-time jobs, the trend of new functional roles steadily increased. After 1951, however, it rapidly increased, as will be discussed later.

4.4.2.5 Infrastructure for Modern Tourism

At the end of the last century, summer tourism was already intensive enough to require a post office with a telephone and telegraph system. The mail was brought daily by mule transport.

Although the chronicler Ruppen (308) lamented the good old times when the post functioned better, there were soon two mule transports per day and the mail was first delivered 3 times per week and then daily. In 1906, there were three daily transports in the summer. Again, the chronicler complained that the post office did not function well. By then, the small bureaucracy might have grown to the size governed by the ubiquitous Parkinson Law so that its efficiency was lost in the muddle of a confused organization.

Step by step, within the timespan of half a century, the village built up its tourist infrastructure. In 1908, a blacksmith in Saas-Grund introduced the electric light. In 1910, the construction of a railroad was discussed, but, as mentioned before, never built. In 1912, the village constructed a cabin for the mountain climbers high up in the mountains. In 1923, Saas-Fee introduced electric light. In 1925, a tourist association was founded and followed by a club for mountain guides in 1927. Between 1929 and 1938, a road connecting Stalden with Saas-Grund was built. In 1930, the village got a water system which supplied the households.

In 1880, the village got its first hotel. In 1931, three family resorts *(Familienpensionen)* were built. In the following years, six new hotels were added. In 1938, a second mountain hotel was built above the village to provide for the better comfort of mountain climbers.

4.4.2.6 Development of the Communal Budget

Up to 1895, the community Saas-Fee had a single budget. After 1895, both the citizens and the municipality had a separate budget. Imseng (166, p. 45) gives an overview of the community budget until 1895 and of the separate municipality budget after 1895 (see Table 4).

Table 4. *Development of the budget from 1849 to 1970*

Year	Income [Swiss Francs]	Expenses
1849	50.67	40.90
1853	457.–	408.27
1854	691.20	271.29
1869	632.08	451.44
1880	1,555.14	949.05
1887	7,527.53	5,135.80
1893	10,792.01	10,904.15
1910	8,399.35	5,109.57
1920	14,597.45	16,564.87
1931	18,864.85	19,540.10
1945	54,000.30	53,395.95
1950	66,674.39	65,312.44
1951 Road construction		
1955	134,449.15	134,030.35
1960	231,778.80	231,234.45
1965	1,564,211.54	1,618,391.47
1970	2,635,204.07	2,597,481.20

Considering the fluctuations of the Swiss currency over the years, the development up to 1951 can be summarized as follows:
– The budget increased at the turn of the century.
– The most important increase occurred between 1880 and 1945, coinciding with the development of the infrastructure. Occasionally, the balance was negative.
– Until 1951, the budget can be considered "healthy."

Summarizing the discussion of the economic development of Saas-Fee, we can state that the socioeconomic change was due mostly to exogeneous factors (i.e., primary conditions) which, however, had to be matched by the endogeneous factors (i.e., sufficient conditions) of Saas-Fee. A major social change without the coincidence of the exogeneous and endogeneous factors would not have been possible.

4.5 Development of the Political Subsystem

Power and political structures determine, to a great extent, the control center of a human system whose development and functioning is crucial for its survival.

This chapter is concerned with the development of the political subsystem in Saas-Fee.

4.5.1 Function of Control Center and Authorities

Saas-Fee and the valley were a single political community for centuries. Given the specific geographical situation, the community was pulled frequently into international power struggles.

Documents report that in feudal times the community had essentially two authorities – the Church and the state – which were often interconnected. Generally accepted norms which should be elaborated by negotiations (133, p. 122) were, for centuries, dictated by Church and state and accepted by the people without major protest. The Church shared and gave legitimacy to the secular power and derived its own authority directly from the Lord. This feudal order was modified only after long struggles in the late Middle Ages.

This system, primarily in the service of the Church and the aristocracy, was of more than only an exploitative character. Consciousness is a late product of human development (177). Lack of consciousness and knowledge are anxiety producing. In such a situation, authority has a logic-structural and anxiety-reducing function. It introduces order into the chaotic stream of events. It gives explanations for the unknown causes of events. Anxiety is high in a population exposed to a wild nature; thus, institutions capable of reducing anxiety gained considerable power. They channeled the needs for regression and protection and developed an ideology which explained that contingencies were created by the intentions of the Almighty and were, therefore, purposeful rather than random. The Lord was a projection of parental figures. The submission of an uniformed majority to a better informed minority was rooted in the "drive economy" of every individual (110, p. 37). This mechanism gave the authorities in the control centers of a society considerable power.

4.5.2 Feudalism

The Count of Huebschburg, also called the Steward *(Meier)* of the market town Visp, was the first mundane authority of the valley and Saas-Fee. Later, the Count of Biandrate connected with the Kingdom of Italy, intermarried with the Huebschburgs, and governed the valley. Both the Count of Biandrate and the Count of Huebschburg received the valley as a feudal tenure from the Bishop of Sion.

There is little known about the relationships between the population and the Counts. De Gingis (cf. 82, p. 19) mentions a riot caused by excessive taxes. The old documents report that the valley became a separate community in the twelfth century. A bill of sale of October 3, 1300, effected between the Count of Biandrate and the valley speaks of a *Communitas* of the Saastal (the valley). In 1365, the Countess *(Majorissa)* of the market town and her son were killed in a riot which led to a battle in Visp between the Episcopate of Sion and the family of the Duke of Savoy and led to a treaty in 1392. From then until Napoleon came into power, some 400 years later, the valley was directly under the dominion of the bishop and free from foreign powers. Basically, however, the feudal power structure was not changed.

Gradually, the farmers acquired more independence. Von Roten (cf. 82, p. 24) reports that the farmers in the Middle Ages already owned seven-tenths of the valley, while three-tenths were the property of the Bishop. The Bishop of Sion organized his territory, the actual Canton Wallis, into ten administrative sectors *(Zehnden)* which gradually gained more freedom over the centuries. The valley was part of the sector Visp. Under the influence of the increasing autonomy of the nearby Italian communities, the sectors pushed towards more independence. In the seventeenth century, the Bishop was forced to acknowledge the sectors as autonomous democratic institutions. From then, the state Wallis had its democratic government and the state council was headed by a "Captain of State" *(Landeshauptmann).*

Thus, the principle of authority which, according to Mendel (250, p. 134), institutionalizes the psychoaffective infantilism from birth to death, had found a new and more appropriate form. The sectors were independent enough to strongly influence legislators and administrators. In 1431, a man from the valley, Antonius Supra de Furum, became a representative of the sector Visp, a fact which demonstrate the increasing political importance of the valley. Several documents of the sixteenth and seventeenth centuries report the development of an increasingly autonomous farmers' guild *(Bauernzunft)*. According to Bielander (cf. 82, p. 32), this was an expression of a new identity gradually replacing the "psychoaffective infantilism," an indicator of an awakening consciousness. It led to questioning the earlier forms of asymmetry and dependency which were no longer accepted as a physical necessity as held by a distorted epistemology (67, p. 77). The new view removed the mask from this "necessity" and revealed its structure as due purely to social constraint. This, of course, was a result of the Age of Enlightenment, as shown by Hacker (134, p. 60). It moved the villagers right into the control center of their life condition.

4.5.3 Autonomy

On February 24, 1673, the four villages of the valley separated, a fact vividly deplored by Saas-Grund which had been the political center of the Saastal. The four villages, up to the twentieth century, kept in common three alps managed by a common valley council. But all the decisions concerning Saas-Fee itself were now made independently.

This autonomy lasted little more than a hundred years. Between 1798 and 1799 the valley got involved in the vortex of the politics of expansion of Napoleon, one of the many powerhungry corporals who terrorized the world in order to satisfy the blind ambitions of a minority. Napoleon's troops reached the valley pursuing the imperial troops of Austria. They plundered and marauded. Between 1802 and 1810, the valley was part of a Reblic under the protection of Switzerland, France, and Italy. In 1810, it became part of a department of the French Empire. In 1815, with Napoleon now definitely banned to the island of St. Helena, the valley became part of the Canton Wallis and entered the Swiss Confederation.

This last change introduced a new political organization at the level of cantonal and communal policy. In 1895, Saas-Fee became a modern municipality and founded two political parties — the Catholic-Conservative People's Party and the Christian-Social People's Party. Although the former was somewhat conservative and the latter more progressive, a fundamental programmatic difference never existed. Membership of one or the other party followed the rules of old kinship battles and political struggles often were the continuation of clan and family feuds by new means.

According to the federalist structure, the valley sent representatives to the State Council (i.e., executive administration) and to the "Great Council" (i.e., legislative administration) of the Canton Wallis, but never to the Council of the Swiss Confederation. It seems that the economic decline of the eighteenth and nineteenth centuries before tourism started reduced, for a considerable period of time, the wider political influence of the valley.

4.5.4 Political Institutions

At the time of the construction of the road in 1951, the village had three political institutions — the municipality, the burgher community, and the political parties.

4.5.4.1 The Municipality

The municipality was made up of all the individuals living in the village. Every 4 years a
president and a community council, composed of four members, were elected. Furthermore, some members of the community functioned as arbitrators; registrars for births,
marriages, and deaths; and land registrars. The community council, together with the
president, decided upon questions concerning infrastructure, taxes, financial policy, and
other administrative issues. Other questions were decided by a communal vote. As a
municipality, the village depended upon the state and the confederation which, as Bellmann et al. (21, p. 121) mention, steer the development of industrialization generally
by means of controlling banking policies.

4.5.4.2 The Burgher Community

The burgher community was made up of all citizens with old vested interests. Composed
of the old families, the members were fewer and more privileged. The burgher community and its council decided questions concerning the common property (i.e., alps,
Almends, forests, and the water).
    The burgher community was essentially independent from the state and the confede-
ration and less involved in restrictions and prohibitions than the municipality because
it was an older form of self-government.

4.5.4.3 Political Parties

Although officially the two village parties were local instruments of national parties,
they were rather instruments of old and new clan politics. This was one reason why the
political parties were mainly active during the election times every 4 years. Each party
tried to push forward its president and its members of council.
    In this context, it seems useful to briefly discuss the function and the power of the
president, as compared with the distribution of power in earlier times. A given power
structure decides the ascription of functions, wealth, and further power, as stressed by
Wurzbacher and Pflaum (376, p. 477). In Saas-Fee, power was concentrated in kinship
systems. There were essentially two family clans who, for a long time and in changing
coalitions, replaced each other in the executive power. Political power means monopoly
of information and decision making which, by its very nature, increases preexisting power. This self-reinforcing mechanism had a tendency to keep the same families in power.
The official carriers of this delegated kinship power were mostly elder men, as is the
custom in patriarchal organizations.
    This custom changed 1948. The village elected a 20-year-old president. This event
had symbolic meaning indicating a basic social change. The road was to be built in the
following years, and the villagers must have anticipated a new era which would need
steering capacities of a new and technological nature. Thus, the old patriarchal system,

in which age decided eligibility, was transformed with one single act into a new and more flexible system.

The young president had an education above average by the standards of the village. His knowledge made him suitable for the resolution of new problems and the management of a village in the process of major changes. He was a symbol for the transition from the agricultural to the industrialized society in which positions are obtained by acquired and not inherited capacities, a mechanism described by Koetter (198, p. 231). As a member of the technocratic elite, the young man's actions and decisions were more often determined by the principles of rationalism and efficiency than by old values and norms.

The new era required a change in the old values and norms, however slowly. New investments were to be made, causing heavy fincial indebtedness for the community, families, and individuals. This might be one of the major reasons for the villagers to elect a young man to the center of power. A young man had the values of the young generation – achievement motivation, willingness to take risks, a certain nonconformism that believes in the blessings of progress. These qualities were shared by his generation which gave the whole process of social change a new calibration, increased its speed, and firmly established its direction. The younger generation and the president decided to utilize, without restriction, the resources of their geography.

Summarizing this chapter we can say that the social change in the political subsystem was triggered by exogeneous factors (i.e., primary conditions) and then steered by endogeneous factors (i.e., sufficient conditions).

4.6 Development of the Religious Subsystem

This chapter briefly reviews the development of the religious subsystem which was intimately connected with the political system of the Roman Catholic Church. It is interesting to note that the change in the religious subsystem was much slower than the change in the political subsystem.

4.6.1 Dependence on the Valley Church

As Ribeiro (294, p. 110) rightly states, the political power of the Roman Catholic Church was crucial for the political and economic development of all the countries with its ideology. Bishops often played major roles in international politics. For instance, Matthaeus Schiner, Bishop of Sion, was involved in the fight against French imperialism and the support of the Pope, who, obviously grateful for rendered services, appointed him as a cardinal in 1515. It is typical of the power structure of that time that Schiner, eventually, lost his power on a local, but not on an international, level. He was expelled by the head of the State Council who supported pro-French politics. This local power struggle illustrates the extent to which Church and State were interconnected and, by the same token, involved in international politics.

Historical sources thoroughly outline the status of the Church. The Church was the carrier of power, ideology, values, and norms whose influence was crucial for the life condition of the villagers.

We do not know when Christianization was introduced in the valley. It is probable that it coincided with the arrival of the Roman legionaries in Wallis in 57 A.D. under the leadership of Caesar.

The first historical documents about the influence of the Church stem from the thirteenth century. In a testament of 1249 (cf. 82, p. 17), Count Jocelin from the market town Visp and the Count of Biandrate inherited in equal parts the *vidumnat Visp* of the Episcopate of Sion. Later, in a treaty of August 2, 1267, the Bishop of Sion and the Bishop of Novarra (Italy) reached an agreement concerning the valley and Saas-Fee which obviously was their property.

The delegation of power from the Church to mundane authorities was not without conflict. The intensity of the power struggle between church and state can be deduced from the fact that in August 8, 1375, the Bishop of Sion, Witschart von Tavel, was killed in his castle by the Baron Anton von Thurn. This was one of the decisive events which, in the long run, led to the gradual autonomy of the valley. It led, for instance, to the purchase of an episcopal property bigger than the valley itself. Much later, in 1785, this region bought its independence from the valley Church, paying six hundred pounds, a large sum of money. Saas-Fee, already politically independent from the valley, received one-quarter of this sum.

On the other hand, the valley Church had to buy its independence from the church of the market town in the sixteenth and seventeenth centuries. The valley, because of its flourishing trade with Italy, had enough money to buy its liberty. This process shows the importance of Ribeiro's (294, p. 140) observation that the Roman Catholic Church loses its power in the countries or regions with a substantial level of mercantile capitalism.

Within the valley, the Church still played a major role. As the chronicler Ruppen (308) reports, the population again and again paid large sums of money in order to rebuild the church of Saas-Grund, destroyed by the outflowings of the Mattmark Lake. Moreover, the families spent money for so-called "family-seasons," i.e., Holy Masses, celebrated each year for all the members of the family. The Church also received many donations by which old people bought their eternal salvation, a belief strongly fostered and exploited by the Church. This can be taken as a local example of a more general policy of the Roman Catholic Church which, as Durant (86, p. 142 ff) describes, drove Luther to protest in the sixteenth century, leading to Reformation and Protestantism.

4.6.2 Development Toward Autonomy

As Duebi (82, p. 48) reports, the valley was a member of the parish of the market town Visp until the thirteenth century. Between 1297 and 1298, it got its own *vicariate*. The valley paid six pounds each year to the parish of Visp — five pounds were paid by the four villages and one pound by the vicar who extracted this pound from the parishioners. This reminds us of the comparable custom of the Roman proconsuls who paid money to the central authorities, getting still more out of the provinces. In 1440, the valley got its own independent parish, paying a considerable fee, but, at least, it did not have to pay any more annual sums.

The clergymen of the valley Church were, with the exception of those of the seventeenth century, citizens of the valley. Up to 1918, the parish of Visp still had the right to propose to the Bishop of Sion every new clergymen for the valley. With great probability these selections were influenced by certain contributions and promises.

In 1534, the Bishop Adrian von Riedmatten gave Saas-Fee permission to build a chapel. In 1666, the village built a second and larger chapel. In the following years, the ecclesiastical institution in the village expanded. In 1709 (cf. 169), a few relatively wealthy families initiated a "chapel path" with fifteen small chapels which soon became a famous pilgrim attraction. The chapel of "Saint Mary to the High Stairs," the center of this chapel path, was soon filled with woodcarved and painted votive pictures showing the hands, hearts, and feet the Virgin had healed.

In 1715, the community and, as the chronicler reports, a few "good doers," founded a rectorate or a chancellery *(Rektoratspfründe)*. In 1746, a tower was erected whose church bells were donated in 1781. Eventually, in 1899, more than 200 years after achieving political autonomy, the village became a parish in its own right with its own clergymen. In 1894, the first church was built. According to the chronicler (308), the new church cost "seventy thousand to eighty thousand Swiss francs, with a main altar, three bells . . . and a harmonium for one hundred francs," an expensive endeavor considering the times and circumstances, although the budding tourism might have instigated an economic optimism. Thus, autonomy was achieved and dependence on the Church became of a more local character.

4.6.3 Role Pattern of the Clergyman

The priest had a privileged position. He could use the Alps and Almends without being a citizen. He had both authority and power and, as the representative of the Church, a conservative ideology.

The chronicler Ruppen (308), a priest himself, deplored the fact that in the valley a barn and a stable were transformed into an Anglican chapel for the British tourists, exclaiming, "if such a thing had happened at the time of our forefathers who built numerous beautiful churches for the Lord!" He predicted confidently that this new institution will have no influence on the people who will simply ignore the Anglican temple. Later, the chronicler's attitude to modern times. He made no comment whatsoever when, in 1889, an Anglican chapel was built in Saas-Fee.

It would be an oversimplication to consider the priest only as the local representative of the ecclesiastial power and economic policy originating in the Vatican. The priest did have this role, but, at the same time, he was at the lowest level of a hierarchical system leading up to dignitaries to the Pope. Therefore, it is probable that he identified more with the villagers than with the splendor of the Vatican.

Generally, the priest pursued a conservative policy, but there was at least one exception to this rule — the priest Imseng who instigated social change by perceiving the economic possibilities of tourism. He died, with the irony of fate, in the Mattmark Lake which was used by his more conservative fellow priest to control the villagers by evoking anxiety and fear of the inferno. This man had the ascetic nature which the Church officially fostered, but which was rarely reached by its representatives. Weber (cf. 314, p.

166) writes that this "intramundane asceticism" is one of the roots of capitalism and a necessary condition for industrialization.

The priest had several official roles, unchanged over centuries. They celebrated the Holy Mass every day and they preached. They sometimes confused "religious shallowness with rhetorical capacity," as Matussek and Egenter (241, p. 87) put it. They preached what the people wanted to hear and the people wanted to hear what they preached — a system of mutual transaction and control. The people looked more for the know-how of preaching than for content which had a tendency to repeat itself, anyhow. Occasional biting remarks from the pulpit, touching the political life of the village, angered the people. In general, he did not interfere with such issues. He painted the ecstasies of heaven and the agonies of hell, he warned and he threatened, and he thundered and begged. The parishioners, knowing the laws of mercantilism, thought it wise to make donations and sacrifices in order to gain celestial ecstasy and avoid infernal agony in the future life.

The priest administered the holy sacraments, especially confession and communion. He organized public and obligatory prayers and the ecclesiastic festivities. He cared for the old and the poor; he gave speeches at births, deaths, and marriages; and he presided over ecclesiastical associations. In general, his life was quiet unless it was stirred up by his own ambitions. He lived comfortably and enjoyed the respect of his parishioners. His power was unchallenged as long as he did not intrude in a forbidden territory.

The priest influenced public opinion through many channels. According to Silbermann and Luthe (327, p. 688), the credibility of a sender of messages depends directly upon his hierarchical position in a social system. We can assume, therefore, that the priest was quite efficient in his control. He had a monopoly of information, enhanced by the frequent confessions of the villagers, stabilizing his hierarchical position.

The status and prestige of the priest were balanced by certain role expectations. The priest was expected to abstain from marriage, sexual intercourse, smoking, and excessive eating or drinking. He was expected to keep secrets, especially those communicated in confessions, and to keep away from the worldly politics of the village unless he was asked for.

The position of the priest, then, was Janus-faced, combining power and impotence at the same time. He was the agent of a normothetic system, bound more than anybody else by its very norms. He was a representative of a power system, often siding with other power systems. This position produced difficult situations and faced him occasionally with incompatible roles — siding with the powerful meant legitimacy for the powerful or siding with the Christian ideology meant to question the legitimacy of worldly power. This normative split became even more important when the state and the Church became independent power systems. The integrative function of the priest became increasingly central when the accelerating speed of social change widened the gap between the contradictions which had to be filled with new interpretations.

4.6.4 Faith, Superstition, and Religious Customs

4.6.4.1 Overflowings of the Mattmark Lake and the Expiation Behavior

The extent to which religiosity, superstition, and the politics of the Church blended can best be studied in the way people reacted to catastrophes, especially to the overflowings of Mattmark Lake. A catastrophe was thought to be provoked by the sins of the people and, therefore, the people had to pay for the expiation of their sins with money and other sacrifices. Each catastrophe strengthened the power and reinforced the financial politics of the Church.

It is interesting to analyze the psychodynamic functions of such reactions to exterior events. Erikson (94, p. 25) describes the basic mechanism of these reactions as follows: individuals and groups who feel threatened, or who are threatened, have a tendency to act as if the exterior catastrophe were provoked by their own intrapsychic qualities. They develop guilt feelings and a bad conscience and, therefore, they expiate. There are, however, other projective techniques for dealing with exterior misfortune, as Mead (247, p. 71) reports. The mountain Arapesh of New Guinea blame the plains Arapesh for causing bad luck because the plains Arapesh do not share their placid and amiable attitude toward life. Both techniques serve the same goal — to find explanations for the vast array of random and mysterious events.

Projective explanations of misfortune and the search for a scapegoat are a common feature of human systems. The mechanism of scapegoating probably originated in Medieval towns where every spring a billy goat was actually accused of all the misfortunes of the previous year and then it was chased out of town in a ritualized way. This outlet for deviant aggressive emotions was, from a sociopsychological standpoint, stabilizing the homeostasis of the human system.

These mechanisms have one common feature — causality is either projected onto the environment in a heteroaggresive way or it is autoaggressively projected upon one's own self. Both mechanisms, in my view, are based upon a distorted epistemology and cosmology which assumes that man is responsible for natural catastrophes. This distorted epistemology, in turn, is rooted in a feeling of overwhelming impotence twisted into its contrary; the illusion of power to control the forces of nature.

Given these theoretical considerations, let us turn back to the people of the valley. Imseng (169, p. 129) reports that the villagers erected crosses at cross roads and along the paths whenever they saw that the water level of the lake was rising. The crosses invited the passers-by to say their prayers and were also the visible symbols of the invisible threat. These omnipresent symbols increased the general anxiety and decreased it at the same time. They fostered the need for regression and the return to infantile expectations and behaviors.

The prayers and donations, however, did not stop the process of nature. In irregular intervals, the overflowing backwaters rushed into the narrow valley and brought death and devastation. The people did not question their model of explanation. Instead, the farmers increased their prayers and donations to the Church and offered sacrifices to expiate their sins. One historical example, reported by Duebi (82, p. 43), may illustrate this process.

On July 14, 1680, there was a terrible overflowing of Mattmark Lake. The intimidated people of the valley promised solemnly to maintain vigils (i.e., to abstain from eating meat on Saturdays or the days before an ecclesiastic celebration) for 40 years. They also promised to abstain from playing cards, dancing at night, and drinking alcohol on Sundays or days of festivities. Freud (105, p. 483 ff) describes this mechanism as follows: misfortune stimulates the "super ego." The super ego demands punishment and the punishment, in our case, is offered by the Roman Catholic Church, the representative of the supreme super ego, God.

The process also demonstrates the well-known observation by Marx that religion is opium for the people (i.e., an anxiolytic and stupefying drug). This shows the complementary sides of the coin — the ideology of the Church not only obfuscates consciousness and understanding, it also fosters a special kind of explanation and, thus, sheds light into a dark spot. Reality is based upon a logical scaffolding (Wittgenstein) and the Church creates such a scaffolding. Thus, the anonymous terror of nature gets a label and a labelled terror is a reduced terror. The floodings were explained as the local version of the biblical deluge.

In this system of religious faith, superstitions, and mutual dependence between Church and believers, the priest had the function which Habermas (133, p. 163) considers to be the basic function of all world-stabilizing systems of interpretation. He had to prevent complete chaos and to divest contingencies of their random character by creating meaningfulness. The flooding, thought to be a punishment from the Lord, bridged the gulf between inner and outer reality; a gulf created by the lack of scientific knowledge. However, when the villagers understood the mechanism of the periodically protruding glacier tongue, blocking the outflow of the lake, the whole system of explanation collapsed. The new knowledge came upon the valley almost simultaneously with the technology for the construction of an evacuation tunnel.

4.6.4.2 Ecology of Religiosity

At this point of our investigation, it is interesting to analyse the deep-rooted sociopsychological reasons for the extreme piety and fear of God which Duebi (82, p. 61) still observed at the turn of the century. It is obvious that dependence and prevalence of superstitious thinking must have their roots in the centuries old ecological system of these people. To study the paradigmatic character of this aspect, I will try to connect the local situation with the general human situation and the universal roots of religiosity.

Freud (106, p. 352 ff) explained religiosity by reducing it to a feeling of impotence in the individual threatened by society and by inner and outer nature. The illusion of providence has a utilitarian and anxietyreducing function. Freud (103, p. 422) also mentioned that he had never had the "oceanic feeling" described by Romain Rolland, a feeling of floating in a limitless ocean of protection. For Freud, religiosity is provoked psychodynamically by the longing for a father. Such longing is increased whenever infantile helplessness increases. The Church knew how to exploit such yearning by threatening the faithful with eternal helplessness. Mendel (250, p. 65) writes that the Catholic idea of hell is defined as the eternal absence of God, the heavenly father. In hell, the damned soul immerges into an "oral-sadistic, anal-sadistic, pregenital inferno."

These explanations are reductionist and make sense only within a certain conceptual framework, to be accepted or rejected according to one's personal and scientific criteria. Nevertheless, they shed some light upon certain aspects of the villagers' religiosity.

Exterior nature in the valley was grim and menacing, as was inner nature. Catholizism viewed sexuality as dirty, thouroughly bad, and to be prohibited. Aggressiveness, another powerful "drive," was controlled by society to guarantee the survival of its individuals. Thus, both sexuality and aggressiveness had to be repressed. The Church, foreseeing the lack of control of both "drives," introduced the cathartic ritual of confession.

Both repression and acting out must have created an intense feeling of helplessness and a yearning for a protective father who could be found in a supernatural being only; a god.

Marx (cf. 111, p. 127), more than Freud, relates the feeling of helplessness and, consequently, the existence of religion to the material conditions of production. He writes in his introduction to the *Deutsche Ideologie,* "Also the formations of mist in the human brain are necessary results of sublimation of its life processes which are connected to material and empirically observable preconditions." The "formations of mist" were morals, religion, metaphysics and other ideologies. They presumably have the function of hindering man's clairvoyance, which could possibly change the situation. Marx (cf. 111, p. 189) makes a similar comment in his *Einleitung zur Kritik der Hegelschen Rechtsphilosophie,* "religion is the illusory sun which turns around man as long as man does not turn around himself."

Obviously, the people of the valley suffered from this "mist" in their brains and the "illusory sun" turning around them. Both mist and sun were provided by the Church which seemed to be interested in maintaining them.

At the same time, religion and superstition were constituents of an ecology of mind with the function of creating meaningfulness where turbulent contingencies frightened the spirits. The chronicler Ruppen (308) illustrates this fact when he claims that the Confederation's apostasy from the Catholic faith has provoked a cold cutting wind *(kalte Brise),* menacing the orthodox villagers. This is a particular case of a general tendency to bring order into the turbulent stream of random events by constructing causality where only temporal coincidence exists.

4.6.4.3 Ecclesiastical Customs

Over the centuries, pagan customs and rituals amalgamated with Catholic ideas and festivities. Just as erosion and human intervention change the face of the earth by multiple transactions, the interactions between the heathen belief system of the old settlers and that of the later Christians created a body of rituals which was both heathen and Christian. A few example shall be mentioned briefly.

The traditional patriarchy, supported by the Roman Catholic Church, which was also a patriarchal system, produced an amazing phenomenon. Whenever a child was born in Saas-Fee, the church bell rang twice for a boy and once for a girl. The same attitude towards women is shown in the old chronicles which mention only the men of the valley and give no information about the number of the women.

In case of death, the villagers said their prayers for 3 days and nights until the funeral. In a special distribution of work, the villagers prayed during the day while the kinship had their wake at night. During the wake, the people not only prayed but also discussed the character of the dead, mentioning only the positive features in a kind of magical exorcism to procure for the dead a good place in the other world.

The mixture of pagan and Christian customs is best seen in the way the Catholic saints and their celebrations were built into the ecology of an agricultural society with its vitalistic and mythological worship of nature. The saints were instrumentalized; they had a protective function in the daily struggle with nature. The following examples will illustrate this.

Saint Antonius the Hermit, celebrated January 17, was the patron saint of cattle. Saint Agatha, celebrated February 5, protected the village against fire. Saint Marc, celebrated April 25, and the "week of prayer" in May were both marked by a procession, the benediction of pastureland, and the demand for protection against bad weather. A week before Corpus Christi, celebrated in June, another procession was held to demand protection against devastations by overflowing rivers. Saint Anna, celebrated July 26, protected the village from grasshoppers. Saint Mary's Birth, in September, was celebrated when the cattle were brought back from the alps. The first sheep were slaughtered October 16, the Holy Day of Saint Gallus. Finally, Saint Nicolaus, celebrated December 6, protected them against avalanches.

These examples illustrate how the villagers tried to control the forces of nature by magic-religious rituals; mobilizing the saints against all possible dangers.

The procession of Corpus Christi, previously mentioned, played a special role in the sociopsychological economy of the village. It was the day when the solidarity, identity, and power of all the institutions in the community were proudly demonstrated. It took place the second Thursday after Pentecost and started, as Imseng (169, p. 179 ff) reports, right after the Holy Mass and led from the church through the village, then returned to the church, and ended at the cemetery. The participants were picturesque and colorful groups representing the different social organizations of the village. In 1845, a brass band with clarinets and drums was formed to play only on this special day. Today, it is called "the old village music." Soldiers in uniform marched with shouldered guns. Women wore rich costumes with a hat ribboned especially for this day. The firemen in uniform and young men in white shirts stepped by. Little boys carried pennons and standards. Little girls, dressed in the white of innocence, carried religious symbols on silk cushions. The president and the community council; the priest and several foreign clergymen, the representatives of ecclesiastic and worldly associations and power; and all the remaining villagers participated in the procession. It was solemn, impressive, and touching. Today, the procession has lost a good deal of its intrinsic meaning and is especially appreciated by the tourists.

After the procession, all the participants were invited to the village hall where the "community drink," a glass of white wine, was offered. While the procession was carried out with stern pomposity, the community drink was celebrated with a pomposity of a more emotional kind. Representatives of the community and the Church gave speeches, both the old and the new music gave short concerts, the mixed choir performed several songs which had been rehearsed throughout the previous year, and all performances were enthusiastically applauded by the villagers. In short, the day of Corpus Christi had a highly integrative function. Everybody was proud and happy, hostilities were forgotten for the time being, and the sense of common strength produced energy for another year of struggle.

All the customs and festivities had one common pattern — they formed a heterogeneous, but integrated unity. This becomes particularly clear in still another custom, existing up to the construction of the road.

It is Lent, the time of fasting. Foreign preachers, mostly Jesuits and Capuchin monks, came to the village to organize so-called holy missions. They climbed the pulpit and gave excited speeches using all the weapons of a well-trained rhetoric. They spoke about heaven which was far off and about hell being threateningly near. They spoke about the right way and warned against the charnal seductions. They painted eternal promises in all the colors of the rainbow and they comforted the poor, suggesting that a camel would sooner walk through the eye of a needle than a rich man enter heaven. They mobilized terror and passed the collection bag through the rows of benches. The sinners made donations to get immediate relief and security in the life after death. The Church organized punishment and redemption at the same time.

Yet another custom with a highly integrative function was the following: twice a year, after the Holy Mass, every family received the *Spaennubrot,* a bread. This bread was bought with the donations of people now dead for whom the villagers prayed during the mass. The bread was distributed by one of the oldest villagers. The selected person had to be a man who had never been president of the village. Obviously, the custom served to satisfy the need of the aged for prestige and status. Since many of the oldest had died, almost every living old man at least once had the honor of distribution. Thus, they reminded the younger people that a premortal donation would give them the benefit of being prayed for in later years. Obviously, this custom served multiple functions.

Summarizing this chapter, it becomes clear that the development of the religious subsystem in the village was almost exclusively due to exogenous factors and that social change in this subsystem occurred very slowly and to a limited extent. In fact, this subsystem maintained its inner structure and rigid boundaries virtually unchanged up to 1951.

4.7 Development of the Sociocultural Subsystem

In the ecological system, the sociocultural subsystem with its values, norms ideas, beliefs, role prescriptions, technical and ritual rules, and its ideologies had the central function of control. Hierarchically seen, the sociocultural subsystem is situated at the top of the pyramid and its governing influence is important. The functions of this subsystem are held by different institutions. The understanding of the village process depends upon a thorough analysis of the institutions and the norms.

4.7.1 General Function of a Sociocultural Subsystem

The sociocultural subsystem is the governor of a human system and an ecological system composed of a human system and nature. To use an analogy, we can compare its parts to a computer, the social institutions being the microelectronic circuits based on silicon wafers and the value pattern being its program or the institutions are the RNA molecules and the electric circuits of the brain, the value pattern is the information stored in the memory, to use a nonmechanistic organismic analogy.

The sociocultural subsystem of a society interconnected with the economic, demographic, political and religious subsystems, and also with the ecological system village-nature and the extra-village suprasystem, although they change at a slower speed and to a lesser extent. Each of the elements of a given system has a certain degree of freedom, resonance, and constraints. A mechanistic view often overlooks the fact that a society does not change in all its features at the same time, the same speed, and to the same extent.

According to Ribeiro (294, p. 31 ff), a sociocultural subsystem is made up of three elements:

1. The adaptive element, i.e., the way a village deals with nature.
2. The associative element, i.e., the way relationships between the villagers and the extra-village population are regulated. The associative and the adaptive system tend to institutionalize the primary formal ways of dealing with each other.
3. The ideological element, i.e., the abstract knowledge concerning the techniques (e.g., agriculture, tourism), the norms (e.g., prescription of submission or achievement), and the symbolic communications (e.g., costumes, customs, rituals).

These three elements will be discussed at some length in this chapter.

From a psychiatric standpoint, it is very important to have a clear view of the socio-cultural subsystem. Contradictions and incongruencies in the arrangement of positions, roles, role expectations, norms, and rules lead to incongruencies in behavior and, consequently, to disturbances in mental health. For this reason, I will discuss the process of socialization with its agents and content. The process of socialization is a process in which a given individual is in-formed (cf. Thayer, 349) about the values, responsibilities, and rights of his society.

4.7.2 Agents of Socialization

4.7.2.1 General Function of the Agents of Socialization

Socialization is an uninterrupted social learning process continuing throughout life. A life process, and with it a village process, passes through different stages. Each stage demands a new subprocess of calibration (i.e., a reorganization and general adaptation to changed circumstances and contexts). This recalibration, and the small adjustments made within a calibration which are controlled by feedback, has to be steered by the agents of socialization; by its institutions, families, and kinship systems; and by the community and the extra-local society.

A successful process of socialization helps to maintain the homeostasis of a human system and its boundaries, structures, and functions. According to Parsons (270-272), there are four major functions which must be guaranteed:

- Goal orientation. In the period of agriculture and cattle breeding, there were different goals to be reached by the villagers. Huts and pasturelands on the Alps, Almends, and in the village had to be built and maintained in good condition; hay had to be collected for the animals to survive in winter; and crops had to be gathered. Each season offered different duties to be fulfilled. The order of the different jobs had to be maintained. Roles had to be exactly defined and the social actors had to be continuously motivated to fulfill their role expectations.
- Adaptation. The villagers had to give money, workhours, and technical skills to reach the goals.
- Integration. To reach the goals, the institutions of the village had to organize the solidarity of its members to guarantee cooperation in the daily struggle with nature. This was the only way to economize the available forces, energies, and means.
- Maintenance of normpatterns. Norms are situated on a metalevel above the actions they control and govern. Maintenance of value patterns guarantees that goal attainment, adaptation, and integration function. If the norms change, contradictions appear which block development. An example of this fact is the above-mentioned conflict between the clergyman and the population of the valley concerning the construction of a mountain hotel. These types of contradictions increased as soon as tourism, with its general social change, increased. It was difficult for the villagers to decide whether or not to give up agriculture and work as mountain guides and in tourist facilities or to continue in their traditional lifestyle.

All these functions had to be guaranteed by the social institutions which I will discuss now in more detail.

4.7.2.2 The Family

(1) General Theoretical Considerations. The family is the basic unit responsible for socialization. In it the social forces, structures, steering mechanisms, and contradictions are focused in microcosm and, thus, become particularly visible. As Koenig (196, 198) rightly states, the family both shapes the structure of a given society and is, in turn, shaped by it. The family is also the "psychological agency" of society (110, p. 17). An agency sells and distributes ideas and ideals, especially to a society which consumes information. Children certainly are part of this consuming society. In order to reach its goal, this agency has to deal with the ubiquitous paradox of the family and the coexistence of the centrifugal and centripetal tendencies of its members (184, p. 15).

In order to analyze the structure and function of the family process and its major transformations during the period of social change, we need a coherent conceptual framework to describe the phenomena observed and to integrate the facts reported by the sources of information. Because the reported facts are insufficient, we will resort to an historical reconstruction, no matter how limited.

My theoretical framework is based upon the concepts developed by Bateson (17), Jackson (171, 172), von Bertalanffy (28, 29), Haley (140, 141), Minuchin (253), Minuchin et al. (254, 255), Miller (251, 252), Ruesch and Bateson (306), Wiener (367, 368), and Guntern (129-131). The concrete information concerning character formation is taken from Duebi (82), Imseng (166, 168, 169), Ruppen (308), and Supersaxo (348).

A family is a kinship system composed of several elements. It is goal-directed and maintains its homeostasis by multiple changes and transformations. It is an open system exchanging matter-energy and information with its environment. Its structure evolves, over time, in a so-called family process. The family process starts with the formation of a couple. This formation involves a period of intensive negotiations in which the two partners try to reach an agreement concerning the way they want to organize their lives together and the general problem of how to run a family. This period demands a mutual adaptation of the individual transactions, roles, role expectations, and attitudes of both partners. It is a period of recalibration for the whole set of individual rules and goals.

Recalibration is needed at every stage of the family process whenever there is a material or informational input (e.g., birth, marriage of a child), output (e.g., death, separation, marriage of a child), or when roles change without a change in the number of constituents (e.g., school entrance, adolescence, midlife, aging). Recalibration is also needed when the suprasystem changes or the relation between the family system and one of its subsystem and/or suprasystems changes (e.g., economic loss, new jobs, population growth, political crisis, change of value patterns in the process of general social change). Since a family process usually starts within two other ongoing family processes, recalibration and synchronization of these two processes is also involved.

Although these rebalancing maneuvres may lead to transitional difficulties, a family system with normal genetic information (i.e., heredity) and normal and continuous input of needed matter-energy and information is able to organize this calibration stage by stage. If the family system is not able to organize the recalibration either because the input is inadequate or the coping capacities are exhausted, crisis occurs. In this case the family homeostasis is disturbed and the development in one or several of its members of pathological signs and stress indicators (e.g., delinquency, psychosomatic symptoms, "crazy behavior") occurs. Although the production of deviant behavior sometimes restores the balance of the family system, it is at the cost of scapegoating one of its members. A better restoration of homeostasis can be achieved through the intervention of family therapy.

The family system has three basic functions or goals — genetic reproduction, socialization, and organization of an economic basis which allows for the maintenance of the family and socializing functions. In order to reach these goals, the family distributes special roles to its members. These roles (e.g., feeding, caring, playing, working) are specific for the sexes, the age, and the specific stages of the family process. The roles are trained during the process of socialization in the primary family of each of its members.

For Parsons (270, 271), the role is the basic unit of sociological analysis. Roles, however, are composed of a certain pattern of transactions (e.g., communications, behavior, interactions). From a syngenetic viewpoint, transactions are the basic unit of analysis. Verbal and nonverbal transactions are embedded in the matrix of roles and in the overriding matrix of the communication process of a given human system, a family, or a village.

I made clear earlier (cf. 129) that each transaction is governed by a hierarchy of determinants (i.e., specific rules and goals and the structure of a given human system) and of metadeterminants [i.e., general principles and antiprinciples (e.g., homeostasis principle, Querencia principle, syngenetic principle)]. The determinants change with a changing context whereas the metadeterminants are universal steering systems and processes always the same, although there are variations as to their quantitative influence.

The semantics of transactions depend upon the context in which they occur and the "world point" (Minkowski) of the four-dimensional space-time continuum of the communication process in which they occur. The semantics determine the pragmatics thus shaping the transactions emitted by the receiver of a message.

Transactions build the web which holds together the social organization of a human system and also of an ecological system composed by a human system and nature. Given this situation, we can assume that the structure of a transactional system is very complex. Figure 8, representing the transactional web of a family with four members, is based upon my theory of transactional topology. For a more exhaustive understanding, the reader is referred to my original paper (cf. 129).

The graph represents a cross section of the family process, a structure composed by only four sets of intrafamilial transactions. It makes clear the transactional web which is formed by the constituents of this family. The abbreviations H, T, Q, A, S, AU, E, and R refer to the metadeterminants. Metadeterminants or principles are of a general and nonspecific character governing all human transactions. The homeostasis principle (H) states that transactional systems have a tendency to maintain their equilibrium. The telekinetic principle (T) is the antiprinciple of the homeostasis principle. It states that a system's equilibrium has to be unbalanced in order to reach a goal. The querencia principle (Q) states that a system has a tendency to realize transactions in a symbolic or physical space which is strategically of advantage. Its antiprinciple, the apertura principle (A), states that systems must generate transactions in a strategically exposed space

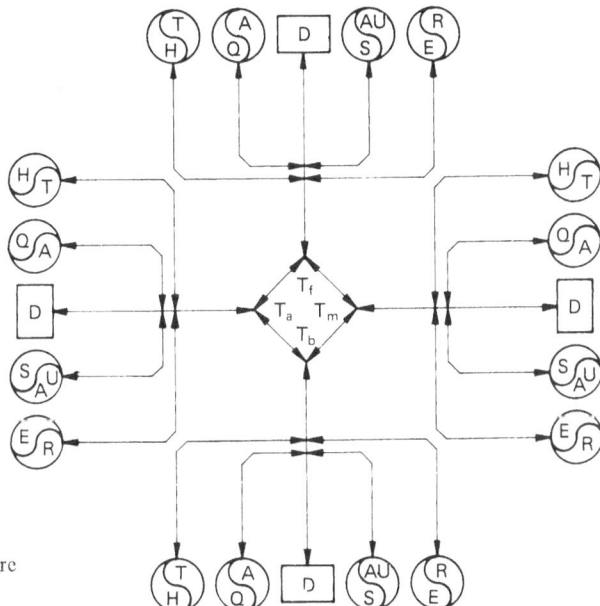

Fig. 8. The transactional structure
of a tetradic family system

in order to permit change. The autonomy principle (AU) states that transactional systems have a tendency to maintain boundaries and its antiprinciple, the syngenetic principle (S), holds that identity and autonomy of a system depend upon its capacity to transcend boundaries (i.e., to build and maintain relationships). The economy principle (E) states that human systems have a tendency to reach goals with a minimum of waste of matter-energy and information. Its antiprinciple, the redundancy principle (R), holds that human systems have a tendency to repeat matter-energy and information outputs in order to be efficient (i.e., to reach a given goal).

Metadeterminants (i.e., principles and antiprinciples) are in complementary relationship and governed by multiple feedback mechanisms. For instance, if a family wants to reach a certain goal, then the interplay of the metadeterminants has to be smooth and well controlled. If the balance of the steering effects of these metadeterminants is dysfunctional (i.e., if the output of principle and antiprinciple is not well-balanced), transactional processes are steered unilaterally into deviation. For instance, autonomy of a person or a family can only be maintained when there is, at the same time, an intensive interplay with the outside world. If this interplay is totally interrupted, as has been demonstrated in the experiments of total sensory and social deprivation, autonomy and identity break down and pseudorelations (e.g., with figures of a hallucinatory character) will occur.

The transactions T_a, T_b, T_m, and T_f, are governed by a set of determinants (D) which has a specific hierarchical structure. For instance, the transaction T_a (i.e., the daughter Ann does not eat) is governed by the rule D_1 (i.e., Ann, don't eat!) which, in turn, is governed by the more general rule D_2 (i.e., Ann, attract the parents attention!). Rule D_2 is again governed by a more general rule D_3 (i.e., Ann, keep the parents from fighting!). D_3 is governed by D_4 (i.e., Ann, maintain the family homeostasis!).

The hierarchical set of rules is finite and the rules governing Ann, brother, mother, and father and, specifically, their transactions are mutually interdependent and governed by multiple feedback mechanisms. Again, the reader is referred to Guntern (129) in order to find a more exhaustive discussion of these complex facts and concepts.

The concept of transactional topology is a map and a map can never be the reality it represents, as Korzybski (202) made clear. The reality of the transactional web of a family system embedded in the hierarchy of suprasystems (e.g., extended kinship, village, valley, Canton, nation, culture) is, in fact, much more complex because the set of specific determinants and the general metadeterminants are interconnected with the different sets of determinants and metadeterminants governing the transactions of the different suprasystems.

Using these general notions, I will now describe the family process of the village.

(2) Structure of the Family in Saas-Fee. The prevailing family structure of the tradition-directed pretourist period was the structure of an extended kinship system. It generally encompassed three generations — grandparents; parents and, sometimes, their single or married brothers and sisters; and children. There were no employees in the household. Separation and divorce did not exist. Catholicism rigidly prohibited both and, therefore, the family structure did not change unless birth, death, or marriage occurred. In some cases, the father was periodically absent when he did seasonal work outside the valley.

Predictably, the extended family with its numerous members shows a high number of interactions. This number can be calculated according to the formula of Bossard (cf. 196, p. 244):

$$x = \frac{y^2 - y}{2}$$

x indicates the number of interactions and y the number of family members. The formula does not indicate anything about the quality of interactions. A high number of interactions in a given system can indicate either overwhelming friendliness or intense hostility.

The family had a hierarchic structure and the influence of the extrafamilial kinship upon decisionmaking was sometimes considerable. This family structure still existed in 1951 and was very much the same centuries before.

(3) Functions and Roles of Family Members. The family had the functions of reproduction, organization of an economic basis, and socialization.

The families of Saas-Fee fulfilled the functions of genetic reproduction rather easily. This role was well-defined and guarenteed. Extramarital sexual activities were strictly prohibited. If they occurred, the chance of pregnancy was high since no contraceptive devices were available. An unmarried mother was ostracized by kinship and village. This rejection, based on repressed intentions, was without compromise.

Notwithstanding the high mortality rate of infants, every family had numerous children. An explosion of population, however, was inhibited by economic factors. Because the economic situation of Saas-Fee did not allow for the formation of more families, only a certain number of the sons and daughters married. The sense of responsibility was high and bachelors were required to give up all claim to the fulfillment of certain needs and desires in the service of society.

Given this situation, the economic base adequately guaranteed the survival and development of population. If this was not the case (e.g., after catastrophes), some families had to emigrate. The remaining led a modest life according to the well-established rules of their society. This situation changed slightly at the end of the nineteenth century when an incipient tourism created a broader economic base. The number of families then increased and so did the population as a whole.

The roles within this system were well-defined. They were sexlinked, agelinked, and linked to the generational level. Sexlinked does not mean that the roles are biologically determined. The work of Linton (cf. 365), Mead (246-248), and many other anthropologists has shown this clearly. The role distribution depends upon the decision of a given society. This decision, in turn, is based upon the nature and history of the social organization. We will see later that the role distribution in the village gradually led to a hidden matriarchy. Some features of matriarchy, a rather rare form of social organization, are described by Mead (248, p. 79 ff) in her field study of the Tschambuli tribe in New Guinea.

In our village, grandparents had considerable authority and often ruled the family until they died. Their ownership of the economic property tended to maintain their authority. They helped the other members of the family in the household and the fields. When they grew old, they did the easier jobs in the house and kitchen and they babysitted. Grandfather taught the skills and technical rules used in the agricultural society. He was the representative of sanctions and the patriarchal authority. Grandmother taught the household technology and the procedures of primitive healthcare and medicine. She represented the principle of social education. Both were responsible for the handing down of legends and myths, traditional customs and rituals, and the ancient attitudes and beliefs from one generation to the next.

Thus, the basic education of children depended to a great extent on the knowledge and activity of their grandparents who derived their authority from their age, the fact that they owned the property, and their narratives in which they connected the present with the past, thus acting as agents of an eternal process. They were not restricted to the altruistic functions of working, giving, and keeping silent which old people, as observed by Chotjewitz (55, p. 21), have to fulfill in modern rural areas. On the contrary, they intervened and directed daily life without hesitation.

The parents were the direct continuation of an authority emanating from the grandparents. They had as much authority and power as was delegated to them. They were, however, responsible for the economic situation.

The father had a well-defined set of roles and obligations, largely in jobs demanding physical strength. He worked in the stables, fields, woods, on the allmends, and alps. He was responsible for the trading of cattle, dairy products, salt, and other objects. Sometimes, in summer, he left the village to to work somewhere in Switzerland or Italy.

The mother had a set of numerous, but not always well-defined, roles in the household, stables, and fields. Since the family was primarily patrilocal, she had to deal with a mother-in-law who delegated as much power and as many roles as she wished. Mother also took over complementary roles when the father was absent, but she was mainly concerned with the kitchen, the production and maintenance of clothes, and the rearing of children. During winter, when there was less work outside the house, she weaved, knitted, and mended clothes.

Both parents were involved in the task of socialization; the father, as the official agent of sanctions, was often the punisher. If he was absent, the mother took over.

The children were involved in different occupational roles from early childhood. Boys worked as shepherds and cowherds or they collected wood and fuel. They helped in the stables and fields. The girls accomplished the same tasks and also took over baby-sitting and other housework. The peergroup, an invention of the industrial era, did not exist at this time. Children were very much integrated in adult life. They trained very early for their later roles.

Children played "agricultural" games, their way of understanding and mastering reality. Once tourism started, children began to play new games appropriate to the new reality. This fact was sometimes deplored by the older generation who did not understand what went on, but assumed that the children heedlessly traded the "good old times" for the "new and dangerous times."

This large multigenerational family structure had the advantage that the same role could be taken over by different members and that inadequate role models could be replaced. Stress also could be distributed among the members. Cooperation between the different roles of the family trained its members for the cooperation in the village. This tradition-directed society produced a firm identity and basic trust protecting the individuals against anxiety, anonymity, and anomie (92). The possible disadvantage of the extended family was the immense social control to which each member was subjected. It did not allow for much autonomous identity and was responsible for an amazing homogeneity of character.

These roles and functions changed slightly when tourism began around the turn of the century. Men started to work as porters, mountain guides, ski instructors, and shop-keepers. Women started to work in the hotels as waitresses, chambermaids, and kitchen-aids. Soon, the number of independent nuclear families increased to the extent that most of the tourist facilities, structurally, grew out of the extended household, a fact which especially affected the mother's roles. As a general rule, she ran the tourist facility and thus moved further and further away from the influence of her mother-in-law. The new times favored a greater flexibility and adaptive capacity of the parents and, with it, the authority of the grandparents gradually decreased. Their tradition-based authority lost its compelling force as the changing life conditions required new value patterns and behavior.

The changing role of the adults also augmented change in the roles of the children. They took over new auxiliary roles in the tourist facilities. At the same time, their independence increased because the adults were increasingly absorbed by activities the children could not share.

The third function of the family was the socialization of its members and the formation of character needed in the context of a harsh nature. Basically, character formation is a result of an interaction process between man and physical and social environment. This has been shown by many field researchers and investigators such as Edgerton (cf. 269, p. 5), Erikson (cf. 297, p. 21 ff), Evans-Pritchard (cf. 291, p. 31), and Fromm (110, 111). Two examples may be quoted. Erikson (cf. 297, p. 21 ff), describing the process of character formation in the tribe of the Yurok Indians, states, "the methods of child rearing are unconscious attempts to extract from the human raw material the behavioral scheme which is the optimum as compared to the special natural conditions and the economic-historic demands of a tribe." In the same sense, Evans-Pritchard (cf. 291, p. 31) describes how the character traits of loyalty and generosity of the Nuer tribe in the Sudan are due to the struggle for survival in an unyielding natural environment.

Before I concretely discuss how the formation of character occurred in the village, it is necessary to explain the conceptual tools I used in my endeavor. There are essentially two models for the description of character formation – the psychoanalytic model and the cybernetic-syngenetic model. The latter is based upon my own research.

The psychoanalytic model was developed by Freud and, subsequently, modified by Reich (292), Fromm (110, 111), Horney (161), Mendel (250), Morgenthaler et al. (256, 260), Parin (269), and other authors. This model has the disadvantage of being built upon the biologic and physical thinking of the last century and of being reductionist, as I showed elsewhere (cf. 130). It also has the intrinsic pitfall, clearly seen by Horn (160, p. 114), that categories developed in an interpersonal context of a dyadic system, the psychoanalytic setting, are transferred to another context for which they are not fit. This, of course, is a clear example of the confusion of foci deplored by Spiegel (337). The psychoanalytic model of character formation was also criticized by Bateson (17), von Bertalanffy (28, 29), Watzlawick et al. (363, 364), and Skinner (329) who claim that psychoanalysts invented a great number of *homunculi* in order to explain the *homo sapiens*. Although such criticisms are justified, the psychoanalytic model remains the most important model used in psychology and most of the descriptions of character formation and personality structure are built upon it.

According to the psychoanalytic model, character is the observable result of the interaction of three hidden psychic elements, or psychodynamic constructs – the ego, the superego, and the id. These three constructs have undergone considerable modification over the years and lack precise definition.

In the early periods of psychoanalysis, the ego was viewed as a relatively helpless entity under the pressure of the forces of drives and instincts (i.e., especially sexuality and aggression) and crushed by the merciless demands of the superego (i.e., of the internalized value patterns). This ego was viewed as the center of consciousness, identity, reflection, and decisionmaking. Later the concept was widened by Hartmann (145) and, still later, by the more encompassing concepts of the self, elaborated by Kohut (201).

The superego was understood as the internalized agent of socialization; it was the incorporated authority of worldly or ecclesiastic origin. The superego contained all the internalized norms, ideologies, beliefs, values, attitude, role prescriptions, and rules. The superego guided the behavior of the individual in order to make it conform to the demands of the society. It is interesting to note that this concept has not experienced any important modification since Freud (107, p. 62 ff).

The id was the representative of "drives," which were supposed to be rooted in the interspace of soma and psyche and, according to Freud (101, p. 410 ff; 103, p. 211; 104, p. 38; 109, p. 70), were basically of a purely biologic nature. This concept was later modified by Fromm (110, 111), Horney (161), and Mendel (250) who emphasized the modification of "drives" by the economic base or the overall structure of society. The drive concept is also used in this sense by philosophers such as Marcuse (237, 238). Basically, the "drives" are thought of as being in the service of self-maintenance and maintenance of species.

I use quotation marks on the word "drive" because of the vagueness of the notion. Even Freud (107, p. 101) admitted that the drive theory is the private mythology of psychoanalysis.

The structure of the triad — ego, superego, and id — was supposed to be built up mainly, if not exclusively, by socialization of mother-child interaction in early infancy. The character formed via identification with the parents was supposed to be basically completed within the first few years of life. This is certainly an oversimplification of reality, as is the rigid developmental model which binds traits of character directly to fixation or regression to the presumably "oral," "anal," "phallic," and "oedipal" stages of growth. Nevertheless, the model has made us aware of many facts and features overlooked for a long period of time. It was modified by Reich (292, p. 176 ff) who views the character as a diachronic modification of the ego or as an armor which the ego builds up against the demands from the id and superego. In this process, three mechanisms are supposed to determine the final structure of the armor — identification with the rejecting person; deviation of aggression from the rejecting person upon the self; and, eventually, reactive defense against sexual "drives," the energy of which is used for this defense.

The major handicap of this model, as correctly critizices by Bateson (17) and Grinker (120), is that it is based upon the energy paradigm, but, as I have shown (cf. 130), it was the only concept available before cybernetics and the theory of information and communication was created. In its most general formulation, as put forward by Lorenzer (227, p. 40), we can agree with this model of character formation even today; it is a process passing through different stages and requiring at each stage the integration of biologic and social demands.

Let us consider briefly the alternative model I formulated for the purpose of this study, which I call the cybernetic-syngenetic model of character formation.

An individual is born into a family. At its arrival, it has certain genetic information. Genetic information determines, as Dobzhansky (75, p. 33) puts it, "the possibility of culture, not its content." Genetic information is a program contained in the structure of DNA. It is modifiable by new combinations according to the principle of probabilistic actions described by Piaget and Imhelder (278, p. 118). The genetic program determines some physical features and the basic biopsychological entities (e.g., "drives," "instincts," and "temperament"). These terms are not satisfactory, but we have no better ones to replace them at this moment, although Jaynes (177, p. 31) has promised to publish some conceptual improvements.

Man has a neocortex which differentiates him from animals and their hypothalamic center; the center of instinct control is underdeveloped compared to animals (285, p. 59). We can assume, therefore, that his neocortex controls his behavior more than the hypothalamus does. On this basis, we can question the claims of the psychoanalytic "drive" model, but also of the reflex model of behaviorism.

The individual starts to transact by laughing, crying, drinking, moving, urinating, and defecating. He has an as yet undifferentiated image of himself, of his emotions and actions. His actions are emitted signals which elicit responses. If the response is specific for an action emitted (e.g., feeding whenever crying is due to hunger; giving a blanket when it is due to the cold; nursing and caring when it is due to unhappiness), the individual begins to differentiate some of his emotions and steering elements. This is the origin of identity. If there is no response, the wrong response, or always the same response, differentiation in the signal pool does not occur and the formation of identity is deficient.

As the child grows, the range and the number of his transactions increase (e.g., he plays, crawls, walks, touches things, and breaks them apart). He explores. He gets in touch with the world and develops the concepts of space, time, and causality, as analyzed by Piaget (275, 276). He develops speech and, again, his transactional range increases (i.e., verbal messages reach distant objects and put him in relation with the world).

To all these transactions the environment responds; sometimes stimulating and encouraging, sometimes rejecting or prohibiting. This leads to a continuous learning process in which the child builds up a list of implicit and explicit rules; specifically, the hierarchy of determinants discussed earlier. In the process of the so-called deutero-learning, described by Bateson (17, p. 279 ff), the child learns different sets of rules according to the different responses he gets from the environment. Even if he interacts only with his mother, which is rarely true, he is interacting with the whole society since the mother's responses are shaped by the whole society. In this sense, we can say that an individual always transacts with the whole ecological system, composed of nature, and a human system. Interaction between nature and human beings shape the character of the latter to a considerable extent.

The learning process continues at school and, later, throughout life, especially when the individual enters a new context. Although the plasticity and flexibility of personality structures sometimes decreases with the years, it can also increase in the process of maturation. This means that life is an uninterrupted learning process occurring in steps and stages and at varying speed and intensity.

In this learning process, there are two major kinds of feedback. Balanced interaction processes are guided by both positive and negative feedback. Unbalanced interaction systems are governed by only one type of feedback which, in the long run, leads to the blowing up of the system. Too much or the complete lack of critizism are equally destructive for human systems. The following examples illustrate how these two types of feedback, alone or in interaction, govern human behavior.

Example 1. A man sits at the bar of a local tavern and drinks. According to his view, he continues to drink because his wife is nagging and criticizes him whenever he is at home. After midnight, he walks home. His wife, furious to see him drunk again, is convinced that she is not firm enough. She scolds, shouts, and criticizes. He decides to leave home again as soon as possible in order to escape his unfriendly wife; thus, the vicious circle continues. In this dyadic system, the transactions are governed by a continuous positive feedback which leads to an escalation of drinking and nagging. Both husband and wife are victims of this process which is controlled by a distorted epistemology. In the long run, this system will lead to a complete schismogenesis, as described by Bateson (16, p. 171 ff).

Example 2. A farmer walks through the fields and passes by an empty stable. He sees a shovel. It is dark and nobody is around. Being a poor farmer he steals the shovel and walks home. He goes to bed but cannot sleep. As a good Catholic, his conscience bothers him. He imagines all the things that can happen to him if his stealing is discovered. He imagines what happens if he unexpectedly dies. Finally, he gets up, puts on his clothes, and brings the shovel back. In this case, the negative feedback from a bad conscience guides a deviant action process back to the norm.

Given the results of this learning process, we can say that the genetic program is completed by the syngenetic program (cf. 131), developed in varying human relationships, composed of information stored probably in RNA molecules (i.e., long term memory) and in bioelectrical circuits (i.e., short term memory). The syngenetic program is "soft" programmed and changes over time, whereas the genetic program is "hard" programmed and remains the same. Both programs control human behavior and, thus, determine character.

The syngenetic program contains the set of rules and determinants which govern transactions. Most of the syngenetic program, stemming from multiple and changing relationships, is never conscious and does not have to be so. The syngenetic program is the hidden code built up by the experiences gained in different contexts. It contains the result of the different types of learning, described by Bateson (17, p. 279). One of its elements of information is the result of metalearning leading to a very important implicit law — that different contexts require different transactions and that all contexts require controlled behavior.

Given this theoretical introduction, let us now use it as a guideline for the description of the process of character formation in the village.

In the extended family system of the tradition-directed society, the process of socialization was essentially determined by all the members of the family. The basic rules and values to be learned were the same for centuries and, therefore, the socialization process did not encounter major difficulties; its authority was unchallenged. Legitimation of power was embedded in a chain of command leading from the parents and the grandparents to the priest and the Lord himself. To teach a firm belief in authority was a central issue of socialization, as were the teaching of conservativism, traditionalism, piety, and the unconditional acceptance of the life condition in obedience and submission to the Lord. Thus, the syngenetic programm was rather rigidly defined and stable, as was the typical character of the people.

A child grew up in a well structured world and encountered a well defined set of rules transmitted in the daily teaching by the adults, the customes, legends and myths, and the ten commandments of the Roman Catholic Church. Since economic conditions had not changed for centuries, neither the expected behavior had changed nor had the rules governing it.

The contingencies and random events which occurred at times were explained away by quoting the old sayings and proverbs, the equivocal meaning of which made them fit every occasion.

As a general rule, the character of the tradition-oriented society was under the whip of a merciless "superego," nourished by the priest who preached every Sunday, *ora et labora* and "in the sweat of thy face shalt thou eat bread." Such a process produced a character which lacked all the "feminine," sensuous, passive, open, and friendly traits. So-called "masculine" traits (e.g., tenacity, control, reserve, and taciturnity) prevailed. Trade with foreigners stimulated some additional traits typical for a mercantile society — flexibility, mistrust, cunning, superficial friendliness, and feigned cordiality. It is interesting to note that some of the latter qualities made up the reputation of the villagers as perceived by the rural population outside the valley.

Human beings are not robots and adaptation to rules does not always occur. Sanctions threatened deviation in order to guarantee the demanded syngenetic program. Deviant behavior was punished physically or psychologically. The main sanction was impending shame. This is a sanction typical for the tradition-directed society, as described by Riesman (297, p. 40 ff). Shame is, as Marx (cf. 110, p. 158) rightly stated, rage detoured from its object and channelled upon the self. This mechanism is partly illustrated by the autoaggressive sanctions at the time of the flooding of the lake discussed earlier.

Once tourism started to change the economic base of the village, it moved from a tradition-directed to an inner-directed society. With it, the values started to change, as did the process of socialization and the sanctions for deviant behavior. The content of the syngenetic program started to be modified. One example of this modification is to be found in the toilet training of children. During the agricultural era, children were not necessarily trained to be clean because, in a farmer's house, different odors from the fields, stable, and kitchen melted into a specific time-honored scent that disturbed no one, but when the household expanded into a tourist facility, the "anal" training changed because certain odors were no longer acceptable. This new "anal" training, based upon a changing economy, produced certain traits of character needed in a mercantile-capitalistic system. Parcimony, tenacity, order, and control were some of the new traits. This character pushed forward industrialization which, in turn, reinforced the formation of these same traits.

At this point, one can ask what this change of programming has to do with the Freudian "anality." In my opinion, there is simply a temporal coincidence, but no developmental "libido" connection, as claimed by psychoanalytic theory. A changing economy demanded a new syngenetic program to guarantee the type of transactions for behavior needed within the new organization of life. Orderliness, cleanliness, and punctuality are the character features an industrialized society needs. The training of children, therefore, changes and, since behavior involving rectal incontinence clearly violates all three functional demands (i.e., rules concerning orderliness, cleanliness, and exact timing), this behavior has to be changed. This temporal coincidence led, amazingly enough, to the postulate of an interconnection between "libidinal" development and character formation.

While these "anal" character traits changed, "oral" traits (e.g., moderate indulgence in eating and drinking) were becoming more acceptable. Also, the preexisting "phallic" traits of fighting, attacking, and domineering were fostered by the growing competition of the tourist era.

This era also fostered innovative-creative behavior in order to match the multiple demands of a new kind. Capacity to take risks, achievement orientation, and spirit of enterprise became highly esteemed. Thus, the rules guaranteeing such behavior had to be encompassed into the syngenetic program. The new socialization was influenced by acculturation (i.e., the gradual taking over of values and behaviors from the tourists who came from industrialized and urbanized areas). The new sanction against deviant behavior was no longer shame, but, rather, guilt, which was the feeling of culpability induced by the pulpit and the daily education. The culpability which already existed earlier was increased and this was not accidental. In a world where rigid social structures began to move all at once, people lost their security. They assumed that something was wrong and the autoaggressive explanation was that they themselves must be wrong.

Culpability mostly concerned aggression and sexuality. Aggression was controlled by the population of the village, since survival in the mountains demanded cooperation and solidarity, but a repressed need remains a need which looks for an outlet. The mechanism of catharsis for aggression was to be found in the village gossip of the old and new society. The hard physical work was another important outlet for aggressions.

In this gossip, the rhetoric celebrated secret fiestas and the art of massive and subliminal allusions was highly perfected. Nonverbal and verbal expressions had to match to be clear enough for the receiver of the message and concealed enough in case of censorship. The stereotype formula for the starting or trading of gossip was, "people say that. . ." or "I don't want to have said anything whatsoever . . . but . . ." In a kind of magic realism, the sender of the message closed his eyes like a child who pretends not to be seen when he does not see the others. Once the gossip was started, it rushed like an atomic chain reaction through the village, bouncing back and forth and creating an avalanche of threat and malicious pleasure. Each person could add, substract, or distort its content according to his own needs which, of course, depended upon the relationship with the subject of the gossip and with the person gossip was directed to. In any case, the result was guaranteed; gossip always damaged the reputation of the victimized person.

Gossip duels were fought over weeks, months, years, and sometimes, generations. Such rituals of aggression were not easily recognizable for the outsider (57, p. 25). This has to be so as not to create too much culpability in the author and the different editors of the gossip and to allow him to regulate his aggressive potential which was not consumed in the physical work of the rural life. The ritual was structured in such a way that inner and outer censorship could be avoided as much as possible.

Sexuality was even more repressed by the Church and sexual activities had to be carefully concealed. Wylie (373, p. 117 ff) observed that in a Catholic rural area in Southern France, the little village Peyrane, extramarital relationships were easily accepted. In Saas-Fee, they were strictly prohibited. As Adorno (3, p. 107) put it, it is the rage based upon sexual repression which fosters a merciless moral sense. This moral (i.e., antisexual) sense was highly developed in the village. It was controlled by the priest, representative, and victim of total sexual repression who sowed the seed for further repression. This repression and embittered condemnation of sex was so massive that even marital sexuality was accepted in an equivocal way, as the following illustration shows.

Up to the 1940s, a pregnant woman tried to hide her pregnancy as long as possible. She was ashamed and tried to avoid undesirable comments. To hide the pregnancy even to the 7th-8th month was easy under the long wide skirts of the traditional costume. However, she did not always escape social control. If she got sick during the celebration of the Mass and had to walk out of the church, the villagers, gloating over other people's misfortune, would repeat for days how this woman had been successfully "caught."

The ecclesiastical attitude toward sex led to grotesque incongruities and contradictions since the conception of children was fostered, but the real or assumed pleasure combined with sex was rejected. This becomes clear in the following custom, still widely displayed in the Canton Wallis until the middle of our century. To bear a child was the duty of a Catholic mother, but, after she delivered the child, she had to go through a ritual of purification – obviously aimed at the sin of sexual pleasure – before being allowed to reenter the church. She would be received by the clergyman on a weekday at the entrance of the church. With prayers and benedictions, she would be led, step by step, into the church and in front of the altar. This ritual accomplished, she was allowed to reenter the church the following Sunday as a purified normal person.

The prospect of reaching heaven was the bait, and the prospect of being damned to eternal hell was the whip. Both constituted strong forces which controlled sexuality and aggression. They were responsible for the deferred gratification pattern which governed the life style of the villagers. This pattern enabled them to undergo the "ordeal of Sisyphos," as Adorno (3, p. 71) aptly put it, which determined the control of their personal and communal "drive" economy. The beginning influence of tourism could not change this pattern because the new ideology of achievement demanded new renouncement and self-control to reach the ultimate goal of the village – to become a famous tourist resort.

4.7.2.3 Kinship System

As Wurzbacher and Pflaum (376, p. 82) state, the kinship system is an auxiliary social system which connects families and society. As Koenig (191, p. 144) points out, a kinship system in rural areas is a system of intensive economic cooperation which fosters solidarity and mutual responsibility. Kinship systems increase the social integration.

In the agricultural society of the village, the kinship system was very important. There were essentially only eight families in the village which, over the centuries, intermarried. Predictably, such inbreeding created strong ties and bonds. There was a distinct kinship identity that governed much of the behavior within the village and its boundaries were rigidly defined and separated one clan from the other.

Within kinship systems, there was mutual help and control which was more extensive and intensive than the control by the village. Late and living members of the family clans were admired models of identification to be followed or bad examples to be avoided. Mutual help made life easier and mutual control tightened the armor around the small area of freedom left for independent decisionmaking. Both heightened the general feeling of trust, security, and identity.

4.7.2.4 Community of Saas-Fee

Saas-Fee was a well-integrated community in which common goals and problems fostered global cooperation and solidarity. Common tasks intensified the network of interdependence, parts of which were already tightly woven by family and kinship.

A community has many goals – integration, control of behavior, socialization, economic survival and development, maintenance of boundaries, and autonomy and identity of the community as a whole and of its subsystems (e.g., kinships, families, and individuals). A community reaches its goals by means of two institutions – the public's opinion, on the one hand, and the Church, school, municipality, burgher community, associations, parties, and professions, on the other. The former type is governed by informal personal transactions whereas the latter type is governed by more formalized transactions often located in a given querencia (i.e., in a specific space-time continuum). Both types of institutions shape, direct, and integrate the transactional web composed by the behavioral patterns of all its members in the different subsystems.

As an example of how public opinion may work, I refer to our discussion of village gossip. Gossip controls the behavior of the person it is aimed at and it integrates the people involved into the common task of trading hostilities wrapped in the equivocal language of gossip. It also maintains the homeostasis of the village by channeling aggression in such a way that it does not become physically destructive.

Institutions are like shells used by short-lived organisms and then abandoned. Shells may serve for several generations or even several centuries. If their basic functions change because society changes, then new shells and new institutions are created. Public opinion is a shell that is as old as mankind. Other institutions (e.g., school, the Church) survived unchanged for a long time, whereas associations and political parties are institutions which were created only when the economic and political situations started to change.

I will briefly discuss the major functions of the institutions characterized by formal transactions and exterior signs and symbols, such as specific space-time; context; customs; and, sometimes, costumes.

(1) School. The village school was originally a communal school in which boys and girls were educated together. All grades were gathered in the same classroom. Later, with the increase of the population, school was differentiated into sex specific classes. Eventually, in the second half of our century, a school for classes of different ages, sexes, and grades was developed.

As Bolte (34, p. 28) and Daheim (66, p. 374) emphasize, the school is a screening device which segregates its members early and decides on vertical mobility. This, however, was not particularly the case in Saas-Fee because there was no possibility for vertical mobility within the village. For generations, the school trained its children during 6 winter months and for 8 years. For 2 more years, there was a course of so-called repetition to be attended a few weeks per year. The content of the learning process encompassed the basic knowledge in reading, writing, arithmetic, geography, and history; the latter subject was studied quite intensively. The dates of the battles of the old Swiss Confederation were dear to the heart of every teacher. History was held in awe and its heroes were highly admired. Thus, the children were prepared for the patriarchal society. This was also stressed by the teaching style. The teacher had not only the right, but the duty, to physically punish his students whenever they did not comply. The school was the drill square for subordinative behavior and the initiation hut for the authoritarian society.

In a tradition-directed society, the child tries to adapt at any price to parents and schoolmasters, as Riesman (297, p. 66) observed. There was, indeed, little conflict between children and teachers according to our information. The schoolmaster was an unchallenged authority who had an admired monopoly on information and often played an important political role in the community. Later, with the changing times, his authority declined, albeit slowly. As Rosenmayr (301, p. 124) points out, the main source of possible conflict lies in the discrepancy between a petrified institution and the vivid youth who pushes toward new frontiers. This situation arose with the budding tourism because the school did not adapt as fast to the social change as the youth did. Still, compared to the modern situation in cities, the decline of authority in the village school can be considered minimal.

(2) The Church and Church-Going. For centuries, the Church and church-going fulfilled an integrative social function. In the church, all the villagers met in a common ritual; sharing time, prayers, and sermons; and also hopes and fears. Before and after church, on the plaza and the way back home, there was time for the exchange of information, chatting, and gossipping.

The social power of an actor depends upon his capacity to create or alleviate states of deprivation and his potential for social control (Hummel 166, p. 1194). The clergyman was a very powerful figure. With the help of the sacraments, especially confession, communion, and anointment, he could alleviate the threat of eternal deprivation. Confession gave him an informational monopoly useful for social control and so was the literal and symbolic metalevel of the pulpit from which he could frighten, threat, or encourage the dependent and often despondent flock. He was responsible to quite an extent for how the villagers experienced their lives and, since the predominant ideas are often the ideas of the dominant individuals, his influence upon their *Weltanschauung* was fundamental.

Fostering a common ideology, the Church was a highly active integrator for diminishing some anxieties by creating new ones which, in a second step, could be alleviated. The Church offered security and, according to the ten commandments, increased the general belief in authority splendidly displayed by the ecclesiastic dignitaries and ultimately rooted in the Lord himself.

The Church also influenced the socialization of the children by teaching the ideas of the catechism which indoctrinated the youngest members in the generally accepted ideology.

(3) The Municipality and the Burgher Community. I discussed some of their functions before. Both institutions organized repetitive rituals at meetings in which people interacted according to formalized patterns. This formalization of the interactional patterns supported the general function of control. Control was of vital importance since the meetings, especially during election times, allowed the display of ritualized aggression, without endangering the coherence of the group too much. If a person lost the election, he was punished for former supposed or real wrongdoing. Thus, the balance of the political subsystem was restored. The loser could maintain that "ingratitude is the reward of the world," saving face and hiding bad conscience and narcissistic rage behind the respectable mask of a well-known proverb. Both the municipality and the burgher community had an important normative function which maintained the homeostasis of the community by controlling horizontal and vertical cooperation and solidarity.

These institutions created the firm basis for development, growth, and transformation of the village as a whole. This is the reason why the two institutions remained virtually unchanged even after the beginning of industrialization.

(4) Associations, Clubs, and Political Parties. In these institutions, as well as in the municipality and burgher community, there was a time limited transfer and delegation of power with one major difference — while municipality and burgher community pursued communal goals, the goals and functions of associations, clubs, and political parties were often more specific and particularistic.

Associations, as Wurzbacher and Pflaum (376, p. 151 ff) state, were products of social differentiation. Being formal organizations, they replace the former informal and personal forms of contact by ritualizing them. They are, therefore, institutions which arise whenever there is a need for formalization.

In the village, the associations, with one exception, started in the 20th century. The sequence of their foundation is the following: old village music in 1854; ski club in 1908; cooperative association in 1908; men's association in 1908; new village music in 1913, dissolved in 1914, and refounded in 1923; Raiffeisenkasse, a form of local bank in 1915; association for promoting tourism in 1925; mountain guide club in 1927; alpine dairyfarming association in 1933; and soccer club in 1937, transformed into a hockey club in 1942, and soon dissolved again.

The old village music, which today is still a great tourist attraction, was obviously founded as a symbol of the turning point between the traditional life and the new life. The uniforms were those worn by the mercenaries, a group the villagers had joined at times. The mercenary lifestyle was prohibited by the New Swiss Constitution of 1848. Six years later, the old village music was founded. This is the time when the first tourists came into the valley and the foundation of this music can be interpreted as a symbol of unity, pride, and identity displayed for a folkloristic purpose to impress the English tourists.

All these associations have one thing in common — they channel and structure some needs and interests into a well-defined organization. This process occurred at a time when the traditional homogeneity and coherence of the social organization began to change. It can, therefore, be interpreted as expressions and symbols of rebalancing maneuvres in the service of homeostasis maintenance.

Associations, clubs, and political parties offered a hierarchy with different roles, each with its own status and prestige. These roles and positions were won or lost in recurrent elections which constituted an immediate feedback for past performance and the way one was socially accepted. Elections and their preparation functioned like computers, calculating plus and minus in a very complex and not always transparent way and indicating the exact position of each member of an association, club, or political party at a given time.

(5) Occupations and Professions. I discussed the development of the occupational structure before, therefore, I will focus here only on the socializing and integrative function of occupations and professions.

People are not only what they think, they are what they do. This means that their identity determines, and is determined by, their actions. These actions, in turn, constitute the structural identity of the system of which they are members. An occupation is composed of a specific pattern of transactions with a specific goal which gives specific status and prestige to its holder. Thus, the occupational structure of a village contributes to its general coherence and social integration.

Occupational roles in traditional Saas-Fee were fairly undifferentiated. Once the social change started, the set of occupational roles started to change and the degree of professionalization increased. The quotient of social mobility is defined, according to Bolte (34, p. 12), by the number of persons with a different occupation from the one their father had. This quotient increased gradually in the village. Intergenerational and intragenerational mobility accelerated. Each of the occupations and professions elaborated a different set of norms in order to check the quality of work and performance. Whoever moved into a new role (e.g., mountain guide, ski instructor, employee) had to learn the rules of the new job and to adapt to the prevailing norms. During social change, general anxiety increases, but the differentiation of norms is anxiety reducing since an ever more complicated world provides clear rules and prescriptions to be followed. Thus, the syngenetic program not only changes, it also becomes more defined.

4.7.2.5 Extralocal Factors

A last group of socializing agents is to be found in extralocal factors and institutions (e.g., trade, seasonal work, emigration, military service, tourism, modern means of communication). The socialization acquired by or transferred through these factors is called acculturation. Acculturation means the taking over of norms and values from another social system which is organized differently from one's own.

To the extent that the village got into contact with the outside world, a flow of information rushed into Saas-Fee. This information flow brought new ideas which often conflicted with the old ones. As Habermas (133, p. 11) illustrates, systemic contradictions and incongruencies are overcome by adaptation. The adaptation has two basic mechanisms – transformation of elements of the system or transformation of the target values. As we have seen, the village adopted both forms of adaptation. For a long time, however, the old syngenetic program was deeply shaken by the process of acculturation.

I shall briefly discuss the six factors leading to a transformation of systemic elements and target values during the process of acculturation.

(1) Trade. The contact with foreign markets and people in the nearby Italian villages initiated the formation of new character traits (e.g., the spirit of speculation and bargaining) which went against the agricultural values of conservation and maintenance. Unlike the farmer, the merchant values property only inasmuch as it is convertible merchandise. The higher the price he can get, the better the merchandise. Good and bad begin to be qualified not in moral terms, but more and more in terms of profit.

This process induced an alienation between man and nature. It also made man more flexible since he slowly learned not to cling too much to the things he possessed. The villagers had to change their attitudes and actions, especially concerning land. Land, a "holy property" for the farmer, had to become a convertible property as soon as industrialization started in order to yield the economic needs necessary for investments. As Znaniecki (cf. 356, p. 78) states, actions have a tendency to build up value patterns in the process of their realization. The action of trading did, indeed, build up new value patterns which, in turn, modified the future actions of the villagers.

(2) Seasonal work. According to Sorokin (cf. 36, p. 28), regional mobility, a form of horizontal social mobility, has two major consequences – loss of security and enlargement of the field of vision. The seasonal workers came back to the village with new technical know-how and new attitudes, beliefs, and values. Seasonal workers were rather achievement motivated people, this being the reason they emigrated in the first place. Their influence on the village was quite important. They pushed forward the process of social change by teaching new skills and values, thus changing the process of socialization.

Being absent for a part of the year, their hierarchical position sometimes changed
within the family. The wife and mother would take over new responsibilities and authority. This, again, influenced the process of socialization. Sometimes the identity of the
whole family was influenced, changing from a tradition-oriented farmer's family to
an open-minded, slightly other-directed family with some money to improve their life
condition and some information about the life styles and the problems of other people.

As Horstmann (162, p. 49) emphasizes, emigration is dependent upon an incongruency between the demographic and the economic subsystem. As expected, it stopped
in Saas-Fee as soon as increasing tourism decreased this incongruency. By then, the acculturation process was fostered by the visiting tourists.

(3) Emigration. Villagers who emigrated definitively to other parts of Switzerland
or foreign countries also influenced socialization. They visited the village once in a while
or they wrote letters. Both mechanisms increased the input of information augmenting
acculturation. Since their narratives were sometimes overdrawn and fantastic, they provoked curiosity and the wish to be like the people they described. These narratives were
the rails along which some elements of acculturation and socialization moved.

(4) Military Service. In earlier centuries, villagers were sometimes hired by foreign
military leaders. They visited foreign countries and brought back the knowledge of new
technical skills, values, and behavior. They, therefore, became agents of acculturation
and socialization.

In 1815, the Canton Wallis, and with it Saas-Fee, joined the Swiss Confederation. In
1848, the constitution made the custom of mercenaries illegal. Switzerland introduced
an obligatory militia and military service for every man beginning at 20 years old. The
military's introductory training has always been seen as a ritual of initiation into manhood. Even in 1970, I would often hear the old villagers say that "only military service
is able to produce a real man."

While in the military service, a young man came in contact with cities and urbanized
people. Being young, he was open to new ideas and brought them back to the village.
At the same time his village consciousness and his regional consciousness were widened
to a national identity. Both processes influenced the socialization of the younger generation.

(5) Tourism. Once tourism had started, the process of acculturation accelerated. The
first English tourists were models of a different life-style, ideas, and values. They seemed
to belong to a superior class of man and, therefore, they were eagerly imitated. They
were urbanized, highly educated, widely travelled, and well-off. They were people who
obviously did not have to work. They created new jobs because they needed mountain
guides, chambermaids, and the like.

The English were a distinguished class, self-confident, noble, and sometimes snob-
bish. To be like them was a goal worth pursuing. The villagers began to learn English,
drink tea, and imitate their behavior in many ways. Tolman (cf. 165, p. 1180) pointed
out that behavioral change occurs in two steps — implicit tendencies of reactions change
first and the behavioral sequence changes later. In Saas-Fee, the people started to identify
with the English who were then at the zenith of their power. It made the villagers more self-
confident and achievement-motivated, leading, for instance, to the high achievements

in ski competition mentioned earlier. These, in turn, produced a kind of communal nationalism; a pride which, in itself, changed the process of socialization.

(6) Mass Media. The mass media of the last century were the newpapers and, later, the radio. Both factors influenced the process of socialization and acculturation.

Mass media influenced the preexisting personal ideas concerning sex, relations, family, groups, and collectives, as stressed by Koenig (196, p. 202 ff). Mass media have a reinforcing rather than a causally stimulating effect, as Silbermann and Luthe (327, p. 693) outlined in their discussion of the outcome of modern mass media research. Nevertheless, the mass media introduced new ideas and stereotypes (e.g., the woman as merchandise, the man as a well-functioning wheel in the economic machinery) which flourished in the cities. They introduced idols and models which often contradicted the traditional ideas. But more than anything else, they connected the village to the outside world, fostering the feeling of interconnectedness and, therefore, changing the provincial parochialism in the direction of a more cosmopolitan consciousness. The mass media were powerful agents of the "rurbanization" mentioned before.

Essentially, the villagers read two newspapers, both of them being mouthpieces of the two political parties. They were regional publications which conformed with the Catholic ideology and were uninfluenced by the crime and sex ideology of modern journals. By supporting or opposing specific local issues, they were an important factor in social control. It is through the formation of attitudes, opinions, ideas, and values that the mass media influenced the process of socialization and the development of a new syngenetic program in the minds of the villagers.

4.7.3 Content and Rituals of Socialization

Socialization is a process by which norms and values are handed down from generation to generation. Once received, this information constitutes the syngenetic program which governs transactions and which is responsible for the coherence of the social organization. The handing down of the information which builds up the syngenetic program is institutionalized. The information is encoded in rituals, customs, legends, fairy tales, and myths. I will discuss both the institutions and the content of the information processing with the implicit ritual rules they contain.

Values are the rules which govern behavior. They determine the extrafunctional capacities of the role carriers. The extrafunctional capacities determine character and personality which enable the actors to play a given role, as Dahrendorf (cf. 68, p. 363) made clear. If the roles change, the extrafunctional capacities have to change and, with them, the values and socialization (i.e., the transfer of values). Depending upon his extrafunctional capacities, a person will choose one or the other occupation. This is especially true in times of social change when alternate roles are available.

A few examples may illustrate this process. A farmer educated in such a way that his character is shy, taciturn, and mistrusting tends to choose a technological profession where he can deal with machines rather than men. If, however, he is openminded, friendly, and outgoing he might instead choose the profession of a hotel manager or innkeeper to deal with people. If he is service oriented and garrulous, he might choose to be a shopkeeper. If he is bold, he might become a mountain guide. If he is aggressive and domineering, he might become a police officer. If he likes to be both friendly and domineering, he might become a ski instructor. In this latter role, which has its own set of rules and values, he is allowed to call each of his guests by the first name which, in European cultures, is a rather unusual and sometimes slightly impolite style of dealing with people one does not know well. No one will protest if a ski instructor shouts to a dignified upper-class woman, "Honey, you are sailing through the landscape like an angry milk cow."

Let us have a closer look now at some of the mechanisms which integrate the social community; especially costumes, customs, legends, myths, norms, and values. They contain the ritual rules which are implicit and guide nonrational behavior. The value patterns (e.g., moral sense, ideas, ideologies, norms), however, are explicit and contain the technical rules which steer rational actions. Both technical and ritual rules are constituents of the syngenetic program.

4.7.3.1 Costumes

Both intensive and extensive social control in Saas-Fee involved the wearing of the traditional costume. Sociopsychological uniformity is simultaneously achieved and expressed by uniforms and the homogeneity of the village created uniform costumes which remained virtually unchanged for centuries. Ethologists, like Eibl-Eibesfeldt (88, p. 509 ff), underline the extent to which uniformity in clothing fosters the smooth cooperation of a given population. Since costumes and social integration are interconnected phenomena, we will have a closer look at each of them.

The classical dress of the men was made of canvas *(Drillich-Hose* or *Trilch-Hose),* a triple-spun and woven fabric which resisted wear and tear. Women wore a skirt made of the same material. It seem that the population was aware of the fact that such uniformity supported social structures and control, an awareness expressed by the chronicler Ruppen (308) who, in 1887, deplored that on "August 15 the last man wearing shorts (short canvas trousers reaching the knee) was buried and with him a piece of simple patriarchic life."

Imseng (166, p. 8) gives an exact description of the costumes still worn at the time of the construction of the road. Women wore a canvas dress consisting of one single piece covering the whole body. They used wooden or low leather shoes, called pitch-shoes *(Pechschuhe),* with a nickel buckle. Their stockings were made of lambs wool, sometimes slightly blue in color. They wore a high collared shirt covered with a triangular kerchief, whose angle pointed between the shoulder blades. On Sundays, they wore a white collar and a white or grey apron. During winter, they covered their head with a white or red wool cap or a hat without *Kress* (cf. Fig. 9). According to Imseng (166, p. 8), all the women had big round earrings "like countesses," obviously a relic of the upper class in feudal times.

According to Duebi (82, p. 64) and Supersaxo (348), the headgear of the woman was especially characteristic of the costume of the valley (Fig. 9). The kerchief was white in summer and yellow-red in winter. On Sundays and holidays, women wore the much admired square hat *(Kresshut)* which was covered with whatever color ribbon was appropriate for the social event being celebrated.

The function of the kerchief and the square-hat and their use were highly regulated, as Imseng (169, p. 174 ff) reports. The following correspondence between a social event and headgear is reported:

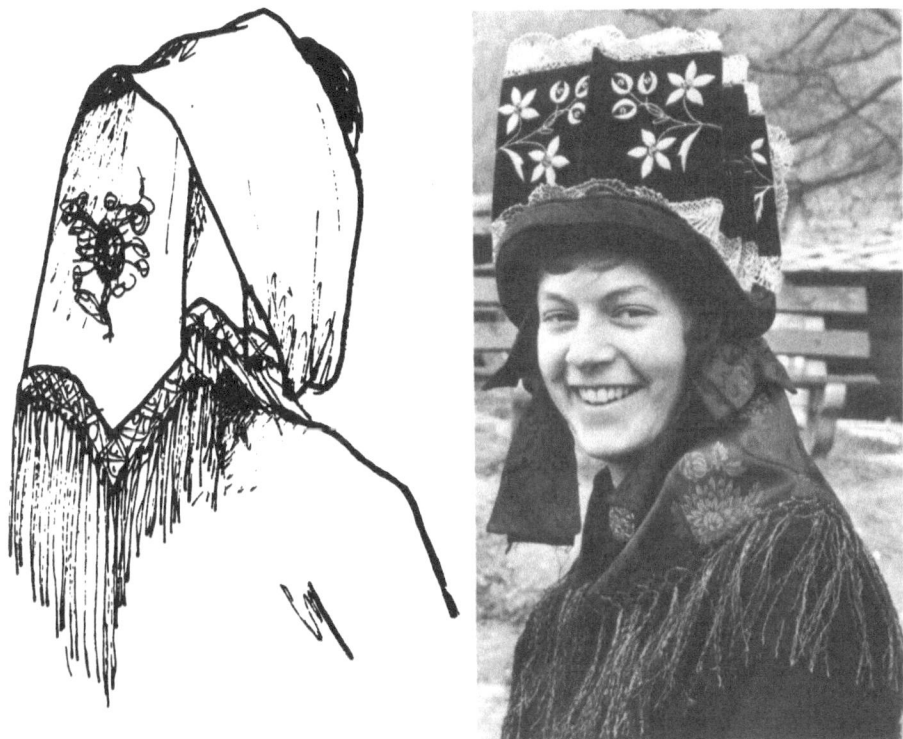

Fig. 9. Kerchief and square-hat. (Photo: W. Imseng, Zeichnung: M. Masini)

- Square-hat with black ribbon, adorned with gold embroidery; worn on the holiday of Corpus Christi and other celebrations
- Square-hat with white ribbon and gold embroidery; worn by the godmother for the baptism of her godchild, the female kinship for the consecration of a priest, or the kinship women for the burial of a child who died before school age
- White embroidered kerchief with fringes; worn on ordinary Sundays by women who had not reached the age of 55, i.e., women able to give birth
- Multicolored kerchief; prescribed for women over 55 and obligatory for ordinary Sundays
- Brown kerchief with embroidery and fringes; worn for burials by women who were not members of the kinship group of the dead, women of the wider kinship wore it for the time between burial and the Mass celebrated after 1 year of mourning
- Black kerchief with black fringes; worn by the women of the immediate kinship group of the dead (e.g., widow, grandmother, sister, mother-in-law, sister-in-law) for burials and during the mourning time. The mourning time varied depending on the degree of kinship, the closer the degree the longer the prescribed mourning time
- Black kerchief with multicolored embroidery and fringes; obligatory for several weeks on Sundays and weekdays for female godchildren after the death of a godfather or godmother and for the nieces after the death of uncles or aunts
- Woolen, red-yellow-green kerchief *(Knerlumpi)* without fringes; worn by old women on all occasions and events not specified in the above enumeration.

It is obvious that the function of the female headgear was far more than protective. It was symbolic and signalized status and social order. This integrative-symbolic function of daily objects has been well analyzed by Levi-Strauss (220, p. 17) who speaks of a *micropéréquation* for primitive thought which integrates every object and every aspect of daily life into a particular class within the "savage thinking." The kerchief signals sex, age, degree of kinship, social relation, social event, state of the life cycle, expected extent of mourning, social status, and position of the female villagers. It transmits the overall message, "I am one of yours, a participant in the daily events of our village." As Eibl-Eibesfeldt (88, p. 126) points out, such signalizing behavior is known in ethology as ritualization.

The kerchief is only one type of ritualization in the village. It is the symbolic signalization which replaces the instinctive orientations and perceptions lost in the process of evolution (Cassirer 52, p. 180 ff). Thus, a simple item (e.g., a ribbon or a kerchief) serves the goal of social integration. They are factors of ordering, structuring, anxiety reduction, and reinforcing togetherness and social identity.

The symbolic function of the female costume was, at least unconsciously, perceived by the chronicler Supersaxo (348, p. 38), a priest who wrote in an enthusiastic tone that, "the white kerchief mirrors the splendor of the snowcovered mountains, the black costume mirrors the dignity of the 4000 meters high mountain peaks." He deplored the fact that the costume disappeared at the time of the construction of the road. He could not yet understand that the upcoming social order demanded new signaling functions and new symbols.

Compared to the women, the men were more uniform in their costumes. They wore wooden shoes or pitch shoes, white or grey wool socks, short tight *Balto* trousers, a red or white vest, a white shirt with a high collar, and a canvas jacket. A black or blue silk shawl replaced the cravat. During the week, they wore a peaked cap and, on Sundays, a low cylinder hat. Every man was bearded and most of them wore small round earrings.

Uniformity in customs, costumes, behavior, and value patterns is important for the social ordering process. Psychologically, order can be a defense mechanism against increasing entropy and its psychophysiological correlate – anxiety.

In Saas-Fee, the level of conscious and unconscious anxiety was high. The unpredictable exterior nature was a constant threat. Repression of sexual and aggressive "drives," the inner nature, created substantial anxiety. Morgenthaler et al. (260, p. 558) described in their analysis of aggression-repression in the tribe of the Agni in West Africa, how this latter process functions. Malinowski (236) analysed a comparable process in primitive societies.

As the incipient social change in Saas-Fee increased the level of anxiety, the ordering function of the costumes decreased. Thus, other mechanisms of anxiety reduction had to be found. The new era provided pharmacologic tools (i.e., alcohol and drugs). Another mechanism was the "obsessionalization" of the predominant character and an increase of armoring which perpetuated the hostile and taciturn character of certain individuals. Alcohol and drugs made this armoring a little more flexible. Technology enabled the villagers to control the exterior nature to a considerable extent, thus, diminishing the impact of one source of anxiety and insecurity.

4.7.3.2 Customs

I will discuss some of the habits and customs which were the most typical for the pre-industrial village. They still existed in 1951.

Habits and customs are formed over centuries; their structure is built up step by step and, once it is completed, customs are so well integrated into the social organization that they become almost invisible. Wein (365, p. 726) reports some hypotheses, developed years ago at the Institute for Social Relations at Harvard, which explain the process of habituation and construction of customs — generally accepted values (e.g., communal solidarity) are transferred to concrete areas of experience (e.g., communal work or the custom of the *Abusitz,* which will be discussed below); in this transfer process attitudes originate (e.g., the basic readiness for cooperation); these attitudes control the actual activities (e.g., sitting together during the *Abusitz* or cooperating in communal work).

Let us now discuss a few of these customs and analyze their socializing and integrative function.

One of the interesting customs, reported by Duebi (82, p. 67), concerned the carnival. On Shrove Thursday, called "fat Thursday," around noon the young unmarried men of the village tried to steal the meatpots of another family. They attempted to dupe the women and catch the *feistu Daru,* a sausage, made from the colon of slaughtered domestic animals, that contained meat, fat, corn, caraway, red radish, and spices. The symbolic function of this custom is obvious — during the time of carnival, when social control allowed for more freedom than usual, young men tried to get a "phallic" object, hidden in a closed container and guarded by women who did not belong to the kinship system. Thus, the transactional setting allowed ritualized acting out of aggressive and sexual needs.

Another customs, connected with Shrovetime, was a parade in which the older boys and the younger men participated. The parade went through the whole village. It was headed by the jugglers *(Goiglera)* wearing carved wooden masks showing demonic, menacing, and rage- and anxiety-ridden faces. They especially chased the young women with tails of horses, mules, or cows. The role expectation of the women was to stay at a corner of the street, provoke the jugglers verbally or nonverbally, and then run away. If they got caught, they were whipped.

Thus, once a year the young men and women could symbolically act out aggressive and sexual fantasies in a ritualized context.

It is interesting to view these two customs in a broader conceptual context. Carnival is a widespread institution in Catholic countries. It seems to be an institution which has the function of a safety valve in a steam engine (i.e., to let steam out when the pressure increases). This "steam" accumulates whenever the repression of vital needs is strong. Ritualized events allow the partial emergence of the repressed needs, although under control and within a well-defined setting. This is a mechanism we can add to the three mechanisms mentioned by Freud (110b, 202) which permit the reappearance of the repressed material, i.e., the decrease of the "countercathexis" (e.g., in the case of illness), the reinforcement of "drives" (e.g., during puberty), and events which allude to the repressed (e.g., observation of copulating animals). The social ritual takes over the control which, otherwise, the individual psyche has to exert.

Repression and sublimation of "drives" diminishes pleasure, but it increases social security, as Freud (105, p. 474) correctly observed. Shrovetime, without endangering social security, allowed a kind of pleasure which was symbolic of the repressed pleasure. Thus, the revolt against sexual repression was organized and channeled by these two customs. As Malinowski (236, p. 186 ff) made clear, the tendency towards incest and rebellion against authority are the two basic dangers which threaten culture. The structure of the two customs (i.e., stealing, whipping nonkinship women) prevented both dangers by alluding to the prohibited reality. This ambiguous character seems to be symptomatic for such customs.

Another custom, reported by Imseng (166, p. 7), was the *Abusitz,* a reunion or meeting occurring during the long winter evenings when people met to play cards, smoke, use snuff, and narrate stories, legends, and myths. Most of the time young men gathered in the families with young marriagiable daughters. Sometimes the meeting occurred within the kinship or with friends. They sat around a table drinking coffee and tea. Alcohol consumption was not known in this context. They gossiped. Often the evening ended with the old people speaking about the old times and telling about myths and legends. Thus, the event was put into a spiritual context which transcended the frame of a simple meeting. It served the function of reminding the participants of the norms of the village and the sanctions whenever norms were violated. As Nietzsche (cf. 365, p. 735) stated, consciousness is formed under the pressure of the need for communication. This pressure was especially great during the winters when the village was cut off from the rest of the world and the farmers had enough leisure time for the *Abusitz.* Clearly, the *Abusitz* was a custom which heightened the consciousness or self-identity and reminded the people of the structure of their ecology of mind.

Another custom was connected with sheep breeding. As we have seen, sheep are connected to the name Saas-Fee (*feia* = female sheep) and, with it, to the origin of Saas-Fee. It is an interesting hypothesis that the sheep might originally have played the role of a village totem. With Levi-Strauss's (222) successful undoing of the totemism concept, however, this hypothesis has lost some of its value.

The sheep were slaughtered in October at a festival whose organization reinforced the coherence of the kinship group. The kinship group was invited to eat the greaves (i.e., *Greibu* = greaves: lipoproteid structures which remain after fat has been cooked for several hours). Greaves, considered a speciality, were eaten together with salt potatoes in the context of a family clan meeting. Often, at this time, the past history and the stories of this or other kinship groups were discussed. I should like to note that, during these evening meetings, young masked men came to visit, often mumbling allusions of a sexual or aggressive nature through the slightly open door.

It seems highly symbolic that the basic biologic structures (i.e., lipoproteid structures) were consumed by the members of the basic social structure (i.e., kinship system) in the context of a ritualized custom in which the members of the kinship group had to literally eat out of the same pot. It would be interesting to analyze this custom in terms of an incorporation of a village totem and to compare it to the two previous customs which deal with the ritualized breaking of the taboos on sexuality and aggression. Because an analysis of this kind would require an extensive discussion of the notions of totem and taboo, as developed by Freud (105) and criticized by Levi-Strauss (223, p. 95), it cannot be included here.

As Duebi (82, p. 68) reports, Saas-Fee did not have any contact with the popular theatre of worldly or ecclesiastic themes. Interestingly enough, the recital of popular drama was well developed in the nearby rural regions. It is not clear whether or not the lack of a theatre tradition is due to ethnic-historical reasons or to the fact that it had been forbidden as one of the sanctions imposed by the Church after the floodings of the lake.

4.7.3.3 Legends and Myths

The science of myths is still in its infancy, as Levi-Strauss (224, p. 3) states in his intro-duction to a science of mythology. A theoretical analysis might, therefore, lack the nec-essary conceptual tools. On the other hand, myths combine a paradox or, as Levi-Strauss (221, p. 209) puts it, they allude to an event that happened a long time ago, and whose pattern is universal and timeless. Myth is the forerunner of history, as Cassirer (53, p. 5 tf) claims. Still, the symbolic meaning of myth is more important than the original so-cial event it is derived from.

I shall take these considerations as the starting point of the following analysis of three myths of the village.

Since the pattern of myth is timeless and universal, it can be assumed that legends and myths teach general norms and they serve social integration; creating identity by binding a given society to its origins. Myths are diachronic sorcerers bringing the past and present times into a magic congruency. This allows the listener to identify with the persons in the myths and legends; what they suffer and experience the listener might suffer and experience at any instant.

Legends and myths preserve and pass on the ritual rules which govern that behavior which is not exclusively rational, as Rex (cf. 356, p. 92) states. In Saas-Fee, these ritual rules were transmitted in a very special context. For the most part, old people narrated the myths and legends in the dim light of a tallow candle or a petroleum lamp, throwing flickering shadows over the faces of the people. In this twilight, the people were highly suggestible, moving together and getting goosepimples as the narration went on.

Legends and myths have themes which both trigger anxiety and, by creating order, reduce it. The latter aspect was clearly seen by Habermas (133, p. 164) who speaks of a "narrative production of a shine of order." Legends and myths build the bridge over the contingencies and give meaning to the world in which the absurdity of random events abound. They have a normothetic function because they indicate the sanctions which punish deviant behavior. Obviously, creation of anxiety and threat of punish-ment belong to the classical weaponry of socialization, as Erikson (92, p. 83) rightly states.

(1) The "Flier Jodern Hansjob". Once upon a time the old Flier Jodern Hansjob, a man from Saas-Fee, boasted that he was not afraid of the *Bozu* (i.e., unredeemed souls who expiate their sins in a no man's land between this world and the next, thus paying for the transgression of a norm). One night, Hansjob walked back from the valley and through the chapel path. It was very late for a man to go home. He was between the twelfth and the thirteenth chapel when, all of a sudden, he heard a whistle. He whistled back. Now, something shouted so that the "mountains and valleys resound-ed," and to demonstrate his courage, Hansjob shouted back. Suddenly, a big billy goat

dashed through the forest, throwing itself from behind onto the back of the old man and holding his shoulders with its forefeet. Hansjob, terrified and struggling to reach the thirteenth chapel, had to drag the buck along. Here, in front of the cross, the old man fell on his knees and promised to improve has bad behavior, to donate money for Holy Masses for the salvation of the poor soul trapped inside the buck, and begged forgiveness for his arrogance. At this moment, the buck leaped off his shoulders and was never seen again.

There is a mixture of pagan and Christian elements in this myth. The unredeemed soul appears in the figure of a billy goat. The billy goat is a symbol of the sexual drive and the voluptuousness condemned by the Church. It is also a symbol of aggression and untamed virility.

There is a transgression of a norm. It is interesting to remember that the hero in the classic Greek tragedy was doomed whenever he displayed *hybris* (i.e., the wrong boldness at the wrong time and in the wrong context) or whenever he missed the *cairos* (i.e., the right time for an action). Hansjob had boasted that he was not afraid of evil spirits, which is a display of *hybris*. He missed the *cairos* because he returned home late, at a time when a good father is supposed to be home.

There is a mixture of magic and religious thinking. The billy goat appears before Hansjob reaches the thirteenth chapel. As Cassirer (53, p. 140) pointed out, numbers, together with space and time, are formal motives found in most myths. In common superstition, thirteen is a symbol of misfortune. Bloch called superstition "the metaphysic of the ignorant" which cannot be extirpated. Such superstition functions according to the mechanism of a self-fulfilling prophecy (e.g., the anxiety of expectation in superstitious people may be stressful enough to trigger hallucinations). Hansjob's anxiety in front of the thirteenth chapel could have been strong enough to produce sensory hallucinations with auditory, tactile, and visual features.

The mythical event occurred in a Catholic region. From a Catholic viewpoint, it is interesting that the punishing event occurs between the twelfth and the thirteenth chapel, which means between the twelfth and the thirteenth station of the Cross. According to Catholicism, Jesus died on the Cross at the twelfth station. At the thirteenth station his corpse was taken from the Cross and put into the lap of Mary his mother. Translated into the symbolism of the myth, the *hybris* of the old man, who wanted to be more than an ordinary human being, died at the twelfth chapel. At the thirteenth chapel, Hansjob had to kneel down and show repentence in order to return to the lap of the Church and, thus, to society and its norms. Since his return is the direct antithesis of his sinful *hybris*, the sanction loses its function and the billy goat disappears.

There was, furthermore, a particular style of interaction. Hansjob perceived a whistling (i.e., a message). He responded to this strange, for the given time and context, communication with a symmetrical interaction (i.e., with shouting) instead of emitting a complementary transaction (i.e., with being silent and submissive). According to the transactional laws governing symmetrical interaction patterns, an escalation started which led to shouting and reached its highest point when the billy goat jumped upon the old man. At this point, a complementary interaction started. The man gave in and the billy goat left the context.

There was a double redemption. Hansjob's display of hybris was followed by his repentance, expiation, and the promised payment for a Holy Mass. He fulfilled the normative expectations. At the same time, Hansjob redeemed the evil spirit in the billy goat whose soul was now freed from wandering.

The then existing lack of knowledge and consciousness needed a projective exteriorization of the psychic state. The event occurred in the loneliness of the night in which Hansjob faced himself. In a state of sensory and psychosocial deprivation, he had auditory; visual, although the legend does not mention explicitly that he "saw" the ram; and tactile hallucinations. Moreover, the interaction between him and the billy goat had homosexual characteristics. The billy goat can be viewed as a projection of the man's own virile spirit which had challenged the norms. There was a dialogue (i.e., whistling and shouting) between the internalized norm, the conscience, and the externalized sanction (i.e., the remorse projection into the aggressive behavior of the billy goat).

(2) The Mother im Brunnji. Once upon a time there was a mother and her only daughter. They lived in a cottage of a little hamlet outside the village, near a little fountain *(Brunnji).* The little girl was often left alone when her mother went for a chat at the *Abusitz.* Usually, she returned very late at night. The little girl was afraid to be left alone and begged her mother repeatedly not to go out because a bad man would visit her and take her away. She asked her mother to sprinkle Holy Water over her. The mother did not listen to the demands of her child. One night, when she returned late, the child was gone. The mother searched desperately for her daughter, but the only thing she ever found was the little shoe of the child's left foot.

A short analysis of this myth yields the following implicit and explicit messages: a mother neglected a normative role expectation which demanded that she renounce her egoistic needs and altruistically fulfill the basic psychological needs of her daughter. She did not care and the child — in a state of emotional and sensory deprivation — hallucinated the punishing element. The bad man was the incorporated sanction for the rejection of a norm and also probably a symbol of the absent husband and father. The mother disregarded both the norm and the repetitive warnings. The warnings were intended to reverse or eliminate the child's deprivation, and at the same time, they were a projection of the child's fantasies of revenge. The mother not only continued to transgress the norm, she also refused to give the child the Holy Water, a magic protection against the persecutor and a symbolic protection she was supposed to provide.

There was a symmetrical interaction, governed by positive feedback, leading to escalation and, finally, to the disruption of the homeostasis of a pathologically functioning dyadic system. The child disappeared, leaving behind her left shoe. "Left" is a symbol of misfortune in the superstitious belief system and also a symbol of the mother's behavioral ineptitude.

In German *linkisch* (i.e., inept) is etymologically deduced from the word *links* (i.e., left). The sanction brought about not only the emotional deprivation of the mother (i.e., the loss of the child), but also a psychosocial deprivation (i.e., the loss of the mother role) which deprived her of her social prestige and status within the community.

(3) The Straw Fire Man. Once upon a time there was a man in Saas-Fee who was so proud and so ambitious that he decided to climb the Dom, the highest mountain on Swiss territory (4554 meters above sea level). Against all warnings of his fellow men, he left the village, taking a bundle of straw which he intended to burn on the peak of the mountain as a sign of his triumph. Three days later, the villagers saw a fire on top of the Dom, but the man was never seen again.

A brief analysis indicates the following mythological content. Mountains were taboo in the old days. The man disregarded the taboo. His *hybris* was so strong that he rejected the warnings of the villagers. These warnings were both a barrier against the transgression of the norm and an expression of social control. He responded to the social control in a symmetrical interaction (i.e., by defiance and rejection). After 3 days, the villagers saw the fire. Three is a symbol of perfection and the number can also be interpreted as a mythological symbol of the triadic system composed of man, social norm, and mountain.

The fire, the intended sign of triumph, was literally and metaphorically a straw fire. In German, the term stands metaphorically for a shortlived passion. The sanction occurred in the form of death in the cold an in solitude far away from any human and social contact. In a Catholic belief system, this meant that the man died without the holy sacraments and, therefore, without grace and mercy. This meant that the man ended in hell. According to Catholic ideology, hell is defined by the total absence of God's love. In the myth, the absence of the human system Saas-Fee was transformed into the absence of the Lord. The myth indicates traces and vestiges of a theocentric-anthropocentric cosmology.

(4) Common Denominator of the Three Myths. All three myths have one common denominator — the transgression of a norm (the authority of which is rooted in God and the function of which is controlled by society, and internalized values) leads to punishment, which demostrates that the norms are not to be disregarded. In all three cases, the victim or the actor runs into the pitfall of *hybris* or he misses the *cairos*.

The efficacy of these myths, which are a metaphoric expression of the normative system, depended upon the fact that such legends and myths were repeated again and again in a highly suggestive context. This repetition from generation to generation created a cognitive structure in the sense of Tolman [i.e., a cognitive matrix leading to a field expectancy which was reinforced by the group process of the narrative and the reception of its content (cf. 165, p. 1222)]. Each listener knew exactly what would happen if he himself transgressed the norm.

4.7.3.4 Value Patterns

As we have seen before, value patterns are elements integrated in the field of determinants which govern human transactions. Values, therefore, are part of the syngenetic program which governs human behavior. These value patterns change over time whenever the behavior changes, and vice versa. Such adaptations occur at different stages of a village process. Whenever the speed of social change increases, a major recalibration occurs. This happens especially when the economic base of a human system changes. In the village, this was the case at the time when tourism began, replacing the old order of the tradition oriented society.

Figure 10 illustrates the cybernetic-syngenetic functional system of value pattern, behavior, and environment and its interdependence with the economic base of a given human system.

The model indicates that the sociocultural subsystem and the economic subsystem are interdependent. The individual is bound to the village which, in turn, is bound to the suprasystem of the extralocal environment. Whenever a change in this cybernetic-

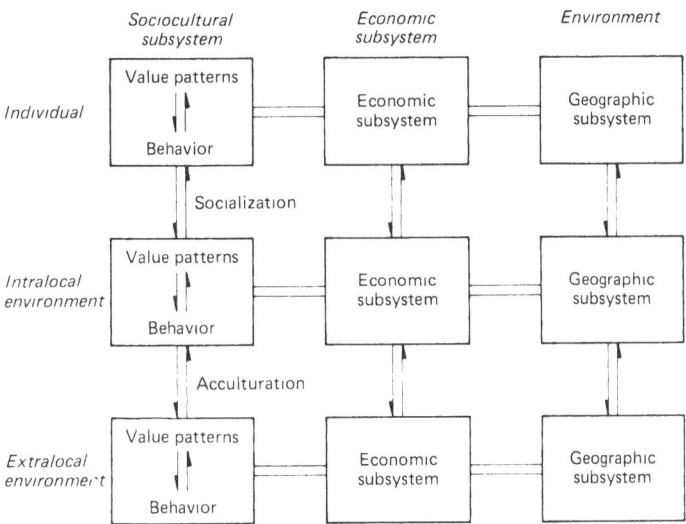

Fig. 10. The cybernetic-syngenetic model of the interdependence of value patterns and environment

syngenetic system occurs, all the subsystems are more or less modified in order to maintain the overall homeostasis. Although in such an open functional system information flows, as a rule, in both directions, the information processing from the top to the bottom of the hierarchy is quantitatively more important. Obviously, the world influences the village more than the world is influenced by the village and, as a rule, the influence of the village upon an individual is more important than the influence of the individual upon the village.

The flow of information from the extralocal system into the intralocal system is called acculturation and the flow of information from the village to the individual is called socialization. We have already discussed how these two processes function and, practically, what kind of sanctions are used in order to guarantee submission to the control of value patterns.

The sociocultural subsystem and the economic subsystem are interdependent and modify each other. Ultimately, the kind of feedback determines to what extent these modifying processes occur; positive feedback increases modification while negative feedback decreases or stops it. The kind of feedback is dependent upon the goal of the human system. The goal, in turn, is computed and reached by transactions and the transactions are governed by the determinants containing the rules and metarules (i.e., the value patterns which govern the elaboration of a hierarchic set of rules). The whole functional system is prodigiously complex. I agree with Habermas (133, p. 18) when he deplores the conceptual lag which makes it very difficult to analyse such complex functional system with the conceptual tools available today.

Pretourist Saas-Fee (i.e., Saas-Fee before the turn of the century) showed the value patterns I have discussed before. With the slow social change in the first half of our century, certain value patterns changed. Seldom did one value completely replace the other. Often they coexisted. The youth moved easily on to the new values whereas the older generations tended to cling to the traditional values.

Parsimony was replaced by the spirit of enterprise, traditionalism by innovative-creative behavior, conservativism by utilitarianism, and the principle of moral integrity by the principle of efficiency.

The economy changed. The village needed money for the construction of the tourist facilities; therefore, land had to be sold.

To sell land was all at once "good," just as holding land had been "good" before. Friendliness towards tourists replaced the former mistrust, with its consequent behavior. Professional competition replaced the former sense of solidarity. Frequent alcohol consumption with the guests, as a sign of fraternization, replaced the highly esteemed value of alcohol abstinence.

A struggle between young and old began. Unquestioned authority of the old and obedience were questioned by the young. The gap between the generations widened. Independent thinking and the utilitarian principle took over. Good was what was efficient to solve the new problems. Rationalism replaced the irrational belief in legends and myths. Born of the traditional agricultural society, they lost their normative value and, little by little, they were forgotten. In 1970, none of the villagers remembered the three myths analyzed before.

Occupational roles created their own sets of values. Each job created a new value pattern which governed the transactions appropriate within an occupational role and a specific context. Mountain guides, for instance, had to be able to take over responsibility. They had to be trustworthy and their behavior predictable and well-controlled. Survival in the mountains depended on their skill as well as on their personality. Ski instructors had to be gentle, funny, attentive, and caring. Hotel managers had to be friendly, hospitable, and easygoing.

The incongruencies between old and new values created stress and insecurity concerning the correct behavior in a given context. In this general confusion, individuals, families, clans, and the whole village split into different camps. More and more people started to act according to their personal interests instead of the communal interests demanded by tradition. Saas-Fee sometimes presented the face of a Potemkin village — friendly and bucolic, but, behind this mask, uproar and boiling conflicts were hidden. Aggressive and rowdy behavior of the male youth in the middle of our century was only one of the symptoms of the time. In short, Saas-Fee was now a system in transition with a set of contradictory values and with a syngenetic program which was very "soft programmed" and in a process of constant transformation.

4.7.4 Synopsis of Sociocultural Development

I have discussed in some detail the development of the sociocultural subsystem which was an integrative part of the village process. We have seen that the structure and function of the agents and the contents of socialization had not changed very much over centuries: however, an incipient tourism at the turn of the century set in motion a process of modification and transformation.

All the elements of this sociocultural subsystem fulfilled one all encompassing function — social integration in the service of goal attainment. Myths and legends, customs and costumes, and belief and value patterns created sense and meaning in the stream of events and guaranteed the predictability of behavior of the individuals. This predictability changed when the village entered the tourist era which required new behavior and new values, thus modifying the syngenetic program which controlled the village as a whole.

In order to clarify the general process of modification, I painted some of the differences and transformations in black and white, treating them as dichotomies rather than complementarities and crystalizing mere tendencies into hard structures. This is an artifact of the analytic approach and it has to be taken into account for the evaluation of the social change before the construction of the road.

5. Construction of the Road in 1951

5.1 Conditions Necessary for Construction of the Road

By the 1930s, the villagers had decided for the first time to build a road from Saas-Grund to Saas-Fee. They agreed to keep the village free from traffic by leading the road only to the edge of the village.

The economic crisis of the 1930s and World War II blocked this endeavor. After World War II, tourism slowly increased, fostering new hopes and leading to the final decision to build the road. In 1951, it was built and the doors for tourism were wide open. In winter 1951-1952, ski fans rushed in and flooded the village for the first time. The former isolation in winter was definitely over and Saas-Fee rose quickly to international popularity, struggling frantically with the events and coping with the new situation as well as it could.

1951 was a caesura in the history of Saas-Fee. The quantitative transformations constituted a quantum leap, an "emergent quality."

The impact on the population was so immense that some villagers don't seem to remember the social changes before 1951 which had helped to prepare the quantum leap on a higher level of complexity.

I will briefly summarize the earlier development which laid the foundations for the radical social change after 1951. I will give, therefore, a condensed overview of all the local and extralocal factors which seemed to transform the village "overnight."

5.1.1 Extralocal Factors

5.1.1.1 Demography

The increase in world population increased the *densité morale,* i.e., the number of interactions. Behaviors were quickly imitated because information traveled fast. The thus produced social control urged the people to do what everybody else seemed to do. Certain behaviors exploded in an epidemic way. One of these was to take vacations.

5.1.1.2 Economy

The process of industrialization and urbanization in Europe and the so-called developed countries of the western hemisphere led to an accumulation of capital, an increased diversification and specialization in the distribution of work, an accelerated work rhythm, and increased leisure time. More and more people, therefore, were eager to take vacations in other countries.

5.1.1.3 Technology

Industrialization led to a rapid development of the means of transportation and communication making it possible to build roads, railroads, cable cars, and skilifts. The invention of skis created a new form of sport. The invention of snowplows made it possible to open roads covered with snow and avalanches, a necessary condition for the adequate functioning of a winter resort.

5.1.1.4 Politics

Once the war was over, the frontiers were open again. The long frustration accumulated during the two world wars and the economic crisis of the 1930s produced a yearning for pleasure and regression; the dialectical awakening of the "pleasure principle" fostered tourism.

5.1.1.5 Religion

The general social change also influenced religious development. The traditional values of the Church, especially the Roman Catholic Church, fostering hard work, duty, abstinence, and ascetism were influenced by modern times. The pulpit gave legitimacy to the new need for taking vacations.

5.1.1.6 Sociocultural Factors

The accumulation of capital and the increase of leisure time created the ideology of consumption. Within this ideology, the behavior of conspicuous consumption (Veblen) arose, often in the service of status display and prestige demonstration. It became fashionable to take vacations in foreign countries.

The increasing speed of the rhythm of life; the growing alienation in the industrial working process; the growing terror of noise, odors, and pollution; and a clouded sky due to the multiplication of nuclei of crystalization escaping from the chimneys of the factories produced an overwhelming demand for a "psychotop" in which the suffering population could regenerate. These circumstances increased tourism.

All these extralocal factors and developments laid the basis for social change in the village, construction of the road, and mass tourism. They had, however, to be matched by the intralocal factors in order to lead to the formulation of goals and to goalattainment.

5.1.2 Intralocal Factors

5.1.2.1 Geography

The extraordinary situation of the village amidst the glaciers and the high mountain peaks of the Alps and the optimal climatic conditions enabled the village to become an object of modern mass tourism.

5.1.2.2 Demography

The increase of the village population, starting at the end of the last century, increased the *densité morale* (Durkheim) and, with it, the number of new ideas. The increase in population also demanded a transformation of the economic base in order to support everybody and avoid emigration.

5.1.2.3 Economy

The early tourism, from the middle of the nineteenth to the middle of the twentieth century, prepared for the passage from agriculture to the building up of a tourist infrastructure. The flexible credit of the banks facilitated the investments made for the construction of the road and the tourist facilities.

5.1.2.4 Technology

The general technological development enabled the villagers to control nature, which was their primary resource. It made possible the construction of means of transportation and tourist facilities.

5.1.2.5 Politics

A new political identity expressed itself in the formation of an elite. The representatives of this elite were the clergyman who built the first two hotels in Saas-Grund, the president of Saas-Fee who built the first hotel in the village, and the 20-year-old president of Saas-Fee who took over in 1948 and organized the village for the definitive leap into the industrialized era. He was an indicator of the power shift from the old to the young.

5.1.2.6 Religion

The contact with the Englishmen and the construction of an Anglican church in the village increased the flexibility of the Roman Catholic Church and its priest, who were forced to accept some new ideas and values. Though not a major factor, this was at least one of the many changes which enabled the villagers to leave the paths of traditional life and move towards tourism. In the overall picture, the Church, however, was a retarding factor for social change. Since the Church's former power was diminished, at least in certain areas of decisionmaking, its impact was not strong enough to block the ongoing process.

5.1.2.7 Sociocultural Factors

The transition from the tradition directed to the inner directed society at the beginning of the century created a high achievement motivation and a general spirit of enterprise. The new identity attained through the victories in the sports world fostered character traits like innovative-creative behavior, self-confidence, and courage to pursue new goals. The acculturation process, set in motion by contact with the guests and mass media, made the villagers eager to adopt the basic values of rationality, efficiency, competition, and utilitarianism.

5.2 Impact of Extralocal and Intralocal Factors

Both, the overall and the specific patterns of extralocal and intralocal factors were responsible for the social change before and after the construction of the road. It was the combination of both which, finally, led to major social change. My explanation of social change in Saas-Fee, therefore, excludes monocausal and reductionist theories (cf.
). The social change involved both the economic base and the sociocultural superstructure with its behaviors and value patterns.

Figure 11 shows the interdependence and feedback of all the factors leading to the passage from agriculture to tourism. The result of the interplay of all the factors was the move, along a diachronic axis, into a new area of industrialization.

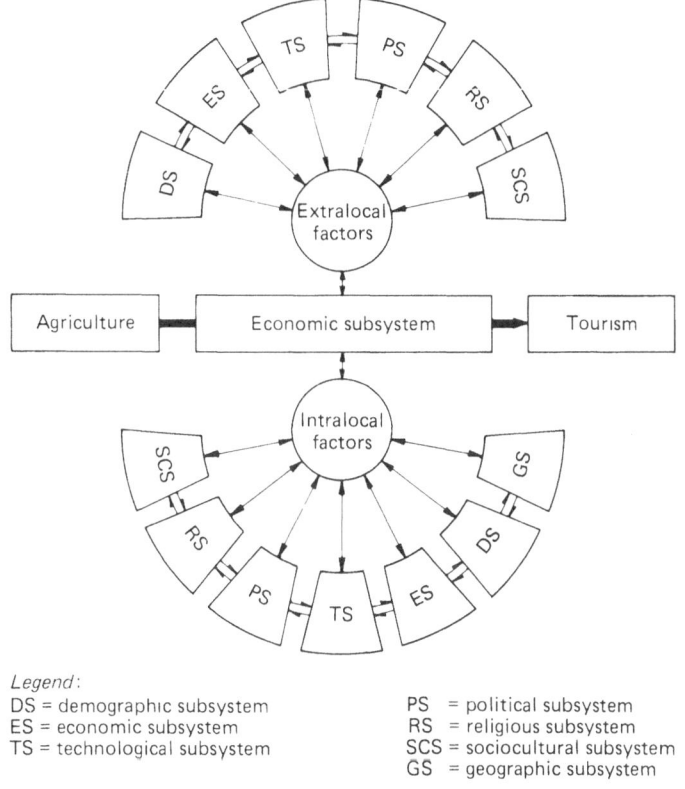

Legend:
DS = demographic subsystem   PS = political subsystem
ES = economic subsystem   RS = religious subsystem
TS = technological subsystem   SCS = sociocultural subsystem
                                    GS = geographic subsystem

Fig. 11. The development of the economic base of Saas-Fee

The same process occurred in the change of the behavioral patterns. Figure 12 shows the transformation of attitudes, ideas, and norms of behavior leading to the transition from the traditional to innovative-creative behavior.

120

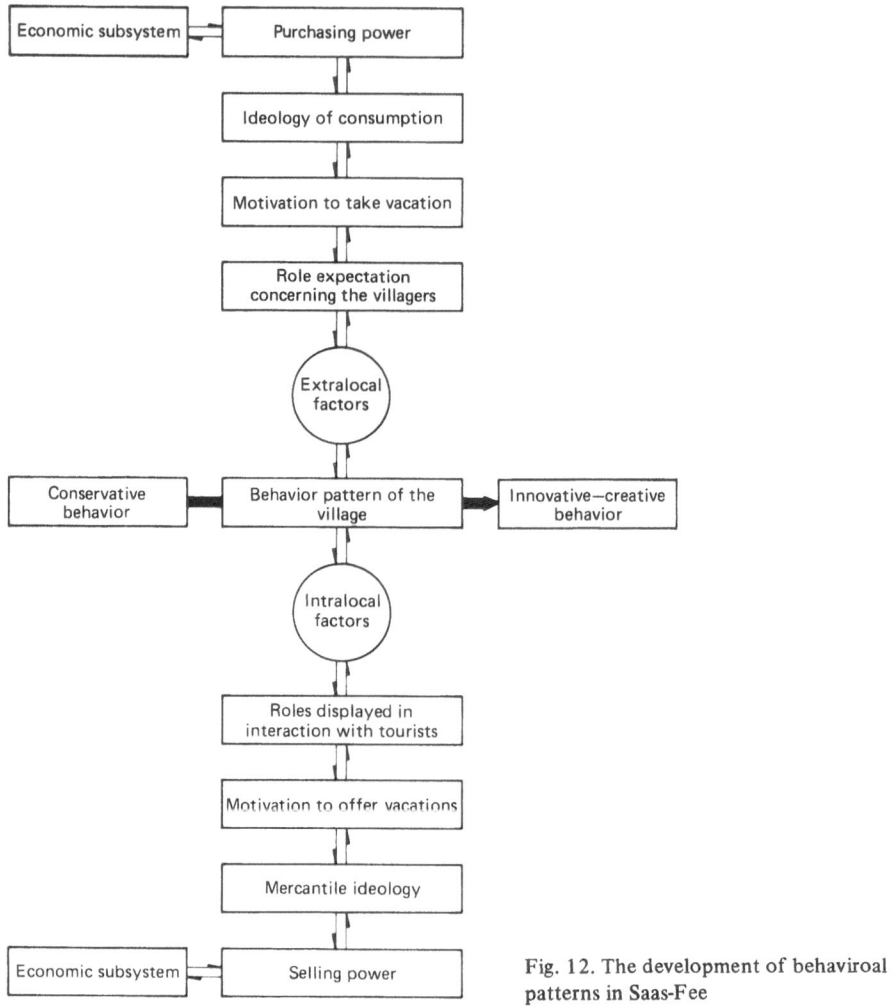

Fig. 12. The development of behaviroal patterns in Saas-Fee

The sociocultural subsystem developed in interdependence with the economic basis. Their speeds of development were equivalent until the end of the last century, then, the two subsystems became disconnected, creating a cultural lag (i.e., a period of time in which the villagers lived in a new economic situation while maintaining the old system of values and ideas).

This cultural lag (Fig. 13) increased in the years to come.

The cultural lag increased whenever the speed of social change increased. The speed varied, as we have seen, over the centuries. The velocity of social change can be measured, theoretically and practically, if we operationalize the elements of our analysis by means of the formula $V = \dfrac{U_s}{t}$, in which V = velocity of social change, U_s = number of structural units changed, and t = units of time.

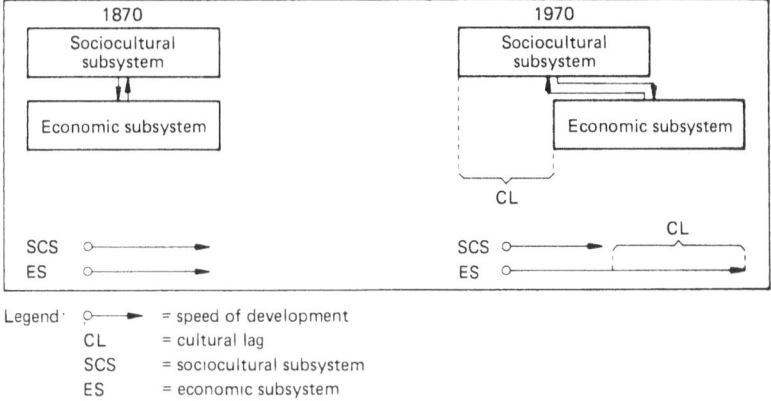

Fig. 13. Phenomenon of the cultural lag

Using this formula we can identify five phases of social change within the village. Each phase is characterized by a specific speed or velocity varying from V_1 (i.e., lowest speed) to V_6 (i.e., highest speed).

The different phases of social change (see Fig. 14) are:

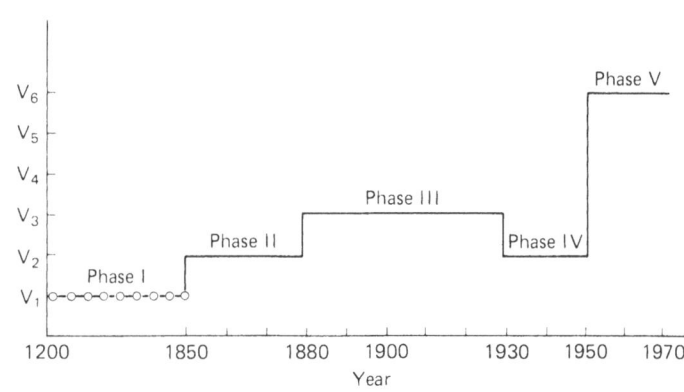

Fig. 14. Different phases of social change in Saas-Fee

Phase I: from the Middle Ages until the middle of the nineteenth century when tourism began. During this period, the developmental speed was very low.

Phase II: from the middle of the nineteenth century until 1880 when the first hotel was built in the village. During this time, the developmental speed increased slightly.

Phase III: from 1880 to 1930, when the economic crisis stopped tourism. During this period the speed of developmen of social change still increased.

Phase IV: from 1930 to 1951. The social change decreased until after the economic crisis and World War II.

122

Phase V: from 1951 to 1970 (i.e., from the construction of the road to 1970), when this study was made. During this period, social change increased to a maximal speed.

The overall impression is that of a more or less linear increase in the speed oc social change with a few major oscillations. The two major events causing the oscillations were the first hotel in 1880 and the construction of the road in 1951.

An interesting hidden sociopsychological aspect is that the initial social change from 1850 to 1880 created a high level of expectation which was projected by extrapolating the present in a linear fashion into the future. The future was supposed to maintain the same speed of social change, but the level of realization, reached in 1951, was lower than the expectation level. The widening gap, at the beginning of the twentieth century, created a field of frustration which constituted a psychological potential for tranforma-tion. This frustrational gap is a phenomenon similar to the more dramatic potential of the revolutionary gap found in prerevolutionary societies, as described by Davies (70) and Tanter and Midlarsky (350). The frustration gap between expectation and realiza-tion level was certainly an important sociopsychological reason motivating the popula-tion for industrialization. This situation is illustrated in Fig. 15.

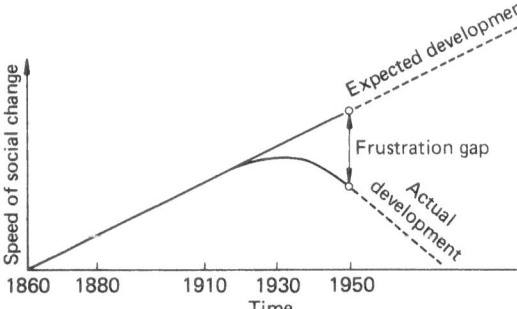

Fig. 15. The phase-specific socio-psycho-logical potential of social change

After enumerating the different aspects, we can state that the interrelation and inter-actions between the discussed extralocal (i.e., necessary) and intralocal (i.e., sufficient) factors built up the structural scaffolding upon which the new social and economic or-ganization of the village was to be built.

6. The Village Process After the Construction of the Road: Increasing Industrialization and Urbanization

6.1 Development of the Demographic Subsystem

6.1.1 General Demographic Development

The development after the construction of the road transformed all the subsystems of the community to an extent never known before. In the demographic subsystem, this general social change led to an important increase in the population and a change in its composition. The increase was primarily due to the rapid development of the economic subsystem, but factors inherent in the demographic process itself also played their part.

The creation of new jobs and occupational roles after 1951 stopped emigration and demographic desintegration which, according to Koetter (200, p. 614), is typical for modern rural areas. The new situation also brought a daily flow of visitors, seasonal workers, and commuting workers of the adjacent villages to Saas-Fee.

The global increase in population from 1930 to 1970 was as follows: in 1930, there were 439 inhabitants; 1 decade later, 475 inhabitants; and 1 decade later, 504 inhabitants. In 1960, the population reached 739 inhabitants and, in 1970, the population had grown to 895 inhabitants. This general increase in population is illustrated by Fig. 16.

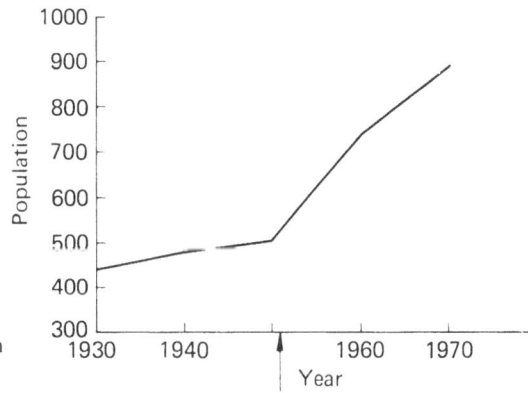

Fig. 16. Increase in the total population

In this and following figures, the arrow indicates the construction of the road in 1951. The graph shows that the increase in population is slow and linear from 1930 to 1950; then a rapid increase occurs. The increase of the 1st decade was greater than the increase in the following decade. This demographic change is due to increasing tourism

124

creating new jobs. The slower increase in the last decade is due to the fact that free valences on the job market were saturated and, partly, to the introduction of contraceptive devices, especially the birth control pill.

It is interesting to note to what extent the demographic subsystem can be influenced by the sociocultural subsystem. In 1968, when I worked in the village for the first time, I prescribed oral contraceptives. Because of his moral convictions, the old doctor had either not done this at all or done it very reluctantly. In 1970, when I returned to Saas-Fee, three of the women who had received the pill were pregnant or already had a child. What had happened in between? The year before, in 1969, the papal *encyclica Humane Vitae* was published condemning the use of contraceptives. In the moral conflict, oscillating between medical permissiveness and ecclesiastic prohibition, the women had given in to the latter.

Comparing the population pyramids of the years 1950, 1960, and 1970, we get the information displayed in Fig. 17.

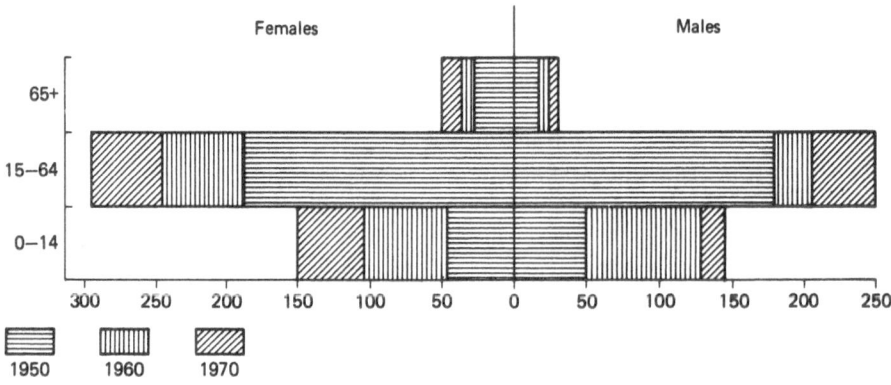

Fig. 17. Development of the demographic structure from 1950 to 1970

The data of figure 22 are global and permit only the following statements: there is a general increase in population over 3 decades, with an increase in females prevailing.

6.1.2 Development of the Generative Structure

The so-called natural development of the population from 1945 to 1970 occurred as shown in Fig. 18. (*N.B.* Different starting points of different figures are due to the available data.)

The generative structure is composed of three structural elements — the marriage structure, the mortality structure, and the birth structure. The combination of all three elements makes it possible to study the architecture of the generative structure and avoid the methodological error of making oversimplified statements, as emphasized by Mackenroth (232a, p. 71).

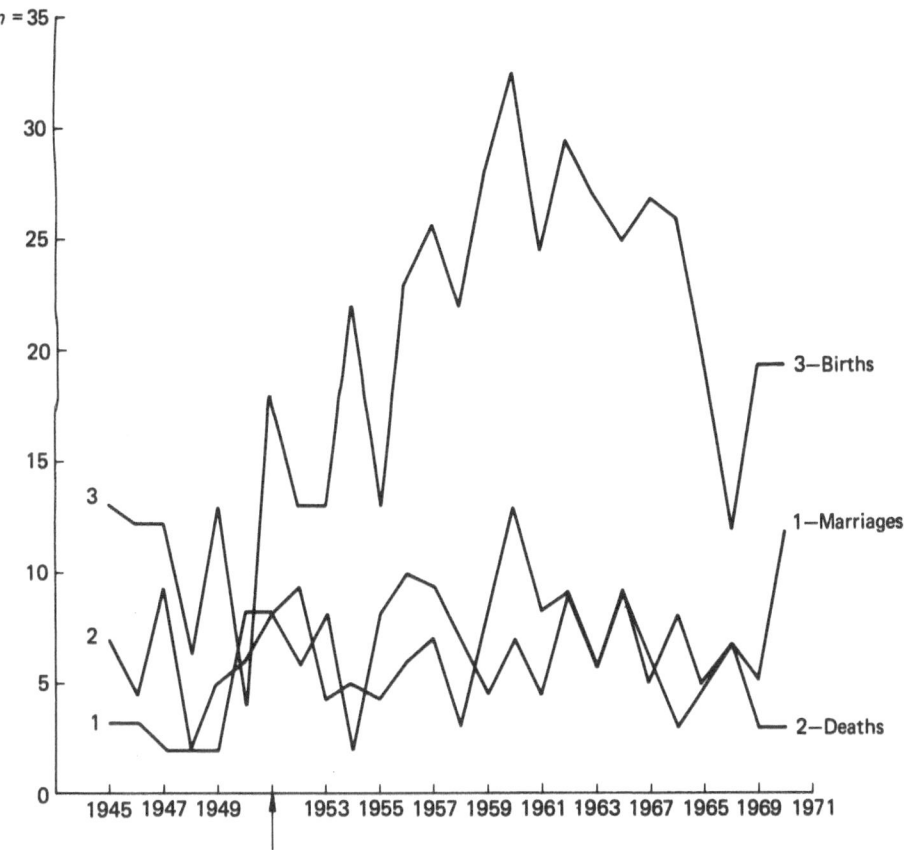

Fig. 18. Development of the generative structure from 1945 to 1970

After the construction of the road, the frequency of marriages increased and, with it, the birth rate. The birth rate reached its peak in 1960 with 33 births. It decreased until 1969, probably due to the introduction of the pill. It increased again after the publication of the *Encyclica Humanae Vitae*. The increase in the birth rate in 1969-1970 occurred before the parallel increase in the number of marriages modified the demographic structure.

The death rate increased very slowly and was primarily due to a general increase in population. The rate oscillated around an average of seven deaths per year.

Observing the population scissor graphically, formed by the development of deaths rate and birth rate, it becomes clear that the scissor opened at the time of the construction of the road, closed gradually around the years 1966-1968, and then reopened. The second scissor phase which, according to Mackenroth (232a, p. 75), was observed by demographers all over Europe, existed in the village only after 1968 and was rather inconspicuous. During the years 1969-1970 the movements of birth and death rates were parallel.

There was a high rate of birth *(Geburtenüberschuß)* until 1966, decreasing slightly thereafter, and increasing again from 1967 to 1970.

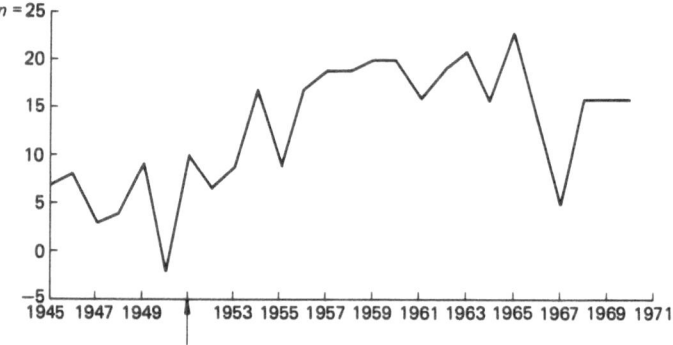

Fig. 19. Development of the high birth rate from 1945 to 1970

The growth rate of the population in 1970 was slightly slower than the world average of 1.9% today (i.e., 1976).

The surplus rate of the population in 1970 can be calculated:

$$\frac{\text{Surplus of birth rate}}{\text{Total population}} = \frac{16}{895} = \frac{X}{100} = 1.78\%$$

6.1.3 Demographic Structure in 1970

Figure 20 indicates the demographic structure of Saas-Fee in 1970. The population structure showed the pyramidal structure typical for a growing population. It was different from the bell-shaped structure which, at that time, was found in most of the rural areas of the Alps where the emigration of the youth led to a superannuated population. The graph illustrates that there was a majority of females, especially in the older generation. No one reached 85 years old. The youngest group (i.e., birth to 14 years) was equally numerous in both sexes. Since the normal sexual proportion, according to Mackenroth (232a, p. 66), is 106 boys to 100 girls, a higher postnatal mortality of boys is probably responsible for the equivalence found.

The group of 15-19-years-old was relatively small, although the birth rate (cf. Fig. 18) increased considerably after 1951. This apparent deficit is brought about by the fact that the younger generation attended boarding schools or professional schools outside the valley.

The demographic stratification of the population in 1970 showed the composition shown in Table 5.

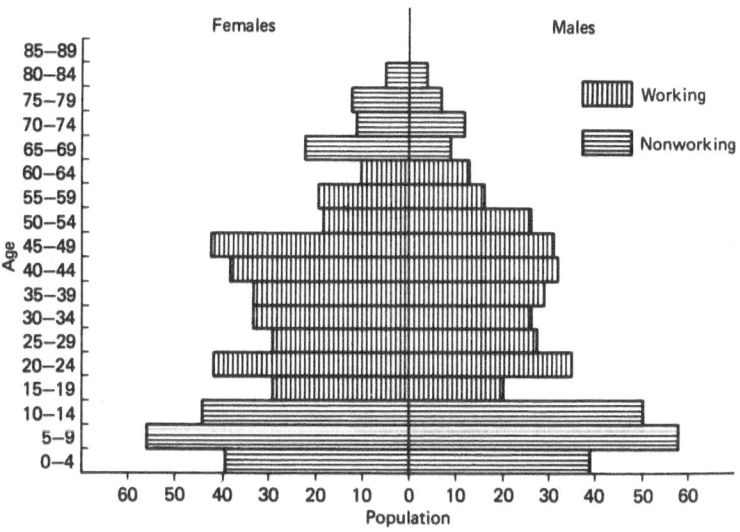

Fig. 20. Demographic structure of the total population in 1970

Table 5. *Demographic stratification of the population in 1970*

1. Sex: 426 men, 469 women
2. Nationality: 851 Swiss, 44 foreigners
3. Language: 858 German, 16 French, 7 Italian, 14 others
4. Religion: 874 Catholic, 21 Protestant
5. Marital status: 475 single (224 men, 251 women),
   391 married (198 men, 193 women)
      7 separated (6 men, 1 woman; not citizens of Saas-Fee)
     27 widowed (4 men, 23 women)
      2 divorced (2 women, not citizens of Saas-Fee)
6. Households: 252 private, 2 others
7. Private households
     38 with 1 person
     56 with 2 persons
     35 with 3 persons
     52 with 4 persons
     30 with 5 persons
     27 with 6 persons
     11 with 7 persons
      0 with 8 persons
      3 with 9 persons

These data, reported in the statistical yearbook (342, p. 136 ff), indicate the exact demographic stratification and need no further analysis for my purposes. I should like to emphasize, however, that in 1970 there were no divorced or separated couples among the citizens of Saas-Fee. This fact, of course, does not allow us to make any assumptions about the quality of marriages. As Koenig (196, p. 270) rightly emphasizes, "overorganized" families do not separate in spite of much conflict. I knew some families in Saas-Fee, whose coherence seemed to be based mainly upon common economic interests.

6.1.4 Fluctuating Population

The overall demographic structure of Saas-Fee in 1970 was complex. In addition to the citizens of the village, there also were the employees and guests. As early as 1960, Supersaxo (348) stated that there were as many tourists in the village as villagers. According to Bellwald and Jaeger (22, p. 21), in 1970, the number of arriving tourists during the winter season was 251,000, while the summer season registered 521,000 arrivals. In the same year, there were 742 employees from outside the village. The three demographic groups — villagers, guests, and employees — amounted to a total of over 80,000 persons per year. The actual figure would be even higher if it were possible to include the many tourists who came just for the day, but, because they do not register anywhere, they cannot be counted.

Table 6 indicates the demographic structure of the employees according to their regional or national origin. Employees from the Canton Wallis and those from foreign countries are almost equal in number. The majority of the employees are women (i.e., waitresses, chambermaids, kitchen aids, shop girls) from the Canton Wallis (i.e., rural areas which, unlike Saas-Fee, did not have a flourishing economy). Table 7 gives a more detailed demographic structure.

Table 6. *Demographic structure of all the employees in 1970*

Origin	Men	Women	Total
Foreign countries	157	151	308
Canton Wallis	93	224	317
Switzerland	35	82	117
Total	285	457	742

Table 7. *Demographic structure of the foreign employees in 1970*

Origin	Men	Women	Total
Spain	52	47	99
Italy	47	10	57
Germany	15	20	35
England	6	27	33
Austria	18	10	28
Yugoslavia	9	2	11
Holland	3	5	8
France	2	3	5
Hungary	1	2	3
Others	4	16	20
Total	157	151	308

The sex distribution of the foreign employees, called "guest workers," is about equal, but the specific distribution per country shows great variation. The composition of the guest workers illustrates the economic situation of their countries and also tells us some-

thing about the customs of their respective cultures. The English workers were employed primarily by English companies who rented chalets for their fellow countrymen.
These chalets were managed by young English people. Spanish couples worked together
while their children, blocked by the immigration law, stayed in Spain in the care of re-
latives. Italian men left their wives and children back home and visited them once a
year.

Statistical figures may appear "value free" and immigration offices permit the influx
of "labor forces," but behind the tabulations and the legal policy is the human truth
put so succinctly by the swiss writer, Max Frisch; "human beings immigrate, not labor
forces."

Summarizing the discussion concerning the development of the demographic subsystem, we can say that the construction of the road induced a major social change in
Saas-Fee. The change which affected the demographic subsystem was both quantitative
and qualitative. Quantitatively, the number of villagers and tourists increased. Qualitatively, a new demographic group, "employees," was introduced.

6.2 Development of the Economic Subsystem

This chapter will discuss to what extent the construction of the road modified the economic subsystem of Saas-Fee.

6.2.1 General Considerations

Technological progress entered a new phase after World War II. It created, as Jantke
(176, p. 97) pointed out, an autonomous and dynamic economic system in many parts
of the world. It brought to Saas-Fee the possibility of the technological opening up of
ski slopes, walking areas, and climbing resorts. Thus, the village had, as an option, an
economic subsystem which made possible a demographic development, bursting the
structure of the traditional economy of subsistence. As a consequence, the primary
economic sector almost vanished and the tertiary sector (i.e., trade and services in the
tourist facilities) increased tremendously.

As Marx (cf. 111, p. 58) claimed, in capitalism, each man speculates how to create
a need in his fellow men. The villagers did not create new needs; they channeled the
need for vacations fostered by the conditions of the industrialized and urbanized areas.
The driving force of the economic development in Saas-Fee were the demands of the
people of these areas for tourist facilities. The fuel accelerating the economic development was the competition with other rural areas which also tried to channel the urban
population into their regions.

The competition in the village itself created contradictory forces – the intralocal
competition controlled by particular interests in opposition to the common goal to
model The Pearl of the Alps into a bucolicly attractive whole. This latter goal checked
the particular interests and encouraged the people to submit to the collective goal. The
instrumental character of neighborhood ethics (266, p. 33) appeared in a new form
which differed from that of the agricultural village in its coexistence of competitive
and synergetic tendencies.

6.2.2 Transportation and Communication System

Right after the road was built, the streets within the village were covered with asphalt pavement. Although mail was still transported by horse and sled, an atavistic relic in 1970, all other transports were made by electrocars. They were almost noiseless and did not pollute the air. Their slow speed of 7-15 kilometers per hour was generally accepted as sufficient. There were three types of electrocars:

— A flat open transportation car
— A car with a driver's cabin for two persons and a flat loading tray (this was the luxury model used by the doctor, a few artisans, and some hotels).
— A big version used for the removal of communal refuse

The price of these electrocars was relatively high. It was about 17,000 Swiss francs in 1970 for an electrocar with cabin and loading battery. Instead of buying a common loading battery, each owner prefered to have his own. This uneconomical custom was a relic of the traditional norm of autonomy and autarchy. It might change one day should the principle of efficiency and rationality completely replace some of the old values.

The narrow streets and paths which had been sufficient for the agricultural village were soon crowded with people and the growing number of electrocars. The original idea of keeping the village quiet and relaxing for pedestrians was soon handicapped by a changing reality.

In the long run, the village will have to improve this system of transportation.

Technology opened up the hillsides and mountains surrounding Saas-Fee. In 1947, the first "lift" was built. In 1952, a second followed. In 1954, the first cablecar transported 16 persons at a time. It gave access to new slopes. It was supplemented in 1959 by a second cablecar reaching an altitude of 2850 meters. In 1962, a third cablecar opened an area to the south of the village and, in 1969, a fourth and a fifth cablecar opened up the north and southwest, an area full of magnificent ski slopes. The highest point reached by the latter construction was 3000 meters above sea level.

In 1970, the village had eighteen cablecars, "gondolas" *(Gondelbahnen)*, and "chair lifts" *(Sessellifts)* and numerous ski lifts which opened a ski arena with a circumference of 200 degrees.

According to Bellwald and Jaeger (22, p. 92), in 1970, the village had the transportation capacities listed in Table 8.

Table 8. *Capacity of transport in 1970*

Means of transport	Transport capacity
	(persons/hour)
Cablecars	2,460
Lifts and *Sesselbahnen*	8,720
Total capacity	11,180

The total length and surface of the ski slopes, according to Bellwald and Jaeger (22, p. 101), were 27,560 meters and 167.8 hectares. Several specially equipped vehicles, so-called snow tracks, maintained the functional state of the slopes.

Furthermore, a network of paths and benches was spread over the whole area inviting people to relax in the woods and on the hillsides.

6.2.3 Tourist Facilities

6.2.3.1 Lodging Capacity

Rapidly expanding tourism demanded a major increase and improvement of the lodging facilities. As Scheuch (316, p. 801) observed, the modern tourist expects a perfect system of services. The demands of the new era were different from the demands of the first period of tourism. The first tourists were members of the upper class for whom hotels were the appropriate lodging facilities. After the Second World War, the middle class started to travel and take vacations. Its members often preferred to stay apartments and chalets. Thus, the so-called "parahotellery" became increasingly important and needed to be built up.

As Table 9 illustrates, "parahotellery" started to become of some importance in the 4th decade of our century, increasing thereafter and bypassing the hotellery in its importance by 1970.

Table 9. *Development of "hotellery" and "parahotellery"*

Year	"Hotellery"	Chalets	Tents
1900	100%	-	-
1935	77%	23%	-
1950	62%	38%	-
1959	56.6%	40%	3.4%
1970	46.6%	51%	2.4%

The development of the "parahotellery" made it possible for almost everyone within the village to increase their income and make investments. Soon, every family had one or several chalets. The family thus continued to be the basic economic unit, a fact which fostered cooperation and social coherence. Extralocal investors were kept away. This policy reversed the original trend of the first tourist period when three of the four existing hotels belonged to extralocal investors. The creation of corporations was made impossible and, thus, a democratic economic situation was fostered. The flexible loan policy of the banks contributed to maintain this situation. After 1945, it had allowed an annual increase of 12% in chalet construction.

I could not get exact data concerning the lodging capacity of Saas-Fee in 1970. Those of 1972, reported by Bellwald and Jaeger (22, p. 7 ff), permit, howevei, an approximate extrapolation. In 1972, the overall lodging capacity was 5995 beds. We can deduce, therefore, that the lodging capacity of 1970 must have been approximately 5700 beds (see Table 10).

Table 10. *Lodging capacity of Saas-Fee in 1972*

"Hotellery"	Beds	"Parahotellery"	Beds
Hotels	1753	Chalets	225
Pensions	67	Apartments	3225
		Vacation homes	150
		Vacation colonies	50
		Other lodgings	45
		SAC cabins[a]	60
		Other cabins	120
		TCS camping[b]	300
Total	1820		4175

[a] SAC = Schweizerischer Alpen Club (Swiss Alpine Club).
[b] TCS = Touring Club Schweiz (Swiss Touring Club).

6.2.3.2 Architecture

The first tourist period had created four hotels which were monumental stone structures that destroyed the esthetic homogeneity of the village. The citizens now decided to change the former policy and give building permission only for constructions which imitated the old chalet. This was a commendable decision, although it led to some strange results.

A given architectural style should be the esthetic expression of a given function. The old chalet fitted the functional demands of the agricultural society. The new "jumbo chalet" often found in the Alps, fitted the new functional demands (i.e., to have maximal lodging capacities in a given space). The esthetic result, however, was rarely satisfying because the old chalet lost its proportion while maintaining its general appearance.

Mitscherlich (256, p. 11), angry about the postwar architecture in Europe, once spoke of an axis of "ruthless demonstration of pecuniary potence" illustrating the questionable taste of haberdashers. This axis was supposed to connect Germany and Italy, obviously passing through Switzerland. This taste did, indeed, affect the village. The tourists from different European countries brought esthetic expectations, combining the desire for red colored lampoons, copperware, and other kitsch objects. They reinforced the preexisting taste of the villagers which, in the turmoil of rapid social change, was rather unstructured and suggestible.

The new constructions were shaped by this taste, by the bureaucratic demands of the fire and police forces, the housing authority, and a kind of fatal autonomy which was aptly expressed in an inscription on one of the new houses in Saas-Fee, *jeder baut nach seinem Sinn* (i.e., everybody builds according to his inclinations). This, indeed, is a statement in stone of the prevailing construction policy.

Interior decoration usually followed a so-called neorustic style, determined mainly by the dictates of conspicuous consumption or the need to demonstrate one's status through one's purchases. Rooms and staircases were often crowded with objects or gadgets, bric-à-brac, copper and tinware, furs, and wood carvings.

There are many reasons for these esthetic aberrations, as well as there are many arguments against my statements. Not everybody will agree, of course, with my evaluation of esthetics because there is no generally accepted system of esthetic evaluation.

Nevertheless, the main reasons for the architectural failures, in my opinion, were the lack of an esthetic education in a school system which was more interested in dates of old battles than in information about a better environment; the lack of general orientation in a period of rapid social change, when all values and ideas were replaced by new ones intruding from all sides; the lack of enough qualified architects to inform the people about contemporary methods and means of construction combining the necessary functions with esthetical aspects; financial considerations to maximize profit, an understandable goal; and, finally, the pressure of conformity (i.e., to do what everybody else did).

Thus, a vicious circle was perpetuated. It led to architectural hybrids combining the old chalet with the monumental structures of the turn of the century, introduced in Saas-Fee by the first four hotels. The same style destroyed the Cote d'Azure in France. Fortunately, exceptions to this rule exist.

6.2.4 Development of Land Prices

The general boom increased the land prices according to the law of supply and demand. Prices also made capricious jumps at times, not explicable by this law.

Demand was great and the available land situated within the construction zone limited. The prices increased to the point where they often equalled those in cities. There was a strange *omertà,* a law of silence, which covered the negotiations so that prices were rarely known publicly. In 1970, a person paid 1,200 francs per square meter for a piece of land at the boundary of the village. According to one of our key informants, the prices rose to 400% during the period from 1951 to 1970.

6.2.5 Development of Financial Policies

The tourist infrastructure (i.e., the construction of a transportation system, buildings, sewers, water supply, and electricity) consumed substantial sums of money. The village was forced to borrow the money from the banks. Mutter (Finanzpolitik in Saas-Fee. Manuscript for personal use, 1975) underlines that the Swiss banks pursued a flexible and generous policy in the years of the economic boom. This situation changed in 1969 when the Swiss government put the breaks on these policies. Generally, economic risks in tourism are high, but since tourism was important to the economy of Switzerland, the banks followed a very liberal policy as long as they could.

The villagers did not encounter major problems obtaining money for the construction of apartments or chalets. Extralocal persons who wanted to buy apartments in Saas-Fee also obtained bank loans easily. The banks supported the parahotellery, which generally showed a positive developmental trend. Hotel finances, however, faced major problems. Explosion of costs, severe competition, and changing tourist customs forced them to survive on a narrow margin of profit.

Mutter (see above) indicates that private investors and joint stock companies who wanted to invest money in the construction of cablecars and ski lifts faced the biggest problems. In 1970, most of the cablecars of the entire Canton Wallis operated on a deficit budget and the banks were reluctant to lend money for more investments in this sector.

6.2.6 Economic Situation of Saas-Fee in 1970

According to Bellwald (24), in 1970, the municipality of Saas-Fee had an income of 2,556,700 francs and expenses of 1,959,700 francs. The difference, a profit of 597,000 francs, was available for further payment of debts or new investments.

In the same year, the total communal obligations were 4,692,700 francs, with a total of 265,000 francs of annual interest due, a sum equal to 23% of the tax revenues. This situation is not alarming when compared to the total revenues and the income of the tourist and transportation facilities owned by the community. Bellwald and Jaeger (Zur wirtschaftlichen Entwicklung in Saas-Fee. Manuscript for personal use, 1975) indicate that the financial situation of the community in 1970 can be regarded as relatively sound.

There was a total indebtedness of 3140 francs per person which, although higher than the per capita indebtedness of a comparable region within the Canton Wallis, was tolerable considering the investments.

An official report (231) indicates that the cablecars transported 669,434 persons in 1970 and produced an income of 2,777,683 francs. For the same year, the tourist association (205, p. 11) shows an income of 365,640 francs and expenses of 386,956 francs. The difference is produced by investments, partly in advertizing.

6.2.7 Economic Situation of Individuals in 1970

Most of the population of Saas-Fee agreed that they were deeply in debt. It is clear that the construction of privately owned tourist facilities was very costly. Ideas about prestige and status, as well as the general competition, induced many families to build more expensively than was necessary. The expected maximization of profit demanded a maximization of investment. Moreover, the construction boom, which radically changed the relationship between supply and demand, increased the costs of construction. The long and complicated transport of construction supplies to Saas-Fee increased the costs even more.

The general indebtedness of the individuals can be roughly deduced from the answers yielded by the questionnaire (Tabel 11). Probands were asked to select from a range of attitudes the view that indicated how they would feel if an economic crisis should occur which seriously affected tourism.

Table 11. *The attitude towards a possible economic crisis*

Evaluation	n	%
No answer	2	2
Great anxiety	47	39
Bearable damage	60	50
Indifference	8	7
Advantage	3	2
Total	120	100

The figure indicates that almost 90% of the population interviewed assumed that they would be severely damaged by an economic crisis, although 50% thought the damage would be bearable. In 1970, the international economic situation played the same role for the village that the Mattmark Lake once played for the population of the valley — it was a constant threat.

The economic situation of Saas-Fee could be changed at any given moment. Tourism is a luxury which is given up by the consumer whenever times are hard.

In 1970, $^2/_3$ of the interviewed sample indicated that their economic situation had improved in the previous 15 years. It is difficult to judge to what extent it had improved. Subjectively, the villagers had an overwhelming awareness of their economic debts and, objectively, their answers were not always congruent with reality I could check in certain cases.

Table 12 lists the answer given by n persons or $x\%$ of the sample.

Table 12. *The economic takeoff since n years*

Takeoff since	n	$\%$
No answer	4	3
0- 4 years	34	28
5- 9 years	15	12
10-14 years	32	27
15-19 years	11	9
20 and more years	24	20
Total	120	100

According to the subjective answers, the monthly individual income in 1970 was as shown in Table 13.

Table 13. *The monthly income of the individuals in 1970*

Monthly income	n	$\%$
No answer	1	1
1000 francs	25	21
2000 francs	43	36
3000 francs	22	19
3000 and more	18	15
3000 and more	11	9
Total	120	100

Given the composition of the sample, which include adolescents and old people, and considering the tendency to indicate less than the actual income, we can assume that the average individual income was probably high when compared to Swiss standards.

136

6.2.8 Development of Tourism

6.2.8.1 General Development of Tourism

The general development of tourism can best be measured by the increase of the number of lodging nights per year, as indicated in Fig. 21.

The graph indicates that the development of tourism stagnated between 1946 and 1951, even decreasing slightly before the construction of the road. Then, there was a steep increase between 1951 and 1970. A microanalysis reveals that the increase showed a periodical rhythmicity. The 5-year periods (i.e., 1946-1951, 1951-1956, 1956-1962, and 1962-1967) had approximately the same angle of increase. The general findings is that the number of lodging nights between 1950 and 1970 increased approximately 10 times.

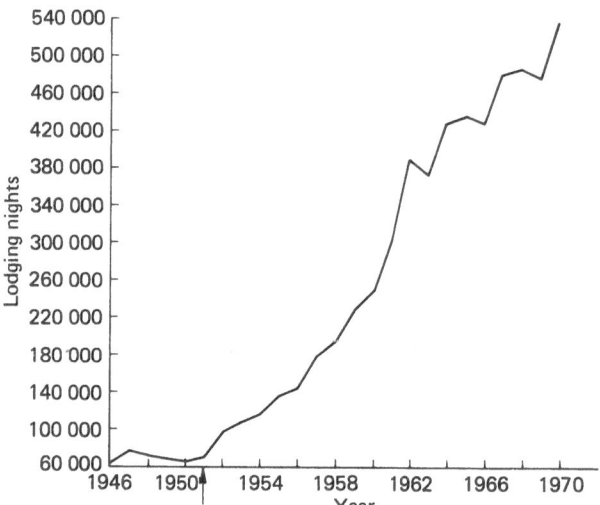

Fig. 21. The Development of the number of lodging nights per year

6.2.8.2 Development in the Winter Season

The development of the winter season, as reported by the tourist association (204), was as shown in Fig. 22.

The hotellery stagnated until 1951, then a rapid increase of the number of lodging nights occurred. Between 1962 and 1968, there was a general, but oscillating, increase depending upon changes in the international currency, political situation, and changing customs in tourism.

The parahotellery increased slowly until 1958, then a rapid increase occurred bypassing the development of hotellery in 1963. In 1970, the development of hotellery and parahotellery was almost equal. Overall, the winter season showed a stable and rapid development.

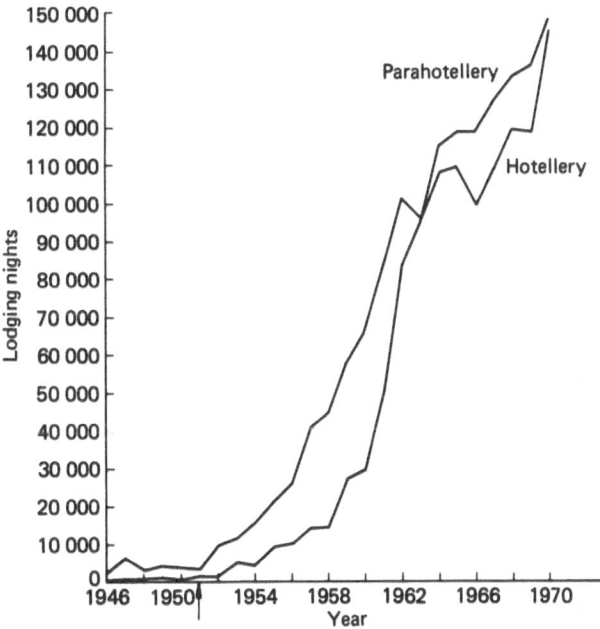

Fig. 22. Development of the lodging nights per year in hotellery and parahotellery during the winter season

6.2.8.3 Development in the Summer Season

The development of the Summer season is more or less comparable to the development of the winter season (see Fig. 23).

The hotellery showed a tendency to decrease until 1951, then an oscillating increase occurred until 1958, followed by a more rapid increase. After 1961, the hotellery showed a stagnating oscillatory development. By 1970, there again was a major increase.

The parahotellery slowly increased up to 1951, then the increase was very rapid until 1967, when the development became retrogressive. Compared to the winter season, the summer season showed a more important development, due to the increasing number of lodging nights in mountain cabins and on camping grounds.

The overall development shows that the number of lodging nights in the hotellery in 1970, as compared to 1946, increased approximately 50 times for the winter season, but only 3 times for the summer season. The winter season had not only the higher rates of increase, but, in 1970, it had also become economically more important than the summer season. The importance of the construction of the road, which made winter tourism possible, is once more emphasized.

6.2.8.4 Nationality of the Tourists

The early tourist era brought mainly Englishmen to Saas-Fee. Modern tourism brings people from many different nations (Fig. 24).

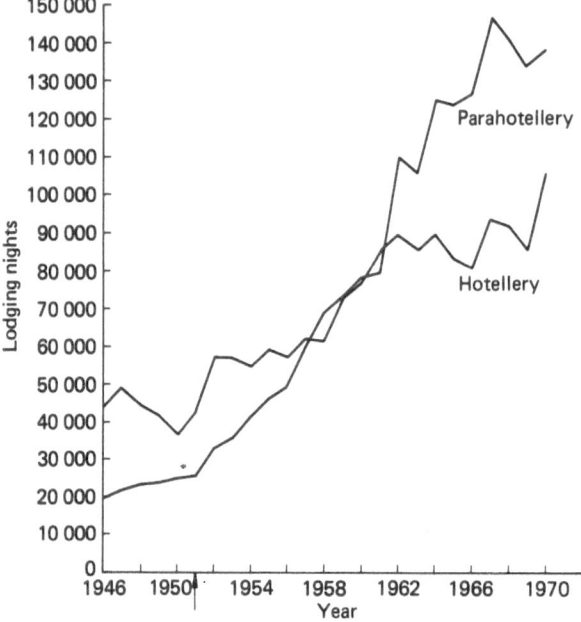

Fig. 23. The development of the lodging nights per year in hotellery and parahotellery during the summer season

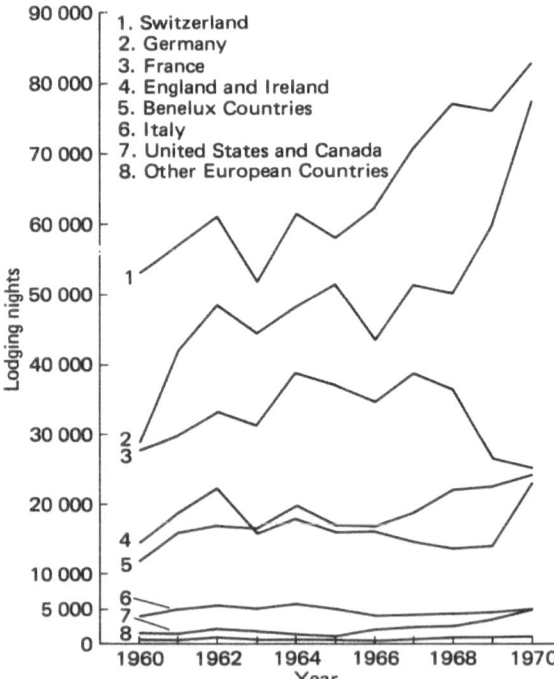

Fig. 24. Development of the lodging nights in relation to the nationality of the tourists

In 1970, most of the tourists came from Switzerland and Germany, both countries having a stable economic situation in the 3 preceding decades. France, England, and the Benelux countries (i.e., the northwest of Europe) provided the second contingent. The development of French tourists was regressive, probably due to their country's monetary situation which was disadvantageous compared to Swiss currency. In 1970, the growth tendency of the three countries converged.

It is interesting to note the developmental curve of English tourists. Currently they seem to take up their old tradition, although preferring the parahotellery. They organized a car service from the airport in Geneva to Saas-Fee to facilitate their arrival.

Italy, Austria, the United States, Canada, and the rest of Europe did not supply many tourists. Austria and Italy were rather poor countries and, moreover, they had their own tourist areas resembling Saas-Fee. The United States and Canada had been neglected by the publicity campaigns. They might provide more tourists in the future because, in 1970, Saas-Fee decided to increase its publicity campaigns in these countries. Until 1970, the American currency was high compared to the European currencies, a fact which allowed the Americans to take vacations in luxury hotels not provided by Saas-Fee.

6.2.9 Development of Occupational Patterns

6.2.9.1 General Development

Increasing specialization and the expanding distribution of work introduced a stratification in the village which completely changed the former homogeneity of the roles in the agricultural society. Many new roles were created and the so-called active population increased (Fig. 25).

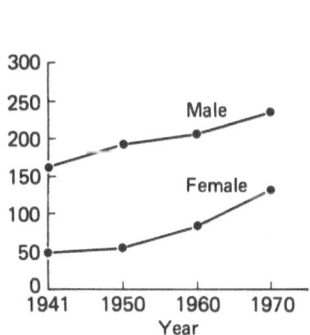

Fig. 25. The increase of the active population

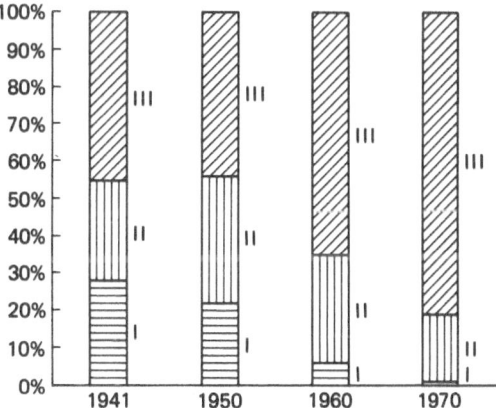

Fig. 26. Development of the three economic sectors

The development of the male active population remained more or less linear in the last three decades whereas the female active population rapidly increased after 1951.

According to official statistics (342), the village had, in 1970, a population of 895, of which 378 were working persons (i.e., 243 men and 135 women). The number of the working women is probably too low because an official declaration would mean higher taxes.

6.2.9.2 Agriculture

As Groth (cf. 199, p. 88) indicates, agriculture as an economic basis diminishes in all the developed countries of the West. This same process started in the village in 1951. As early as 1960, Supersaxo (348, p. 39) reported that "today the produce of the agriculture does not contribute much more to the income of the village Saas-Fee than a thin soup contributes to a dinner." He also mentioned that many people remained in the agricultural sector for purely traditional convictions.

More and more pastureland and fields were left uncultivated and fallowland increased, a process typical for industrialized rural areas (199, p. 141). Thus, the efforts of generations were destroyed within a very few years. By 1970, the village did not even produce enough for the basic needs of its population. According to an informant, it produced only half the potatoes and a third of the vegetables needed.

Importing goods became cheaper than producing them because all the labor was tied up elsewhere. Agriculture became increasingly a remnant of old times, a shrinking monument of the old way of living. This, as Bellman et al. (21, p. 110) reports, seems to be typical for many rural areas in the Alps. Imseng (168) indicated that the alpage above the village was used for the last time in 1969. In 1970, during the main tourist season, the village imported 1000 liters of milk daily.

The development of the various economic sectors is illustrated in Fig. 26.

Agriculture (i.e., sector I) rapidly decreased. In 1970, only 1% of the population worked in agriculture. The development of the other sectors will be discussed below.

As Bellwald and Jaeger (22) report, the decrease of the agricultural sector of Saas-Fee corresponds to the general development in the Canton Wallis (Fig. 27).

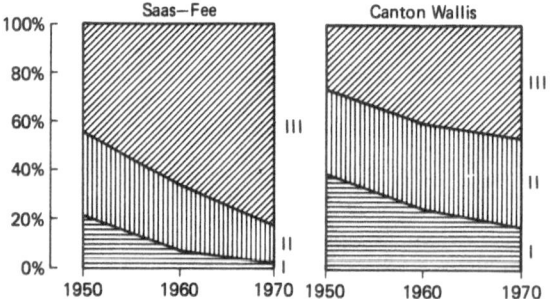

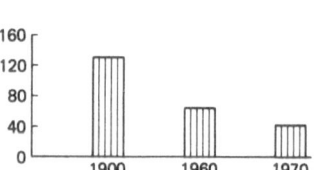

Fig. 27. Development of the three economic sectors (indicated in percentage of the working population) in Saas-Fee and the Canton Wallis

Fig. 28. Decrease of horned cattle

The statistical yearbook (342) indicates that, in 1970, only 19 economic units with cattle were operating in Saas-Fee, and no one identified himself as being fully employed in agriculture. Figure 28 indicates the decrease in horned cattle.

Although the cattle decreased by about 35.8% from 1966 to 1970, the number of sheep increased during the same period by 4.4%. I discussed earlier that this increase transcends the purely economic function and is an indicator of hidden nostalgy for "the good old time." Shepherds were well paid. As Imseng (167, p. 180) indicates, in 1966, a shepherd received a salary of 4500 Swiss Francs for a period of 5 months, a high salary compared to standard wages and the skills and intensity of work demanded.

6.2.9.3 Trade

As figure 26 illustrates, sector II increased during the time of the major constructions and decreased afterwards. The development of the village trade was quite different, as compared to the corresponding development of sector II in the Canton Wallis (cf. Fig. 27). As soon as the village started to build up the infrastructure for tourism, the number of occupational roles in sector II increased. There was a growing demand for masons, carpenters, roof makers, joiners, plumbers, electricians, painters, mechanics, and many others. Most of these jobs were taken by villagers, many of them being apprentices. Once the lodging facilities and the infrastructure were built, the need for these skilled workers decreased and many changed their occupational roles. While in 1960 29% of the working population were active in sector II, their number decreased to 17% in 1970.

As Ribeiro (294, p. 145) states, the industrial revolution liquidates remainders of the trading sector. This clearly happened in Saas-Fee. By 1970, almost half of the artisans had changed over to the services of economic sector III.

6.2.9.4 Services

The major economic development occurred in economic sector III, as Fig. 26 illustrates. This process was more important than the corresponding change in the Canton Wallis, as Fig. 27 shows. Once both the winter and summer seasons flourished, there was a great demand for mountain guides; ski instructors; employees in shops and transportation facilities; men to maintain the slopes, pathways, and streets; and people to work in restaurants, hotels, chalets, and bars.

There were quantitative shifts within certain occupational roles. As Imseng (166, p. 42) reports, the village had 65 mountain guides after the construction of the road. Thus (348, p. 33), it supplied $1/_8$ of all the mountain guides of Switzerland, but the times rapidly changed and, with them, the customs and demands of tourists. The classical time for mountain climbing was soon over because the ambitious pioneers were attracted by greater challenges in the Andes and the Himalayas. Moreover, there were now climbing courses all over Europe where young people learned the necessary skills and became independent of guides. By 1959, there were only 25-30 mountain guides left in the village, and their number decreased to 20 in 1970. The glamour had gone and what remained was an ordinary or sometimes even boring job.

In 1951, a ski school was opened. Supersaxo (348, p. 25) reports that in the first winter it gave 5,735 half day lessons. This number increased to 25,660 in 1958-1959 and to 87,800 in 1969-1970. Saas-Fee's importance had proceeded from the 26th position in Switzerland to the 5th. It boasted 50 ski instructors in 1970. Many auxiliary instructors from outside the village were hired in order to meet the growing demands.

The professional roles moved from the "undetermined" to the "determined" (Mack) positions. This implies (Daheim 68, p. 364) that there were now clear demands for the apprenticeship of an occupational role and the role expectations were explicit, clearly defined, and known by all the constituents of an interactional system. This was the case for mountain guides and ski instructors. The roles were less clearly defined for employees in the transportation sector, where apprenticeship was not required, although the role expectation was clear. Apprenticeship, demands, and expectations were even less clear for women whose occupational roles showed only a small degree of professionalization.

By 1960, 65% of the working individuals were occupied in the service sector. The number increased to 81% in 1970. This shift in the occupational roles was only one of the many indicators of the profound social change leading from the tradition directed to the inner-directed society.

6.2.10 Distribution of Work

6.2.10.1 General Aspects

Tourism introduced a new distribution of work, a greater number of workhours, and an accelerated rhythm of work. In 1970, 42.5% of the sample indicated they worked more than 10 hours per day, 7 days per week during the season (Fig. 29).

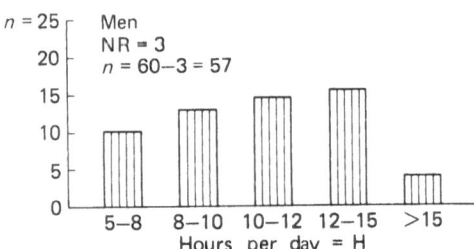

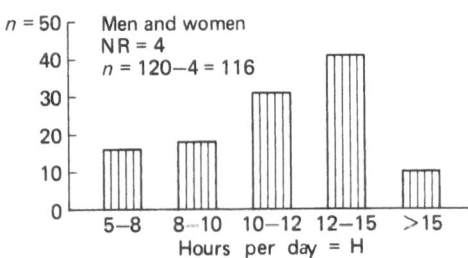

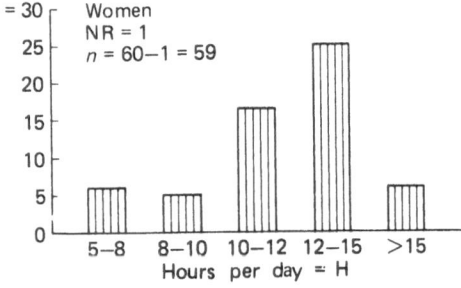

Fig. 29. Distribution of the work hours during the season

Fig. 30. Sex-specific distribution of the work-hours during the season

The long workhours were typical for the preindustrial society (316, p. 742) since work and spare time were not strictly separated. Many of the occupational functions belonged to the area of the so-called *semiloisirs* (i.e., the administrative work had to be done during spare time when all other duties were finished).

It is interesting to look briefly at the sociological theories concerning the distribution of work. As Fromm (111, p. 137 ff) shows, the economists from Smith to Marx had different ideas about the function of the origin of distribution work. For Smith (cf. 111), the distribution of work was a function of the general exchange of goods while, for Marx (cf. 111), it was rooted ultimately in the primordial distribution of work during the sexual act. Wyss's (375, p. 15) witty comment on the latter statement is that it was obviously deduced from a limited knowledge of the different technical possibilities of sexual intercourse. The sex linked distribution of work, observed all over the world, is certainly not biologically, but socially, determined, as Mead (247, 248) showed in her interesting comparative studies on role patterns in primitive societies.

Mayntz and Ziegler (242, p. 475) stated that the contemporary theoreticians of organization see the *raison d'être* of every organization in the distribution of work. The distribution of work in Saas-Fee was definitely brought about by tourism (i.e., by the demands of guests concerning food, lodging, shopping, sports, and recreation). Schelsky (314, p. 162) observed that the introduction of technological installations also increases the distribution of work. The village acquired many such installations. The new distribution of work was the specific form of organization the inhabitants developed in order to satisfy the demands of their guests. It had three main features – a sex-specific asymmetry, a class-specific asymmetry, and a season-specific asymmetry.

6.2.10.2 Sex-Specific Asymmetry

The women experienced an accumulation of roles and functions which often were not clearly defined, while the roles of men were clearly defined but quantitatively less demanding. This asymmetry certainly cannot be explained by reducing it to male supremacy, as Adler (2, p. 116) does. In fact, there are many reasons for it, a few of which are:

– The part-time emigration of many men in the preindustrial era forced the women into an accumulation of roles.
– The tourist facilities often originated in the extended household and, since the household was the traditional domain of women, they took over certain functions which arose with the advent of tourism.
– The new occupational roles of men (e.g., mountain guides, ski instructors) led to the fact that they were often absent during the day or for several days in a row. Again, the women had to take over the responsibilities of household and tourist facilities where their uninterrupted presence led to a monopoly in information and authority.
– In 1970, over 50% of the couples were composed of a man originally from the village and a woman from an industrialized and, often, urbanized area.

Often the wife's education and technological know-how were superior to the knowledge of her husband. She spoke different languages and she adapted more easily to the required social functions in the interaction with guests; one reason more to make her central.

A social system within the technological society always has a certain power aspect, as Marcuse (237, p. 18) pointed out. The distribution of work in the village, with the role accumulation of women, led to an increase in their power and, with it, to a specific form of *hidden matriarchy* that I consider to be typical for Saas-Fee. Although the men officially "wore the breeches," as the villagers say, everybody seemed to be more or less aware that women ran most of the tourist facilities. Women collected and screened information; made most of the decisions concerning the guests, employees, artisans, and suppliers; dealt with the needs and complaints of everybody concerned; and reached an autonomy which was more extensive than that of women of the middle class in urbanized areas, as described by Scherhorn (315, p. 874). The women, however, paid for their autonomy; according to my inquiry, more than 50% of them worked more than 12 hours per day while only $^1/_3$ of the men did so (Fig. 30).

The number of sleephours showed an asymmetry which mirrored the workhours. Women generally slept fewer hours per night than men, yet women rarely complained about their work situation. Probably, the feeling of being overloaded with responsibilities was assuaged by the pleasant feeling of autonomy and authority.

6.2.10.3 Class-Specific Asymmetry

Already, in the rural village of the pretourist era, there was a stratification of the population. In the traditional era, more than 90% of the population were farmers. There were differences of money, status, and power between the clergyman and the villagers. There were similar differences, although less important, between the few wealthy farmers and the poor farmers. This social stratification changed during industrialization. By 1970, there were four social classes in Saas-Fee.

- The upper class was composed of the priest, the president, and the wealthy hotel owners.
- The second class was composed of the school teachers, mountain guides, ski instructors, merchants, artisans, and employees of bureaucratic institutions.
- The third class was composed of employees of the transportation facilities working on the slopes, on technological constructions, and in hotels and restaurants.
- The fourth class was composed of unskilled workers, mostly foreigners, employed in auxiliary jobs in hotels and restaurants.

Status and prestige of these four semidefined classes was also influenced by their origin. Villagers of any class had higher status and prestige than extralocal employees of the same or even higher class. The status differences between class one and two were not very important. The important status boundary was between class two and three.

The extralocal workers, called *Pendler,* commuted between Saas-Fee and their villages. They came in the morning and left at night. As a rule, workers enter into only partial relationships with the system they work in (199, p. 150). Moreover, they did not pay taxes in the village and thus were distinctly separate from the native population. They entered the village in groups, they walked through the village in groups, and they left the village in groups. Even in the restaurants, they stayed among themselves and rarely mixed with the native population. The boundary between the villagers and the commuting workers was maintained by specific interactions. It was based upon an implicit mutual agreement with hidden rules and the villagers did not consider it as something special or extraordinary.

I discussed earlier the demographic distribution of the employees. Two-thirds of the employees were young women working in hotels, restaurants, and shops. If they liked the work and the spirit of the facility, they stayed longer. If they did not like it, they left it after one season and, in some cases, after a few days. Generally the turnover of employees was high. Their status in the interactional system of employee-employer depended upon the general economic situation. If this situation was good, their position was strong because they were badly needed; if the situation changed for the worse, they could be let go any day. In 1970, their position was very strong. They earned wages up to 3000 francs monthly, plus food and lodging. The employers generally assumed that they treated their employees very well — in my inquiry, 33% indicated treating them in a friendly manner whereas only 16% indicated treating them in an authoritative manner.

As Touraine (357, p. 419) rightly claims, common goals foster social integration. The common goal of running a successful tourist facility and having satisfied guests brought employers and employees together. What separated them was the fact that a well organized tourist facility brought much money to the employer whereas the employee received the wages agreed upon. The surplus profit, therefore, was earned by work in common, but kept by the privileged owner of the facility alone.

The employee's status was also dependent upon his origin. Foreign employees formed a subculture of their own with its rules, styles, and behaviors. They only adapted partly to the culture they were in. This seems to be an ubiquitous phenomenon, observed by Horstmann (162, p. 57). They were treated rather nicely as I repeatedly observed. Nevertheless, they had to adapt to the demands of the employers because their immigration permission depended upon their "good" behavior (i.e., upon submission and unilateral adaptation). They were the exponents of a horizontal regional mobility which could be reversed at any given moment. The accumulation of capital in Saas-Fee directed this mobility towards the village, replacing the former centrifugal mobility. Foreign employees and the commuting workers from the nearby areas were oncall individuals living on a shaky economic basis and never knowing how long they would be needed.

6.2.10.4 Season-Specific Asymmetry

The tides of international tourism are such that tourism reaches peak times or decreases virtually to zero depending on the time of the year. This uneven rhythm had always been a major source of stress for the population of Saas-Fee. The villagers had to adapt to the rhythm of tourism just as they had to adapt to the rhythm of nature in the agricultural era. Marcuse (237, p. 22) stated that the freedom of the enterpreneur produces hard work, insecurity, and anxiety. In the village, the inhabitants were mostly enterpreneurs and they took their share of consequences. They had to adapt to the peaks of Christmas and Easter and suffered from understimulation in October and November.

In 1970, four major periods of tourism divided the year:
— The interseason. This was essentially November and, to a lesser degree, May. During this time, Saas-Fee was very quiet. There were no tourists. With one exception, all the hotels, dancing halls, restaurants, chalets, and most of the shops were closed. The streets were almost empty. The native population stayed at home. Some did the administrative work neglected during the passed year and some took vacations in foreign countries, but most of them had children who had to go to school. The school was one of the institutions which had not adapted to the demands of the new era. Children had their holidays when their parents were most absorbed by tourism.

—	The preseason. This started at the beginning of December and lasted 2-3 weeks, depending on weather and snow conditions. During this time, the villagers prepared for the near season. All the tourists and their functional state were checked. New employees arrived and were instructed for their jobs. The time was busy and full of expectations.

In the years before 1970, the preseason slightly changed because special inexpensive arrangements brought the first groups of ski fans to the village. This tendency might grow if effective advertizing campaigns get to change the tourist customs, which are rather rigidly determined.

—	The season. The winter season started officially around Christmas. All at once, the streets were crowded with people. The native population of 895 had grown by over 15,000, composed of residential guests and tourists visiting during the day. There was life, noise, and turbulence. The shop windows were illuminated and stayed open until late. The village vibrated and the flow of matter-energy and information reached a peak level.

In the second week of January, the scenery reversed into its previous state almost as dramatically. Most of the guests left and the so-called January hole began, a time when the villagers tried to overcome the Christmas shock.

In February, tourism increased again. Hotellery and parahotellery were practically booked out. Now the composition of the guests was different. At Christmas, mainly young people came to the village, but now middle-aged people would be the main representatives. They were called the "good" guests becaused they consumed more and stayed longer, sometimes until Easter. Easter time was a new peak of 2-3 weeks with practically no vacancies.

The former gap between winter and summer season was now increasingly filled with tourists attracted by special arrangements. The summer season lasted 4-5 months, depending on weather conditions. Its importance, however, had been bypassed, since 1951 by the winter season.

—	The after-season. This lasted from the beginning of October to the beginning of November. During this time, the village was closing down the tourist facilities and cleaning up. The employees were paid and left. The balance of the season was being drawn and the village slid gradually into the general understimulation of the interseason.

6.3 Development of the Political Subsystem

According to the theory of historical materialism, a changing economy is supposed to introduce a change in the ideological superstructure and its subsystem. This was, indeed, the case in Saas-Fee, but the two processes were not synchronized. The superstructure was in a cultural lag and, with it, its political subsystem. The political subsystem had changed, but very little since the construction of the road.

In 1948, a 20-year-old man was elected president of Saas-Fee. He was reelected every 4 years until 1968. He influenced the course of the village process to a considerable extent. Skilled in the art of persuasion, he was a technocrat who had the necessary charm to motivate the village for the accomplishment of his own goals and ideas. His education made him open to the needs of the time and he planned for the future, defining goals and motivating the population to make the necessary sacrifices in order to reach these goals. He was a man who fell right into the lap of *cairos*, the right time, and made the best of it.

Opponents accused him of indebting the village in an irresponsible way. His supporters emphasized that the construction of all the tourist facilities and transportation systems was necessary as a long term investment which would provide for present and future generations. The image of a tourist resort is difficult to build up and easy to destroy; dissatisfied tourists would harm the reputation of Saas-Fee. A costly technological and human machinery was needed to satisfy their demands.

As Wurzbacher and Pflaum (376, p. 275) stress, the power of the president rises in industrialized areas because more and more information is centered in his administration. Unlike traditional times, the decisionmaking now demands a supply of special information the man in the street usually does not have. This fosters a dangerous credibility gap, leading, as Habermas (133, p. 95) showed, to a motivational crisis which can throw a human system out of balance. The young president of Saas-Fee mastered this difficult task well and this is one of his greatest merits.

History is easily personified and we should be aware of the fact that the control center in the village was composed not only of the president, but also of the community council, and both, in turn, were controlled by the whole population. The president, therefore, was only the personification of a general spirit of enterprise formulating and articulating communal ideas.

In 1970, there was still the two-party system in Saas-Fee; a political couriosity since, in Switzerland, the two parties were only two wings of the same party — the Christian People's Party (CVP). The two parties in the village had no alternative ideas to offer since they had an almost identical program. The "blacks" were more conservative and the "yellows" more progressive. As we have seen before, membership of one party or the other was mainly motivated by old kinship politics. In 1970, this situation had changed slightly; more and more of the younger generation had become "yellow."

Generally, the young took more power: they wanted rapid development. The old had a tendency to put the breaks on. The generation gap widened. The differences and origins of the conflicts were symbolized in the way the two groups referred to each other. The old called the young "young grapes" *(jungi Tribla)* and the young called the old "old testicles" *(alti Seckla)*. The first expression was aimed at the immaturity and the potential of fermentation of the young; obviously perceived as dangerous. The latter expression denoted the castration fantasies aiming at the removal of the biologically determined power potential of the old. This conflict was rarely brought into the open, it was, rather, discussed when the two groups were among themselves.

The political life in the village was usually rather quiet, but a political fever broke out every 4 years when elections were held. Then, the temperature increased and so did the number of rashes — the eruptions of verbal violence. The exploding forces of particularistic interests were, however, checked by the common goal to make the village a successful resort. Once the elections were over, the emotional waves calmed down.

The growing complexity of the administrative tasks demanded that the community council (i.e., five men, including the president) employ assistants. In 1970, the number of supplementary employees was five. They excecuted the orders of the president and the community council. These orders had to fit into the general framework of the cantonal and federal policies. In some areas, the communal administration collaborated with the local police which was directed by the cantonal administration.

As a rule, collaboration with higher political centers ran smoothly. Sometimes, local decisions and intentions collided with decisions made on the cantonal or federal level. One example may illustrate such a collision which upset the villagers for some time. In the 1960s, Saas-Fee planned to build a cablecar leading to an altitude of 3500 meters above sea level.

The ambitious project was torpedoed on the federal level by interest groups representing Cantons with a similar tourist industry which were not willing to give up any advantage in the competition with Saas-Fee. Most of the villagers were furious about such interference in their internal affairs and deplored the good old times when such things were unheard of. Others agreed with the federal decision, arguing that the village had already expanded enough and had more than its share of communal debts.

Women did not play an official political role. Their right to vote was introduced on a cantonal level in 1970, with an amazing majority of 72.6% of the votes. In Saas-Fee, 84 men voted for and 42 against it. Since the women played an important role in the tourist industry, however, they had indirectly influenced the official decisions made by their husband and sons. The *hidden matriarchy* was active behind the superficial cover of female discrimination.

The political course of the village was also influenced by interest groups and associations. Their function will be discussed later.

Summarizing this chapter, we can say that the political subsystem did not change very much compared to the period before 1951. In fact, the political, religious, and sociocultural subsystem developed more slowly than the demographic and economic subsystems.

6.4 Development of the Religious Subsystem

The religious subsystem of the village was strongly influenced by the general development of the policies of the Roman Catholic Church. Pope John XXIII, elected in 1958 and obviously thought to be a pope for a short transition time, amazed the world and shook a petrified Catholizism. His *Encyclica Mater et Magistra* (1961) opened new avenues for the social policy of the Church, and his *Encyclica Pacem in Terris* (1963), addressed not only to the members of the Roman Catholic Church, but to all Christians, concerned the Catholic peace policy and theory. It spoke a clear language which was different from the often nebulous rhetoric of his conservative predecessors. Pope John XXIII also organized the Vaticanum II, which was terminated by his follower Paul VI, elected pope in 1963.

The *Vaticanum II,* the 21st ecumenical council, produced an astonishing number of new decrees and decisions. It changed the liturgy, the education of priests, the pastoral duties of Bishops, and Christian education. It also dealt with the function of mass media, the relationships to non-Christian religions, the freedom of practicing religion, the position of the Church in the modern world, and other fundamental problems.

These events influenced the religious subsystem of Saas-Fee. The younger generations welcomed the changes in general and the changes in liturugy in particular. The older generations – the most frequent churchgoers – did not. They were used to the traditional procedures of the priest reading the Holy Mass in Latin and they never questioned the fact that they did not understand the texts. They prayed in German, the priest prayed in Latin, and God could understand both of them. Although the priest and the chaplain intellectually convinced them that the changes were positive, emotionally they rejected them.

All the other reforms, however, were just too much. The priest no longer turned his back to the community while celebrating the Mass. The Holy Communion could be received after having eaten breakfast. Eating meat on Fridays was suddenly allowed. The vigils no longer had the old importance. Mixed marriages, formerly forbidden by the sanction of excommunication, were allowed. The "eternal truths" were invalidated and replaced by a new set of obligations and prescriptions. Up to now, the Church had been the only institution not involved in social change. Their guarantee of stability and security began to falter. How much the older people were angered and shaken is expressed in the words of an old man I asked, in 1970, about the new Easter liturgy. He shrugged his shoulders, sighed, and said in a resigned voice, "Now they have carnival in the church throughout the year."

In 1970, the Church in the village was represented by a priest and a chaplain. The latter was younger and had some modern ideas which attracted the youth. Both representatives had the integrative function of stabilizers in the process of social change. Sometimes, they put the breaks on and intruded in the affairs of the tourist resort. For instance, the old priest announced from the pulpit that the dancing hall was "an instrument of the devil, a pitfall of the lascivious, and of prohibited concupiscence." He did not accept that a tourist resort needed dancing halls, just as a church needed an altar, for purely functional reasons.

Sometimes, the two clergymen functioned as integrators when the coherence of the social system was threatened. In the 1950s, the ski instructors got into a fight about competence and autonomy. One group, feeling neglected, founded a new ski school which attracted the best of the young instructors and expanded rapidly. The peace of the village was disturbed and the social homeostasis threatened. The boundaries between the groups rapidly petrified and the priest intervened. He achieved the closing of the new ski school and the reintegration of its members into the old one without losing face. The integration of the village was reestablished and the priest won prestige.

The Church had explained the overflowings of Mattmark Lake as dependent upon the Lord. Now it explained the hardship and the economic risks brought about by tourism as dependent upon the Lord who could be moved by prayers and donations. Thus, the situation of the village could be controlled by the pious villagers and steered in the right direction.

In other cases, the Church produced confusion and anxiety. This was the case when Pope Paul VI published the *Encyclica Humanae Vitae* (1969) in which he formally forbade the use of contraceptive devices. Fromm (110, p. 100) claimed that the Church is a traditional source of anxiety and guilt, threatening damnation for transgressions of her *ex cathedra* prescriptions. The women were put into a double bind whose nature was analyzed by Bateson et al. (18). They were put into a you-can't-win situation.

Whatever they did, they were punished. If they used contraceptive devices, they felt culpable towards the Lord; if they did not use them, they risked having more children than they wanted; and, if they refused sex, they threatened their relationships with their husbands.

It is difficult to judge the degree of relegiosity and adherence to the Church. This is a basic problem for the sociology of religion, as Fuerstenberg (112, p. 104 ff) emphasizes. We can observe the churchgoing and the development of the institutions. We can also evaluate the conscious attitudes and opinions by means of questionnaires. These methods yield some answers, but not enough.

In 1963, a new church was built in the center of the village, an expression of the central position of religion in the psychosocial economy of the village. The inquiry, accomplished in 1970, indicated that 77% of the population believed that their confessional binding to the Church was not influenced by the social changes after 1951, 9% (mostly older people) indicated that their binding had even been reinforced, and 13% (mostly the young) indicated a decrease. They were also questioned about changes in the frequency of the churchgoing of the interviewed person, his or her partner, and his or her parents. The overall result was the following:

- There was no significant difference in the frequency of churchgoing.
- The highest frequency was found among the older generations and in the female group. Older women were the most active churchgoers, often assisting Mass every day. This corresponds with the findings of Hoselitz and Merill (164), who emphasize the greater conservativism in the female sex.

The economic takeoff in the village led to an increasing competition which is a source of potential desintegration in a social organizations. Churchgoing was an important ritual of integration which can partly explain the high frequency indicated in the questionnaire – 69% of the sample went to church every Sunday, 22% went to church during the week as well. This is a high frequency compared to studies made in other rural areas (112).

Sunday, on the way to church or after church on the plaza, was about the only regular time that all the people of the village met and visited together. For a period of time, churchgoing was combined with another ritual involving and integrating the men of the village. In front of the church was the old hotel, originally built and owned by the community. It was now owned by a man who was respected and liked by everyone. After church, the men gathered around this man and had a drink together. They enjoyed each others company surrounding a man who was able to create an experience of solidarity. In the 1960s, the owner died and the ritual vanished. The people mourned and deplored the loss for the community.

The continuing centrality of the Church's position was further corroborated by the results of an investigation concerning the evaluation and appreciation of the two clergymen. Both were perceived as God's representatives by 81% of the sample, as an authoritative father figure by 9%, and as a trustworthy person by 7%. Only 6% saw the priest as a neutral or indifferent functionary and no one evaluated him as a negative symbol. This confirms the observations made by Gehlen (114, p. 33) that technological progressivism and cultural conservativism coexist. The village did not change much in its attitude towards the Church.

Predictably, these attitudes and customs will not change as long as the village is in the period of cultural lag. As Freud (106, p. 352 ff) made clear, God and religion have an auxiliary function for a threatened narcissism. The identity and narcissism of people living in a period of rapid social change is threatened. Freud (105, p. 432) claims that man needs at least three devices to make life bearable – important diversions, substitute satisfactions, and drugs. In the village, hard work and interaction with tourists constituted the diversions; religion was an anxiety reducing substitute for other satisfactions; and alcohol and drugs came into use, as we shall see later.

6.5 Development of the Sociocultural Subsystem

6.5.1 General Aspects

Social processes, being related to the subprocesses of the different subsystems of a human system, are of a stochastic nature. In the case of Saas-Fee, the demographic and the economic subsystem changed rapidly while the political and the religious subsystems lagged behind, creating the cultural lag. This same desynchronization could be observed in the institutions and agents of socialization which changed more slowly and unevenly than the demographic and the economic subsystems.

The following chapter deals with the transformations – their speed and direction – of the different elements within the sociocultural subsystem and with their interdendence upon the processes in other subsystems.

6.5.2 Agents of Sozialization

After 1951, the agents of socialization were responsible for the general goal orientation (e.g., to become a famous tourist resort), adaptation (i.e., to organize money, people, and skills necessary for goal attainment), integration (i.e., to motivate the social cooperation of all the population), and the maintenance of value patterns (i.e., the norms taught in the family, at school, and in church which should fit the behavior necessary in the new era). The sociocultural subsystem was able to fulfill these functions with varying success in different areas of concern, depending upon the functional capacities of its agents of socialization.

6.5.2.1 The Family

(1) Family Structure. There were few patrilocal families left in 1970. The general tendency was for couples to move away and found their own households and tourist facilities. Neolocality, with financial independece, constituted a general trend towards the breakdown of the extended family pattern, a trend also observed by Koenig (196, p. 220).

The typical family of 1970 was the nuclear family with from two to four children. The couple was heterogameous. In more than 50%, the wife came from an industrialized and/or urbanized area. In some cases, she was Protestant. Grandparents and single kin sometimes helped in the family, but the nuclear family was essentially autonomous.

Generally, the extralocal women had a tendency to emphasize and strengthen the boundaries between the nuclear family and the kinship group. They did not want to be influenced in their way of thinking and acting, which was sometimes quite different from the custom of the village.

The economic situation and the accumulation of roles by the women fostered the formation of small families. Frequent pregnancies would have made it impossible to fulfill all the roles and functions needed in the modern tourist facilities.

The number of intrafamilial interactions decreased because the number of family numbers decreased and the distribution of work led to the separate functioning of the family members. Children spent a great deal of time outside the family since the parents did not often have the necessary time to deal with them. The family cycle had become shorter [cf. Koenig (196, p. 45)] because many children left at the age of puberty in order to attend school outside the valley. This development was brought about by the fact that the technological progress made the school system of the village more and more insufficient for dealing with more sophisticated problems. This seems to be an ubiquitous phenomenon today, as Koenig (191, p. 124) observed.

The results of the investigation indicated that 23% of the population believed that modern tourism had an integrative function upon the family because there were common problems to deal with, 67% of the sample felt that tourism disturbed the family because the distribution of work did not allow for enough exchange and communication, and 7% indicated that tourism had a clearly detrimental effect upon the family structure.

(2) Roles Within the Family. The modern family, centering upon the economic function and reproduction, delegates the role of character formation more and more. This, of course, changes the roles of all the family members to quite an extent.

The role repertoire of the woman generally showed the features of a concentric continuity within household and tourist feacilities, whereas the role pattern of the man can be described as having the features of an eccentric dispersion. Eccentric here means the range of activities transcending the extended household.

This asymmetric role distribution led to the structure of the hidden matriarchy. although very young couples tended to organize their role distribution towards more symmetry, this process was just beginning. Both partners suffered from the asymmetry. Generally, they would have liked to change it, but they felt unable to do so.

The man functioned as husband, father, and had an occupational role in the mountains or on the slopes. In addition, many of them worked part-time in shops and restaurants. Although they officially owned the tourist facilities, the women usually ran them.

The woman functioned as wife, mother, and organized for the household and tourist facilities. She was the center of information. Requests and demands were brought to her. She managed the conflicts and problems between employees and tourists. She was generally overburdened, worked harder than men, and put in longer hours.

Grandparents helped in the tourist facilities and with babysitting. Their influence upon the youth had diminished. The children preferred the neomyths of the mass media to the old myths and legends of their grandparents. The TV gained in importance as an orientation to the new world. Still, the old people were not without status and prestige, but, little by little, they were excluded from the transactional circuit of the nuclear family. My investigation indicated that 98% of the population welcomed the presence and help of grandparents and other old people, while only 2% seemed to perceive them as an additional burden. This means that the older generation was still well integrated, as compared to other industrial and urban areas, even though their roles had changed or were completely discarded.

In the modern family, which was still the economic unit, the children did not have many roles left. They helped here and there, but, generally, they were rather disruptive to the smooth functioning of the economic units. Since parents were completely absorbed during the tourist season, children were left more and more on their own. They often were on the the streets and they integrated with peer groups, whose social importance was clearly increasing.

(3) Functions of the Family

Reproduction. The major change in the family's basic function (i.e., reproduction) was a shrinkage in the number of children. The modern family was small. Although this decrease occurred despite the demands of the Church and the old customs, it was in accord with the universal principle of utility and rationalism (i.e., the maintenance of a congruity between the size of the population and the economic subsystem).

Socialization and Formation of Character. Ribeiro (294, p. 186) claims that a basic social change requires a complete transformation of the educational system in order to adapt the traditional norms and values to the demands of a changing society. Saas-Fee did not change its educational system radically. The standards of child care had not changed essentially, but they seemed to be enforced with less intensity, consistency, and effectiveness.

Some key informants went even so far as to say that the process of socialization in the village showed signs and symptoms of anomie. Objectively, this was not the case, but, quite obviously, something in the effects of the education had changed. It did not always change for the better. The new situation demanded that values be transmitted which fostered the qualities of personality needed in a village depending on tourism. Such qualities were friendliness, openmindedness, flexibility, independence, capacity to organize, capacity to speak several languages, and to empathize with different attitudes and beliefs. These qualities should be integrated in a multilevel identification process which creates the final identity of a personality, as described by Erikson (92, p. 108). Such identity was not built up easily in the village where the models of identification were incongruent, often contradictory, and quickly changing.

As Schwanenberg (321, p. 215) points out, the child builds up his motivations playing out the multidimensional roles of the significant figures of his environment. Motivations, in turn, are responsible for the input of norms and values. In Saas-Fee, relations between children and significant persons were often fragmented. A mother did not have much time for her child, at least not during the season. The father was often absent and the employees changed every few months. Continuity and congruence of the in-formation (351) of socialization was no longer guaranteed. A shaky self was sometimes the result.

The guests had priority. Consequently, children were only intermittently educated. They were punished only when it did not disturb the guests or when the coping potential of the parents was exhausted. Children were often rewarded with money because it was the resource the parents always had available. Thus, relationships were robbed of affect, instrumentalized, and increasingly rarefied. This, of course, influenced the syngenetic program and, with it, the attitudes and transactions of the children. My future followup studies might reveal to what extent this process influenced the general character formation. Predictably, these children will be grownups with little coping potential under stress.

My observations contrasts with the self-evaluations of the sample. More than two-thirds indicated that their children were educated mainly by the parents, while only 12% thought that they were educated mainly by the employees and 8% indicated that kinship played an important role in education. However, when asked in an informal context, most of the same individuals indicated that the parents no longer had much influence upon character formation. Furthermore, they thought that the educational style of parents was ineffective, because positive sanctions (e.g., money, presents) prevailed, while the time-honored negative sanctions (e.g., physical or psychosocial punishment) had been lost.

The arguments for these assumptions were that approximately 15% of the youth failed when going to nonvillage schools. This relatively high percentage can be explained by the fact that the children, in general, were not motivated to leave the village. Their parents wanted them to be prepared for modern times and delegated their own desires for prestige and certain goal attainments to the youth. They also wanted their children to be off the streets and away from the tourists who displayed behavior patterns for vacations rather than for their daily struggle with problems of a tourist resort.

Finally, there was the pressure of conformity. If the neighbor's child was going to a boarding school outside the village, their own child must go too.

One could expect, after all, that these children would show a high number of neurotic symptoms and behavioral disorders. However, the number of such problems was almost equivalent to the number of problems the adults suffered from their own young, as indicated in the questionnaire. The symptoms were biting of finger nails (20%), enuresis (18%), pavor nocturnus (17%), educational problems (11%), stuttering (8%), and stealing (5%).

The direct field observations showed that couples were often in conflict because their different cultural background did not allow successful negotiations about values and norms. There was, however, a discrepancy between the field observations and the results of the structured interview. Only 15% of the couples indicated tensions, whereas 59% described their marriage as harmonious. Again, the limits of the structured interview become apparent.

The direct field observations showed that parents who disagreed about values and norms often avoided teaching anything to children to prevent conflicts with their partners. This left the children without leadership. Consequently, they developed a character which became increasingly other-directed, in the sense of Riesman (297). Value patterns were no longer internalized. They changed from context to context and from event to event, according to the principle of the highest pressure. The behavior displayed by admired persons was imitated readily. This youth displayed the "shrunken inwardness" Horkheimer (159, p. 95) spoke of.

After all, who was this youth according to the results of the questionnaire? The judgments were prevailingly pessimistic and the relation of indicated positive to negative character traits was one to three. These judgments were, of course, subjective and it is well-known that the older generations tend to assume that the youth of today is worse than the youth of yesterday. When Socrates described the youth of Athenes he did so in very negative terms. Watzlawick et al. (364, p. 51) report the following engraving in a clay slate 3000 years ago, "the youth of today is putrified unto its roots. The youth is bad, without religion, and lazy. It will never be like the youth of times passed and it will be incapable to maintain our civilization." Indeed, Athens and Babylon perished, but not because of their youth. They perished because their social systems were unable to maintain their boundaries and substance in a changing historical context.

In Saas-Fee, the young generation grew up in a technological environment, with parents who were overburdened, and with role models offered by employees and tourists. They underwent an intensive process of acculturation. They took over bits of behavior here and there and they took over the implicit and sometimes explicit rules of their idols. At the same time, they maintained many of the old behavior patterns, which I could observe especially in the boys.

On the one hand, the boys were eager to behave like the guests — to pay bills with pompous gestures, use a picked up language, walk like urban people, consume drinks and other things like wealthy holiday makers, and so forth. On the other hand, when coming in direct contact with the foreign guests, they fell back into their old behavior patterns of the traditional virility. They inhaled deeply, expanding their chest; put on a stern, almost hostile, expression; and spoke in a choked voice. They displayed the behavior patterns of the threatened and mistrusting mountain dweller.

There was an important gap between the older and younger generations. The older generation exhibited the traditional and inner directed character traits. They were directed at successful professional careers and increase of income. They had a high achievement motivation and they acknowledged the old values of self-control and parsimony. The younger generation, however, was other-directed (297). They were interested in fun and having a good time with peers. For a youth to be successful meant to be accepted by his peer group, to avoid major struggles over opinions and attitudes, and to display a high degree of freedom in all behaviors as well as in hairstyle and fashion. In short, he had to assimilate. Where the older generation was competitive, the younger generation often showed indifference. In 1970, the village did not have a single youth who was a champion in sports, although it had had many at the time of the early industrialization. This seems to be an ubiquitous law; scanning the participation charts of winter sport competitions one becomes aware of the fact that the champions come from upcoming or totally unknown villages, while well-established tourist resorts seem to lack the necessary achievement motivation in this field.

Parents were often amazed and alarmed by the enormous speed with which the youth adopted and gave up certain behaviors and models which were "in" one day and "out" the next. They did not understand the extent to which this was a normal reaction to the rapid social change in the village and the children were responding with high flexibility, while the older people often responded with discomfort and rigidity.

All the described features of the new character have to be understood as ideal types (Weber). Each actual individual showed deviations from the general model and was composed of an agglomerate of more or less different and contradictory features. The only fixed pattern, unmistakenly present, was the intergenerational difference in character traits.

The Economic Unit. In 1970, the family of Saas-Fee fulfilled, better than ever, the function of being the economic base. The flow of cash was high and, notwithstanding the substantial indebtedness of many families, they all had the money to provide for their members, send their children to expensive boarding schools away from the village, and buy everything needed.

6.5.2.2 Kinship

The role of the extended kinship group changed dramatically. The women, often coming from urbanized and industrialized areas, refused the intrusion of the kinship group. Generally, with a higher education than their husbands and kin, they felt independent and prevented or ignored the possible influence of the clan whenever they could. This was relatively easy because the nuclear family was independent, to a considerable extent, in its organization as an economic unit and this inhibited social control from outside. Whenever members of the extended family were needed, they came into the household only upon request and for clearly defined functions.

6.5.2.3 Peer Groups

To the extent that the parents were absorbed in their occupational roles, the peer group became increasingly important for the youth. Role expectations rules, and behaviors were worked out in the peer group rather than elsewhere. The peer group derived its norms from comic strips, mass media, and tourists rather than from their families.

The first peer group which was clearly recognized as such was observed shortly after 1951. It was composed of young men displaying rather aggressive behavior and boasting, quarreling, and entering restaurants paraphrasing the sun king of France, *"Saas-Fee c'est nous."* The villagers were alarmed. The group's demonstrative behavior vanished shortly after.

The prevailing adolescent peer group of 1970 was of a more agreeable kind. The youngsters were fun oriented; they drank considerably, danced, and had sex if they had the courage to do so. They rarely quarreled and were an instrument of social integration. Within their rituals they overcame the old gaps between the different family clans. Whoever behaved according to their rules and shared their attitudes and beliefs was welcome, independent of his family background.

The boundaries between adolescent peer groups and adults were rather rigidly drawn. Discussions between the generations often ended in silent conflict avoidance. The authority of the parents was less effective than the authority of the peer group. The pressure of conformity within the group was enormous, as was mutual help whenever conflicts with parents led to sanctions. The youth preferred to be on bad terms with the parents rather than to be excluded from the group. This meant that the peers became self-regulative agents of socialization, transmitting values and norms and shaping the behavior of girls and boys.

6.5.2.4 School

With the general social change, the structure and the functions of the school, within the process of socialization, changed. In 1970, there were two male and three female teachers for 73 boys and 77 girls in eight grades. The kindergarten was run by two female teachers in two parallel grades with 22 and 23 children. All the following schools were away from the village — 27 students attended boarding schools, 17 apprentices attended specialized schools, and a number of students attended language schools.

The trend towards higher education prevailed. The parents, subjected to the Peter Principle, had reached their stage of incompetence within the tourist era. They pushed their children into specialized education. The children were delegated to realize the ideal self of the parents, a psychosocial mechanism mentioned by Richter (296, p. 168 ff).

This led to an unfavorable situation, since too many doctors, engineers, and other academicians were produced for which the village had a limited demand. The overeducation also led to the fact that the village lacked increasingly what it needed most for its survival (i.e., skilled workers to take over the occupational roles of the tourist industry).

Generally, the over 35 population, in an informal context, complained about their education which had prepared them for the functions and roles of the new era. They especially deplored the fact that they did not speak foreign languages which would facilitate their contacts with the guests from many different countries. In the questionnaire, however, only 12% of the sample indicated that they considered their education as insufficient. Again, one is amazed by the discrepancy between the results of the two methods of investigation.

Given the number of youths attending schools away from the village, their influence upon sozialization was important and positive. These adolescents soon learned that the local values were not absolute. They learned to adapt to different lifestyles. They became more flexible and those who returned to the village were prepared to function more smoothly with the guests. More of the "overeducated" villagers might return in the future because Europe produces more academicians than this specific labor market can absorb.

6.5.2.5 Church and the Church Going

I refer to the previous discussion (cf. p. 148) about the functions of these institutions in the process of socialization and social integration.

6.5.2.6 Associations and Clubs

As Wurzbacher and Pflaum (376, p. 152) state, associations are a feature of urbanization and replace informal patterns of interaction by formalized patterns within rational organizations. We have seen (cf. p. 99) that the associations and clubs were founded after tourism was introduced (i.e., with industrialization, urbanization, and new models and patterns).

In 1970, the village had a large number of associations which can be devided into four major groups:

- *Ecclesiastical associations:* mothers' association, men's association, youth association, Cecilia association (i.e., choral society dedicated to Saint Cecilia), blue ring association (girls), young sentinel associations (boys).
- *Cultural associations:* costume association, old village music, brass band association, choral society.
- *Associations based on commercial interests:* tourism association, hoteliers association, trade and commerce association, cattle breeding association, dairy farming association, fire brigade.

— *Sport clubs:* ski club, curling club, gymnastic club for women, gymnastic club for men, mountain guide club, ski instructor club, military shooting club, nonmilitary shooting club, small caliber shooting club, hunters' club, bowling club, gymnastic club for girls.

The criteria for the above typology are overlapping. One fact becomes apparent, to the extent to which competition had changed the interactional pattern of the population, a clear trend for formalize interactions within the growing number of organizations became apparent. These clubs and associations had an integrative social function which was more or less conscious to the population.

Different local institutions had different integrative effects. The sample indicated the following hierarchy: 73% thought churchgoing as socially integrative, 71% assumed that the music associations were integrative, and 48% indicated that the ecclesiastic associations were integrative. Commercial interest associations ranked lower; only 27% of the sample thought them to be socially integrative. Obviously, this hierarchical ladder was constructed according to the individual satisfaction of emotional needs, rather than according to general functional principles. Political parties ranked very low; only 13% of the probands thought that parties were integrative.

Two-thirds of the population were members of associations and many were members of several associations; 43% indicated participating occasionally in the activities, 47% participated regularly, and 10% either did not participate at all or did not give any indication.

The clubs and associations offered positions and functions for the display of status and prestige. This had nothing to do with the financial status of the members. Instead, the value of social cooperation and integration was gratified. This was especially true during the festivities of these associations and during their rituals of elections when aggressions were channeled and the centrifugal tendencies of a competitive society checked and controlled.

6.5.2.7 Occupations

Different occupational roles elaborated their own code of ethics. The construction of the code was goal oriented. There was a common systemic goal and different subsystemic goals to be reached. The systemic goal was to give the tourist resort a positive image. The subsystemic goals varied according to the occupational roles. The mountain guide, for instance, had to guarantee the safety of his expedition and to demonstrate the beauty of the mountains and the thrill of self-control during the climb. The ski instructor tried to introduce the guests to the elegance of a dancing style on skis. The hotelier wanted to produce excellent service and a first-class kitchen.

The attempted goal attainment shaped the ethical code, which controlled the behaviors and, thus, the occupational roles had a major impact on socialization. Despite a certain competitiveness between the members of the different occupational roles, the common systemic goal demanded cooperation and mutual restraint from selfish behavior patterns.

6.5.2.8 Extralocal Agents of Socialization

(1) Guests. Malinowski (cf. 274) emphasized that acculturation has a great impact upon social change. This could be clearly observed in Saas-Fee. The high number of

tourists increased the influence of acculturation as their technologies, behavior, and value patterns were taken over by the inhabitants. Tourists exhibited styles of behavior according to their cultural background and adapted to the setting of a tourist resort. They came to regress, relax, and have fun. They offered the youth a model of behavior easy to imitate. Hummel (165, p. 1197) writes that only such persons are imitated who consume gratifications to a great extent and who have many resources available. The tourists in Saas-Fee fitted into this picture. For the time being, they were literally and metaphorically on the sunny side of the street.

No wonder that the youth of the village tended to choose their models of identification among the tourists who gave the impression that this was their usual way of life. Compared to them, their parents lived a hard and undesirable life. The youth preferred the sunny side of the street and, thus, slid into a motivational crisis. The achievement motivation decreased or, rather, changed in direction. The new goal was having fun and not performance.

It is difficult to evaluate the influence of tourists upon socialization. I have data only concerning the interactional style, not its content. In my inquiry, 75% of the sample indicated that they had very friendly relationships with tourists, 17% indicated that they shared purely commercial interests with them, 5% indicated a certain distance, and 3% were completely indifferent toward the guests.

It is interesting to confront these data with the data of an investigation by Bellwald and Jaeger (22, p. 52) who questioned 853 tourists. According to this study, 37% indicated that they had friendly interactions with the villagers, 25% judged the villagers to be eager for contact, 36% believed them to be uncommunicative, 8% thought they were rejecting, and 4% indicated other opinions.

Whatever the style of interaction, as punctuated by one or the other partner of this dyadic system, we can assume that the mutual influence was intensive and that the villagers, especially the youth, took on a set of new behavior patterns. Thus, acculturation led gradually to a certain degree of urbanization.

(2) Extralocal Schools and Colleges. We have already discussed (cf. p. 156) the influence of these schools upon the socialization of the inhabitants of the village. Although only a small number of the population was directly influenced, they were the potential leaders. If the top of a hierarchy is influenced, sooner or later the whole pyramid will be.

(3) Military Service. Although military service had a socializing effect before 1951, its impact had considerably decreased by now. On the one hand, people did not believe so strongly in the benedictions of the military machinery and, on the other hand, the youth had encountered the new values and norms in the contact with the tourists long before the military service.

It was no longer generally held that military service "makes a man a real man." Instead, the service interfered with the eonomic interests of the male population who did not like to leave their work during the tourist season.

(4) Modern Mass Media. My methodological approach does not allow me to give quantitative data concerning the influence of mass media upon the village; however, the direct field observation yielded some results indicating the extent of its influence.

In 1970, the kiosks and newsstands sold a wide range of international journals and newspapers, including the few regional traditional newspapers. The former brought the concerns of the international world to the village and the latter reflected the traditional way of life shaped by Catholicism to a considerable extent. The German sex-and-crime magazines were widely read. An old taboo seemed to falter. The Catholic values concerning sex and aggression had changed and the village had adopted a permissive attitude towards the passive consumption of sex and aggression.

Every household had a television. Adorno (3, p. 70) assumed that television makes people "to what they already are." In my opinion, television, in its actual form, offers a wider range of different styles of life and models of identification. It reinforces the conspicuous consumption of a mercantile society.

Summarizing this chapter, we can assume that the mass media reinforced the general transformation of the process of socialization and acculturation. The village gradually moved away from local and toward universal norms and values.

6.5.3 Contents and Rituals of Socialization

Redfield (291, p. 4) suggested that homogeneity and slow social change are typical for rural areas. In Saas-Fee, on the contrary, heterogeneity and selective rapid social change had influenced all phenomena of the social organization. A few of these phenomena shall be discussed briefly.

6.5.3.1 Costumes and Customs

After 1951, costumes and customs rapidly changed. In 1970, the old costumes had almost vanished. The old women still wore them and, for a few very special events in the village, many other women would put them on. Gradually, this habit became part of the tourist folklore and the costumes practically lost their former symbolic and signalizing functions.

The traditional canvas suit for men was replaced by the modern uniform such as jeans and pullovers or the modern ski fashions. The official costumes were universal. Only a few subgroups (e.g., mountain guides, ski instructors, and employees of the transportation facilities) had specific professional uniforms that are found today in the whole region of the Alps. The former local uniformity was replaced by a uniformity which did not distinguish the village from the outside, but only the subgroups in the village and tourist resorts in the Alps from the rest of the world.

The old customs had vanished too. The *Abusitz* was forgotten. Now, the families gathered around their television and, instead of the old myths and legends, the consumed neomyths, international sports news, and political news. The *mother zum Brunnji* (cf. p. 111) was forgotten and replaced by more trivial magazine stories. The "Flijer Hansjob" and the "straw-fire man" vanished into the grottoes of oblivion.

The procession of Corpus Christ and the Carnival parade were kept, but the events no longer had the almost atavistic depth. They were now folkloristic events more in the service of the tourists. The animal tails used at Carnival to whip young women were replaced by plastic carpet beaters, devices lacking the symbolic content. The costumes worn for Carnival became increasingly unauthentic.

Ancient customs are not abolished or modified without good reasons. The customs in Saas-Fee had an integrative function. They were also ritualized outlets for the population's repressed aggressions and sexuality. These functions were obviously not needed any longer. The modern Saas-Fee provided new rituals with integrative functions and its attitude towards aggression and sexuality had become more permissive.

The new customs were sometimes less obvious than the old ones, which were striking for their highly ritualized formality and their sometimes atavistic aspect. One of the new and more obvious customs was the ski descent at night. All the ski instructors of the village, carying burning torches, glided down a steep and rocky mountain, forming a flickering and mysterious snake in the dark night. As they descended, they were more and more descernable until they arrived in the village where a crowd expected them on the central plaza. They were cheered and received like heroes. They were introduced and introduced themselves in several languages to the waiting crowd. This modern folklore was produced mainly for the tourists.

Another, less obvious, custom was a drinking ritual displayed by a certain group of male villagers. This ritual was called "to pay a round" *(as tournée zalu)*. Generally, it started with one man sitting alone at a table in a bar or restaurant. Another man entered and was asked by the first, "do you pay a round?" To answer "no" would have been a display of hostility. As a rule, the second man agreed. They drank "a round" together. Then, the first man had to pay another "round." This process was sometimes repeated until both were drunk.

It often happened that the pattern ran differently. A third man entered the room, was invited, accepted, and paid a round. This meant that each of the first two men had to pay another round. More men entered, joined the group, and paid rounds which increased in a spiralic way. During these drinking rituals, the men joked; slapped each other's shoulders; and, if it was not election time, they were generally cordial according to the scheme "if you are my buddy I am yours." At the end of the ritual, all had drank more than intended. In general, only villagers were invited to this ritual.

This ritual served several functions, but it was mainly integrative, binding latent aggressions in a competitive village, where everybody tried to have more guests than his neighbor. Another function was to break the isolation of the individuals. In the agricultural era, they often worked together in the fields and on the alpages for days and weeks. In 1970, everyone was involved with his own tourists and facilities, which left him little time to visit with his fellow men. Another function was the reduction of anxiety and stress, produced by their financial indebtedness, the hidden matriarchy, and the uneven working rhythm of the tourist resort. Drinking together was a ritual of catharsis and alleviation. The ritual also functioned in the service of controlling sexuality. The temptations were great. Many female guests were eager to organize a little holiday adventure with one of the suntanned mountain dwellers; however, the social control was still very strong and who entered which house and at what time could easily be checked. Catholicism was still strong enough, at least for the older generation, to demand repression of extramarital sexuality. To drink together and tell dirty jokes and invent erotic stories helped to keep their sexual drives under control. It banished anxiety, fostered togetherness, and also simultaneously allowed each man to show, amidst all this fraternity, that he had as much cash in his pocket as anybody else.

162

What did the villagers do with their spare time? There was not much of it during the season, but there was October, November, and the time between the summer and winter season. During these periods, the men drank together and did "business," a label that covered a whole lot of different activities from chatting, gossiping, boasting, and brawling to negotiating, buying, and selling. A few men were busy with woodcarving or sheep raising. The weather was usually poor and outdoor activities came to a halt.

Women continued to fulfill their various roles and functions. They had more time for their children in the off-season, but were usually preoccupied with questons of management, personel, and new investments in the tourist facilities. They visited the clubs and associations more frequently and took more time to talk with their fellow women. They also tried to get some rest to be prepared for the stress to come.

6.5.3.2 Legends and Myths

The old legends and myths were dead. Meanwhile, they had been collected by writers and, in many a house, there was an anthology of these traditional messages. Most of the people, however, ignored them and, even when narrated by an old person, they had lost the vigor and suggestive strength they had in passed times. Time moved fast and the right mood for listening and getting involved was lacking. The old legends and myths no longer served the functions they had in the old world.

The new world needed new values. The mentality of submission was not needed any longer. On the contrary, it was hindering for progress. The children, pacemakers of new trends and indicators of change, were thrilled by Tarzan, Batman, Barbarella, Asterix and Obelix, Lucky Luke, and other contemporary mythical heroes who successfully fought against the intricacies of the modern world. This enthusiasm was an expression of the qualities demanded in a world where cunning, flexibility, and the spirit of enterprise were requisite and growing complexity fostered dreams of magical grandeur. Creative-innovative behavior was more appreciated than the traditional submission under "eternal laws."

There were, however, some legends from the pioneer epoch which were told, especially, in the bars and restaurants and aimed at the formation of a strong identity. People liked to tell, for instance, about a mountain guide. He was in the middle of an icy mountainside when his exhausted guest became hysterical. The mountain guide, of course, mastered the dramatic situation by calming down the guest with a firm hand. Another story was the extremely dangerous rescue mission of a foreign lady who had fallen into a crevice and could not be saved in time because a dense fog covered the glaciers. The men shuddered when they imitated the sound of the frozen corpse being lifted out of the crevice by a helicopter. In these cases, the neomyths became the vehicle for self-representation, often leading to boasting and, with it, depreciative criticism of other villagers who were not friends of the narrator. This, of course, provoked conterattacks. The neomyths were challenged and the spirit of reverence, present when the old myths were told, was lacking.

Another neomyth dealt with the glorious triumph of the Oliympic Games in St. Moritz in 1948 when the villagers won the gold medal. One of the winners later met a tragic death in the mountains, where he was lost in a snowstorm. The villagers spoke with deep respect of this man and the possible heroic acts he might have accomplished had he not been killed. In this story, the atavistic fear surfaced again and the old taboo, so well formulated in the myth of the straw-fire man, still seemed to hold true, although held in check by their confidence in modern technology. Other, more trivial myths were about drinking and foolhardiness. For instance, a villager, after consuming his 36th whisky, walked on his hands, dead drunk, on top of the railings of a small bridges leading over a wild mountain torrent, boasting, "and I tell you, I will not learn to swim tonight." Or, a cunning realtor treated a "stupid" guest for several hours with cherry brandy before he sold him his heritage, a piece of land he had no use for and for which the guest, after days of heavy bargaining, was now ready to pay an enormous sum.

Such were the neomyths, too young to provoke deep interest and almost exclusively turning around the display of cunning, pride, and spirit of enterprise. They fitted, however, with the modern life situation which demanded such qualities. They had a socializing effect upon the youth who tried to copy, especially, the drinking habits of the new village heroes.

6.5.3.3 Value Patterns

Value patterns are dependent upon the stage of the process of a human system, its economy, and its ecology, as Bateson (16, 17), Daheim (66), Fromm (110, 111), Mead (246, 247), Morgenthaler et al. (259, 260), Parin (269), and many other authors correctly pointed out. Value patterns change more slowly than the other elements of a human system. This guarantees the maintenance of the system's boundaries and its identity; it preserves a viable homeostasis.

I made clear (cf. p. 112 f.) that values are part of the rules which govern human transactions and that they are determined by these transactions, goals, and metadeterminants (i.e., by what I call principles and antiprinciples of transactions and also by the systemic structure of the human system which produces them). Although there is a clear hierarchy in this explanatory model, multiple feedback processes give this hierarchy a circular structure. Since the social structure of Saas-Fee and its goals and transactions had changed and, since the quantitative and interconnected steering output of the governing principles had changed, the value patterns, predictably, had to be changed. Thus, the syngenetic program of the youth in 1970 was quite different from the syngenetic program of the middle-aged and older generation.

The values which governed the former behaviors (e.g., taciturnity, solidarity, modesty, achievement motivation, sexuality, aggression) had changed. The changes occurred to a varying extent so that old and new values coexisted. Moreover, there was a gap between the official values and the actual behaviors. This gap led to contradictions influencing the governing process of transactions. These transactions, in turn, were often symptoms of the general cultural lag due to the varying speed of change.

One of the values in the syngenetic program of the older individuals was taciturnity and reserve. It was needed in the old times. Taciturnity and reserve were a handicap in the tourist era. The guests wanted to be welcomed and to feel at home. Bellwald and Jaeger (22) reported that almost half of the guests (i.e., 47%) indicated that the villagers were reserved, rejecting, and unfriendly. This was, however, not the way the villagers described themselves. Their self-image illustrated the gap between officially acknowledged and actually governing values.

Another old value was solidarity, needed for survival in an unyielding nature. In 1970, competition in the village was a central value. Everyone liked to be more successful than his neighbor. Although the individual competition was covered over by a common competition with other tourist resorts, it was still there. Aggressive-competitive behavior was often labelled as being necessary in the service of the guests. The universal principle "business is business," a far-reaching statement which allows many different hermeneutics, had been introduced in the village. Thus, solidarity was threatened, but its maintenance needed, to be attractive for the guests. The Pearl of the Alps had to be a happy place where the myth of the Arcadian paradise was a reality. The new type of solidarity was controlled by drinking rituals and a surprisingly active participation in associations and clubs where aggressions were channeled into formalized rituals.

Modesty and self-restraint had been replaced by an expansive and aggressive spirit of enterprise, a value pattern needed in the industrialized societies. The young maverick pursuing an aggressive and expansive business policy, transcending the old limitations of a financial or social nature, was basically accepted, sometimes publicy attacked, but always secretly admired. The man who diversified his business according to the capitalistic rules was a model of identification as long as he reached his goals. To be successful was a top value. When this value was not achieved, social ostracism was often the consequence. A loser dropped out or was partly pushed out of the network of communications and transactions. He became a marginal figure. He was a threat to the new mythology of winning at any price and, therefore, a threat to the values governing this kind of goal directed transaction.

Formerly, the culture was prohibitive. Now, permissive value patterns replaced many of the former prohibitions. To have fun, drink with the guests and with his fellow men, and adapt to the new values coming to the village was admitted or desired. However, some taboos were still existing. Although sex and crime magazines were available, Adorno's dictum (3, p. 100) that sexual liberation in actual society is a myth held true, to some extent, in the village. The guests displayed some libertinism, as did the single foreign employees who were mostly isolated from their own social context and social control. The latter's libertinism was accepted by a repressive tolerance, as described by Marcuse (237). The employer tolerated almost any behavior of the employee as long as it did not interfere with the work ethic. Satisfaction of emotional and sexual needs regenerated the motivation for daily achievement within the tourist facilities. For the native population, however, the old prohibitions governed their actual behavior. The village was small and social control very efficient.

In the pretourist village, the values governing daily work were very demanding. It was a generally accepted norm to work to the point of exhaustion, especially during the summer months. Money was earned by hard work; easy profit was not possible. In the new time, the principle of *ora et labora* changed to "organize your resources and work only as much as you need to." Still, the major part of the population, especially the women, needed to work hard. Work, however, was no longer experienced as freely chosen and liberating, but rather as a burden.

Achievement motivation and success compelled many a villager to work more than needed. The success of his neighbor kept him going when he would have relaxed. The universal principle "good is what is useful for achievement," governed the village. It changed the work and the work attitudes and demanded new achievements daily. Achievement became a status symbol conferring prestige (Koetter 199, p. 173; 376, p. 44). The new work ethic was only one of the many signs of the upcoming otherdirected society.

Other values had not changed at all. Autonomy and pride were actually reinforced by enterprise and achievement motivation. The we-have-made-it mentality soldered the village together and glossed over many basic contradictions. Pride as a value and behavior was part of the narcissistic armor of the modern character. Behind this armor, however, was the face of anxiety which increases when aggressions are not adequately detoured, as Morgenthaler et al. (260, p. 558) showed in their ethnoanalytic study of the Agni tribe in West Africa. Anxiety also increases when sexuality is repressed. The more anxiety increases the more the armor rigidifies.

The coexistence of contradictory values upset individuals and families. They had the alternative of going with the new times and feeling guilty or of going with the old times and feeling like dupes because they did not achieve what their neighbors achieved. The principle of utility and efficiency was often the catalyst which decided in the battle between old and new values. This principle derived from the economic subsystem which was more advanced than the sociocultural subsystem with its confusing patchwork of old and new values.

In the middle of this trouble, however, was a firm feeling of identity. The economic achievements, as well as the frequent compliments from the guests who admired the "natural" villagers and envied their "healthy" life, were welcome gratifications.

At this point, the question arises concerning what will happen to the sociocultural subsystem and the identity of these people if, one day, the tourists keep away? Will their identity collapse when it is no longer nourished by the admiration of the guests? Will anomie occur? Will there be an increasing rate of suicide? Will there be other pathological symptoms?

Hopefully, the syngenetic program, with its new values of efficiency and adaptation, will be congruent and hard programmed enough to help the villagers cope with such a crisis always lurking in the background of every high risk enterprise.

Social Change and Stress

7. General Stress Concepts

This chapter is concerned with one basic question — what are the possible concepts which can explain the interconnection between social change and stress? How do the manifold stressors, created by social change, affect individuals, families, and a village as a whole?

The stress indicators (i.e., the health disorders found in Saas-Fee in 1970) will be discussed in detail later. The following discussion is based partly upon concepts developed by Lazarus (207), Levi (213-215) and myself (Guntern 128, 132).

7.1 Stressors Due to Intrasystemic Contradictions

I conceive of symptoms as being codified sommunications, indicating a structural unbalance or disturbance or, more precisely, indicating the loss — actual or threatening — of homeostasis in a given human system.

In a human system, there are many hierarchical levels of organization with many subsystems which can lose their homeostasis and which, therefore, can show symptoms. In a village, there are two major levels of organization — the level of psychobiologic organization (i.e., organisms and population) and the level of social organization (i.e., social institutions). This differentiation into two major levels does not mean that there are no important interconnections between the levels. For the sake of analytic clarity, the levels are treated as being separate. We have to be aware, however, of their interconnections.

The level of psychobiologic organization consists of several subsystems (i.e., individual, couple, family, and kinship), as does the level of social organization (i.e., demographic, economic, politic, religious, and sociocultural). It is a question of logical typing and of a theoretical vantage point whether or not we describe many or few subsystems and whether or not we define one system as a subsystem or a suprasystem in relation to another. The interested reader will find a excellent discussion of this theoretical problem in Miller (251, 152).

Whatever logical typing we choose, it leads to a descriptive framework which creates a system of coordination in which we can describe transactions and communications; feedback processes; recalibration and step functions; homeostasis; and, finally, symptoms. The hierarchy, in such a descriptive system, ist not linear. It has a circular configuration. What is a stressor from one point of view is a stress indicator from another point of view, and vice versa.

Levi (215) proposed a stress model which explains the production of stress indicators or symptoms in an individual (Fig. 31).

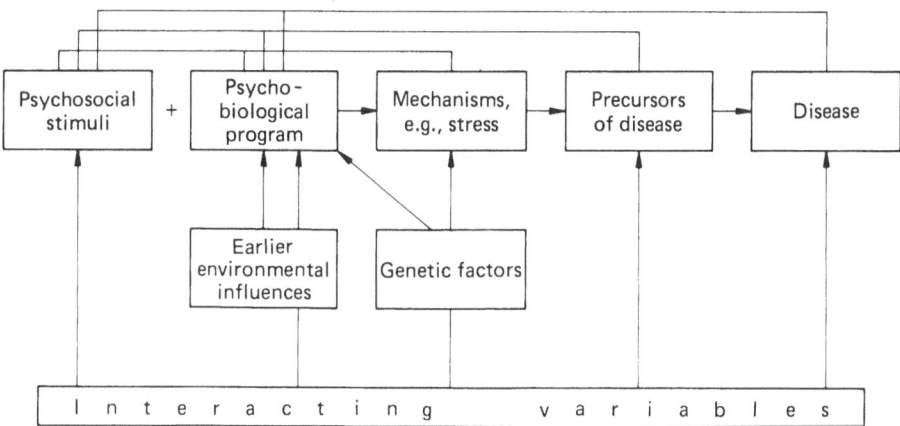

Fig. 31. The stress model by Levi

This concept shows how psychosocial stimuli (i.e., stressors), originating somewhere in the social organization, lead to the production of stress. It indicates how stressors, together with a specific psychobiologic program, trigger certain physiological mechanism (e.g., stress), thus leading to precursors of disease (e.g., vasoconstriction), and eventually to disease (e.g., hypertension). The model does not explain, however, the creation of stress or the loss of homeostasis in an entire community (i.e., on the level of the social organization). I therefore propose a different stress model which helps to explain the complicated process of the genesis of stressors in a social organization (Fig. 32).

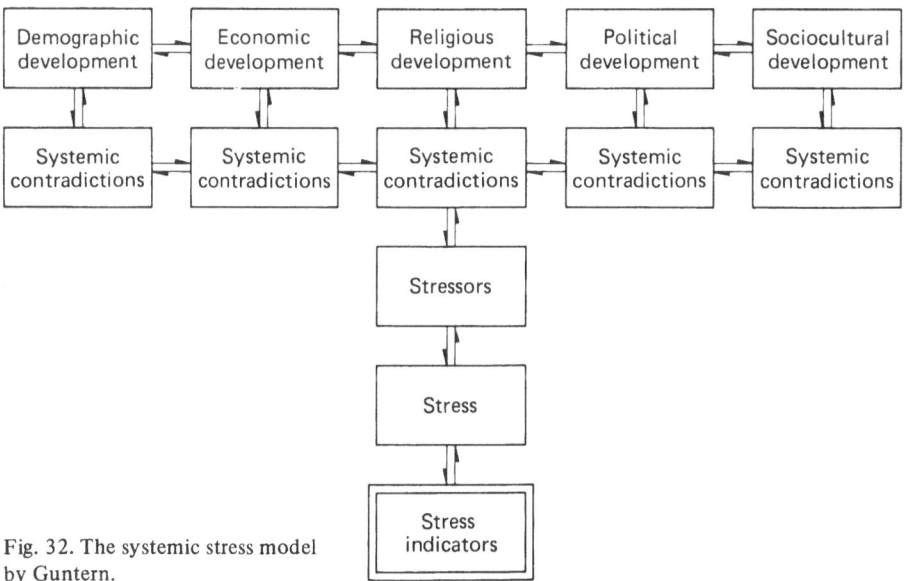

Fig. 32. The systemic stress model by Guntern.

Several basic observations and inferred assumptions led to the formulation of this model:

- The diachronic process of development of the different social subsystems within a village leads to intrasystemic and/or intersystemic contradictions and tensions, thus, pushing the subsystems and/or the system as a whole more and more out of balance and leading to the loss of intrasystemic homeostasis.
- The system as a whole and, also, the different subsystems may or may not be able, according to the principle of Le Chatelier, to counterbalance this loss of homeostasis via adaptive coping processes.
- If the socioeconomic or sociocultural stimuli are too strong (i.e., qualitatively, quantitatively, or in duration) for the elasticity or the capacity of the intrasystemic coping mechanisms, they become psychosocial stimuli (i.e., stressors).
- These stressors, indicating a loss of homeostasis on the level of the social organization, lead to stress and, potentially, to stress indicators on the level of the sociobiologic organization (e.g., alcoholism, psychosomatic symptoms) only if they transcend the psychobiologic system's capacity of coping.
- These different propagation processes are not unidirectional, but are embedded in two-way processes which are situated in a network of relations controlled by multiple feedback mechanisms. The overall pattern ultimately determines the type of stress indicators we observe; the organizational level where they are to be found; and, if they are to be found on the level of psychobiologic organizations, which are the reactions of risk, the groups at risk, and the situations of risk for a given human system. The human system, by the way, will determine the preventive and therapeutic strategies of a health care program.

The next chapter will briefly summarize the different intrasystemic contradictions discussed in the previous chapters.

7.1.1 Demographic Development

The social change after 1951 destroyed the former homogeneity of the demographic subsystem. In 1970, there were three major demographic classes — the native population, the employees, and the guests. All of them displayed different kinds of official status and prestige. Even within the group of employees, there were distinct differences. Swiss employees had a higher status than foreign employees. German, Austrian, and English employees had a higher status than the employees from the south of Europe. All these differences created tensions and intrasystemic contradictions in the demographic subsystem affecting the villagers.

7.1.2 Economic Development

By 1970, the homeostasis of the former agricultural economic basis was destroyed. The village depended upon the flow of international tourism. Individuals, families, and the community were financially in debt and, at the same time, the tourist industry was extremely dependent upon the international economic and political situation. This fact created anticipatory stress, as has been analyzed by Lazarus (207).

There were asymmetric patterns in the structure of the economic subsystem; there was a season-specific, class-specific, and sex-specific asymmetry in the distribution of work and economic roles. This asymmetry constituted a stressor. There were also the conflicts and contradictions between the former family and kinship centered economy and the modern and more interest centered economy that were run mostly by nuclear families.

The extent to which the season-specific asymmetry of work can lead to stress is best illustrated by the concept of Levi (213, 215), which correlates the genesis of stress with the degree of exterior stimulation (Fig. 33).

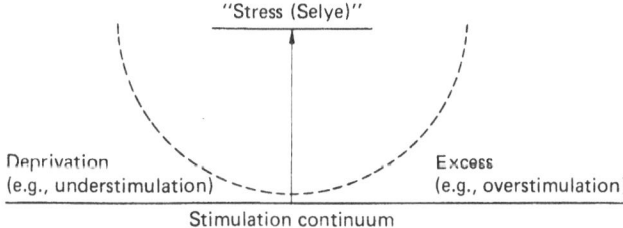

Fig. 33. Stimulation and genesis of stress according to Levi

Although the rhythm of work during the main season, especially Christmas and Eastertime, led to overstimulation and, thus, to stress, the psychosocial understimulation of the interseason and, partly, of the afterseason also led to stress.

7.1.3 Religious Development

In 1970, there were conflicts between the formerly homogenous and traditional Catholicism and the modern libertinism introduced by the tourists from different religious backgrounds. There were also the conflicts and contradictions between the old "eternal" truth of the pre-*Vaticanum II* and the new "eternal" truth of the post-*Vaticanum II*. All these contradictions constituted a major source of stressors.

7.1.4 Political Development

There were only minor tensions and contradictions within the political subsystem which sometimes created stress. There were, however, contradictions between local and extra-local politics (e.g., the case of the cablecar whose construction was prohibited by a federal decision) which functioned as stressors.

7.1.5 Sociocultural Development

There were conflicts between the old and the new values and the old and new type of socialization, due to the general acculturation. Also, acculturation was influenced by the fact that, in almost two-thirds of the native families, the mother had originally come from an industrialized and/or urbanized area while the father was a villager.

In short, there were the conflicts between the beliefs, attitudes, role expectations, and behaviors of the tradition directed society, held by the older people; the inner directed society, held mostly by the middle age groups; and the other directed society, partly held by the young generation. All these contradictions were important sources of stressors. Moreover, there was a battery of stressors due to intersystemic contradictions between the different subsystems or between the village and the outside world. Since they were numerous and have been discussed in the previous chapters, they will not be enumerated here in detail.

7.1.6 Speed of Social Change

In 1970, the village was in a cultural lag which was brought about basically by the different speeds of development of the different subsystems in the village. The economic subsystem had changed very fast while most of the other subsystems were in a developmental lag. This situation is illustrated by Fig. 34. The effect of the cultural lag was partly decreased and partly increased by acculturation, a fact illustrated by the next figure.

Figure 35 illustrates the multiple interconnections between the different subsystems which are influenced by the process of acculturation. Whenever a stimulus transcended

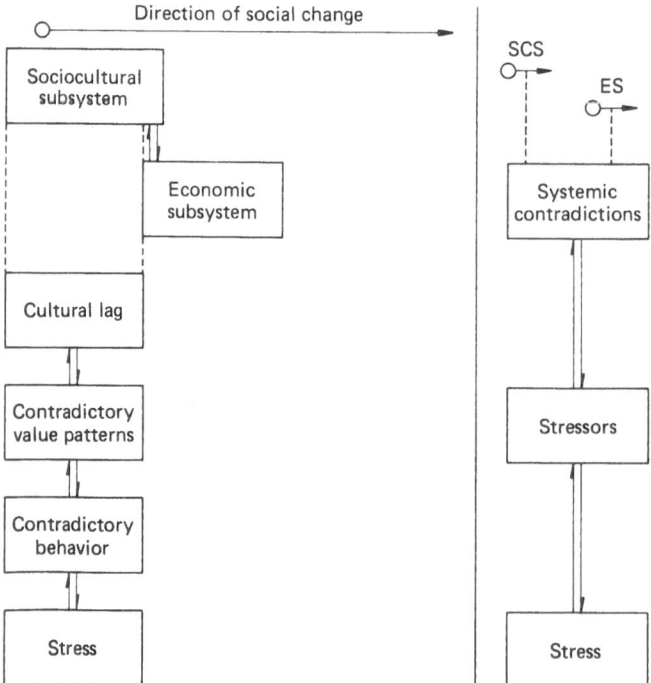

Fig. 34. The stress producing effect of the cultural lag

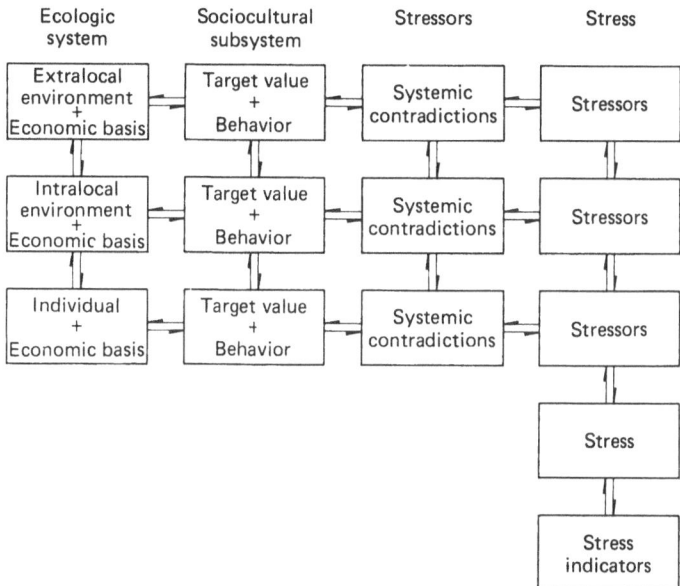

Fig. 35. The stress producing effect of acculturation

the capacity of the system's coping mechanisms, there occurred a significant input into the stressor pool of the village.

7.2 Stress

According to Selye's (cf. 214, p. 31) well-known definition, stress is "the unspecific re-action of an organism to any demand made upon it." Stress can only be observed indi-rectly by measuring stress indicators of a physiological-biochemical or a behavioral nature.

For a more complete discussion of stressors, stress, and stress indicators, the reader is referred to the next chapter.

7.3 Stress Indicators

Stressors lead to stress. Stress can be measured by the presence of stress indicators. The village showed a series of stress indicators (e.g., psychosomatic symptoms and syndrom-es, consumption of alcohol, drugs and tobacco, criminality, neurotic and psychotic dis-orders).

These stress indicators pertain only to the level of biopsychological organisms. There would also be a set of stress indicators on the level of social organization (e.g., dysfunc-tional processes in different subsystems) which I neglect here, although I am aware that

174

they exist. Their description (see previous chapter) in this context would require a more general stress concept with a set of more general definitions and we would have to define stress as an actual or threatening loss of homeostasis and not as "the unspecific reaction of an organism to any demand made upon it," as Selye (323) does.

Figure 36 simplifies a complex reality. There is, indeed, a steady state between the different indicators of stress. An individual who is an indicator of a disturbed systemic

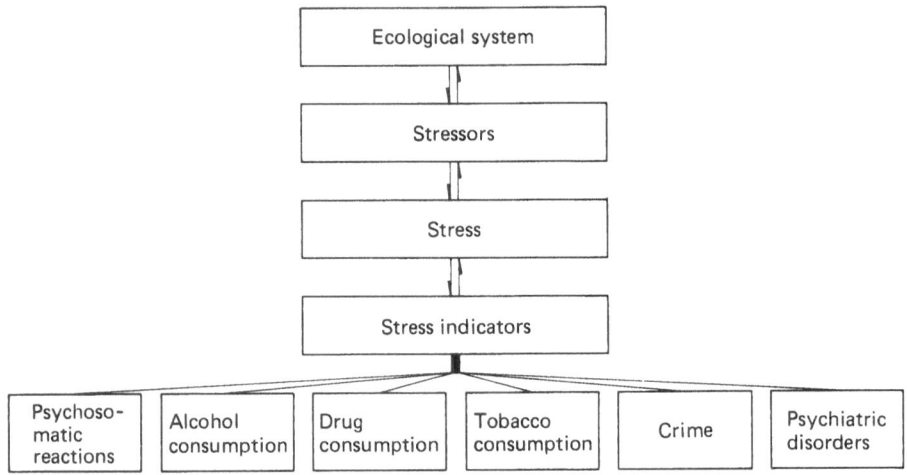

Fig. 36. Stress indicators in Saas-Fee

(e.g., family, village) homeostasis often indicates stress by different means and ways. The same individual can communicate stress by drinking excessively, developing psychosomatic symptoms, or becoming depression. The same individual can express stress differently at different times and in different contexts. There are also generation-specific and sex-specific ways of expressing stress which I observed in the village (e.g., alcoholism in men, tranquillizer consumption in women, certain psychosomatic symptoms in adolescents).

Figure 37 illustrates this steady state of stress indicators.

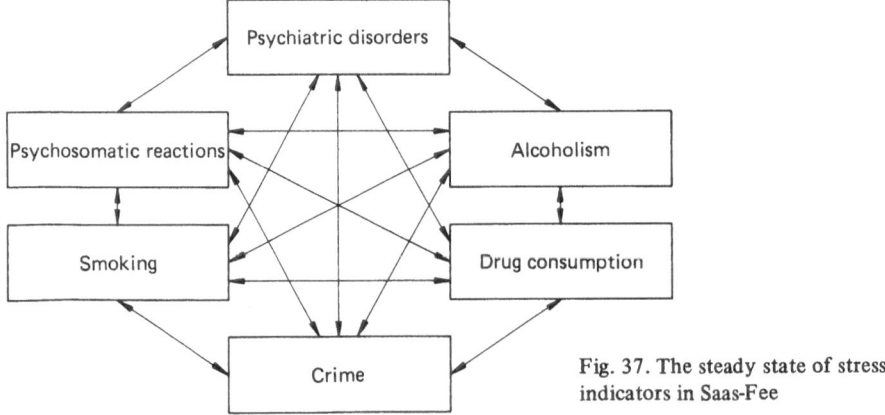

Fig. 37. The steady state of stress indicators in Saas-Fee

8. Social Change and Stress Indicators

It will be the goal of the followup study Saas-Fee to investigate whether or not there is an interaction between social change and stress and how this possible interaction functions in the different phases of the village process. The first cross-sectional study, discussed in the following chapters, describes the state of mental health in 1970. The future cross-sectional studies (e.g., 1980, 1990) will hopefully show to what extent the health situation is modified by further social change. Predictably, the number of stress indicators decreases because the population will have had time for a general readjustment or a better recalibration.

Not all the possible stress indicators of the village are described in this study because the methodological approach allowed gathering only a certain set of data which, however, are typical of the general health situation of the population. As desirable as it might have been, it was not possible to clinically examine the whole population, or even a representative sample. Such an endeavor would have required a team of trained investigators and more financial support. Still, the present results can be regarded as representative for the health disorders of the population. They are sufficient for the purpose of the followup study since the same stress indicators will be investigated in the future cross-sectional studies.

It seems to be impossible to show a causal relationship between stress and social change. What can be demonstrated, however, is the correlation and the temporal coincidence between changing social structures and stress. A causal relationship could be shown only by means of controlled interventions in human systems. Such interventions are not possible because ethical responsibilities limit the technologically possible interventions.

Stress Indicators Observed in 1970: Physical and Mental Health Aspects of the Village Process

9. Psychosomatic Disorders

9.1 General Questions and Problems

Du Bois (81) recently claimed that in an average middle European general practice, approximately 60% of the patients suffer from psychogenic functional disorders and that, therefore, they come to a practitioner with complaints he is not trained to deal with. Similar statements can be found in international literature, usually made by psychodynamically oriented authors. Rarely, if ever, do the authors indicate how they arrived at such quantifications and claims. For this reason, their assumptions have to be regarded critically.

It becomes even more important to be cautious when we consider the low reliability of psychiatric diagnosis, as illustrated by Dohrenwend and Dohrenwend (79, p. 82). They compared 25 epidemiologic investigations concerning the frequency of nontreated psychic illness in different populations. The difference in rate of incidence oscillated between 0.8% and 64%, a tremendous discrepancy which is obviously more due to the difference in diagnostic reliability than to differences in the populations investigated.

Working as a general practitioner in the village, I had the impression that the number of functional psychosomatic disorders was rather high. For the above mentioned methodological reasons, I did not want to make any quantitative statements about the frequency of these disorders. There were, moreover, other reasons which prevented me from doing so:

- Since the old village doctor was chronically ill, but did not want to give up his practice, he was often replaced by up to five substitutes within 2 years. Therefore, many of the villagers preferred consulting practitioners outside the valley.
- The case register of the practice, therefore, was insufficient and could not be used for my purpose. The diagnoses were not reliable since the substituting doctors were of different levels of training.
- The frequency of consultations of the native population varied according to the season. It was low during the high season when the villagers did not have the time for medical consultations and increased during the interseason and afterseason, but, for the above mentioned reasons, many villagers did not consult the village doctor.
- Sporting accidents are frequent in a tourist resort. It was, however, difficult to evaluate to what extent these accidents were purely "accidental" or due to chronic stress, fatigue, or other psychosocial factors.
- In the general practice of a small village, the technological installations are limited and, therefore, the diagnostic reliability is restricted. It is very difficult, for instance, to differentiate somatic troubles of the musculosceletal system from purely functional disorders.

For these reasons, I decided not to use the case register of the general practice. Instead, I used the symptoms and syndromes encountered in my daily work as a guideline for the construction of a questionnaire to get a reliable picture of the complaints and symptoms of the whole population. In a second step, I expected to find one or more clusters of symptoms which would be typical for the state of health of the village population.

Basically, the villagers assumed that tourism and social change were responsible for the onset and frequency of most of their symptoms. They attributed their chronic fatigue, irritability, sleeping disorders, and a certain asthenic-hypersensitive disposition, especially apparent towards the end of the season, to the seasonal stress.

The flow of patients in my practice gradually increased and the overall picture became clearer. It seemed that the subjective attitude towards stress was more related to the number and intensity of problems and symptoms than to the objective amount of work. It also seemed that at the end of the season the number of female patients increased more than the number of male patients. Moreover, women complained more about psychovegetative, not clearly defined, troubles and disorders while men came with well-defined somatic complaints.

I was faced with some basic questions:

- Did the social change, seen by the villagers as the culprit, play a pathogenic and/or pathoplastic role for the onset and frequency of symptoms?
- Was there a correlation between the type and number of symptoms and syndromes observed in the practice and the type and number of symptoms indicated by the representative sample?
- Was there a correlation between the sex distribution of the symptoms and syndromes observed and the sex distribution indicated by the representative sample?
- Was there a correlation between the frequency of symptoms and syndromes and the amount of workhours or, instead, was there a correlation between the frequency of symptoms and syndromes and the subjective attitude towards tourism and the new mode of life?

Before discussing these questions we need a brief overview of the international literature dealing with the major theories and concepts of stress and psychosomatic disorders.

9.2 Stress and Psychosomatic Disorders: Brief Overview of the International Literature

9.2.1 Notion of Stress

9.2.1.1 Historical Aspects

Stress is a term which was introduced in the scientific discussion by Selye (323). Selye, a physiologist, basing his theory upon his own experimental work, observed that different stressor agents (e.g., effort, trauma, infection, rays, operative interventions) produce stress in the organism (i.e., they create a certain state of reaction). He labeled the sum of all the nonspecific reactions upon a stimulus as the general adaptation syndrome. He also described, for the first time, a so-called stress axis which interconnects the pituitary gland and the adrenal glands which, under stress, produce the ACTH and adrenal hormones which constitute the physiological substratum of the stress response.

As Lazarus (207) rightly critizises, Selye (323) used the term stress to describe different aspects of the stress process. Thus, since the very introduction of the term, it has lent itself to a confusion which does not facilitate communication between the members of different disciplines interested in the phenomenon of stress.

This terminological confusion has been enhanced by the fact that the term "stress" quickly entered the everyday language and was used for labeling all kinds of different phenomena. "Stress" was often confused with "stressor," thus, "stress" became a label with a negative connotation. To equate stress with a negative phenomenon was not the intention of Selye (323). Levi (213) makes clear that stress has the positive result of preparing an organism for achievement. He (213, p. 12) mentions the work by Frankenhaeuser et al. who proved that individuals with a high adrenaline excretion (i.e., a physiological stress indicator) show greater achievements in certain types of problem resolution (e.g., conflict of perception, decision behavior, understimulation) than individuals with a low adrenaline excretion. Stress prepares the organism for flight or fight, the two basic strategies to cope with a potentially dangerous situation.

9.2.1.2 Definitions

There are a number of definitions and circumscriptions of stress by several authors especially used in the context of psychosomatic problems.

Satin (313) describes as "life stress" a change in the emitional, physical, or social milieu of an individual who has an insufficient coping capacity. Dohrenwend (79) reports as stress producing the objective events in the life of an individual which interrupt or threaten to interrupt his habitual activities. Dohrenwend (78, p. 168) mentions the view of Froeberg et al. who describes change in itself as stress producing and the view of Brown and Birley (42) who think that events are stress producing which, according to the general opinion, produce emotional disorders in people.

These definitions and circumscriptions imply the reaction of the concerned individual as a criterion of stress. In this context, Dohrenwend (78, p. 168) asks whether or not desirability or undesirability of an event determines its stressing character. Studying the physiological results of measurable indicators, he emphasizes that the individual responds to the event itself rather than to its emotional impact.

Holmes and Rahe (154) measure stress indirectly by measuring the work of adaptation an individual has to do when facing a change. In this case, stress is a process which demands adaptational efforts, measurable in the so-called life-change units (LCU). Coddington (60), investigating children, holds a similar position.

Groen (121) offers a more detailed definition. He labels as stress a change in the inner and/or outer situation of an organism, whereby the change is of such a duration and/or intensity that the organism has to adapt in an extraordinary way in order to maintain its homeostasis for its life. Depending upon the different stimuli, Groen (121) differentiates between a physical, chemical, emotional, microbiologic and interhuman (i.e., conflicts or deprivation) stress. A social stress arises when the life condition of an individual or a group is frustrated or threatened to be frustrated by social circumstances or a culturally determined prescription.

All these definitions are heterogenous and they have a limited operational range. Moreover, the differentiation between stressors and stress is rarely made.

In 1971, Selye (cf. 214, p. 31) clarified the issue by defining stress as "the nonspecific answer of the organism to any demand made upon it." In accordance with this, Lazarus (207) proposed to use "stress" onyl as a general term describing the different answers and reactions of the organism to a tissue damaging stimulus (i.e., physiological stress), or an exterior threat (i.e., psychological stress).

9.2.1.3 Stressors

For Selye (323), a stressor is a noxious stimulus. Lazarus (207) differentiates between psychological stressors (i.e., threat) and physiological stressors (i.e., stimuli which damage body tissue).

As Levi (214) emphasizes, the connection between physical stressors and stress has never been seriously questioned, but the correlation between psychosocial stressors and health disorders has been questioned for a long time. Interesting research in ethology, however, proved that there is a correlation between psychosocial stimuli or stressors and stress and illness.

According to Cronholm (65), the scientific work of Lorenz, Tinbergen, and Von Frisch instigated a series of interesting studies, a few of which are noteworthy in the context of my research. Von Holst (cf. 65, p. 26) studied the behavior and physiological reaction of the species Tupaja. He showed that threatening and aggressive behavior, which is blocked by a transparent net, triggers stress in the threatened animal in the next cage, who was defeated in earlier fights. This stress leads to renal insufficiency and to coma with uremic exitus. Lapin and Cherkovich (cf. 65, p. 27) isolated the male with the highest rank within a pavian group and let it observe how lower ranking animals were fed or how lower ranking males copulated with females. The isolated male showed signs of rage and anxiety and after 4-5 months, it suffered from "neurotic symptoms" and somatic symptoms (e.g., arterial hypertension, coronary insufficiency, myocardial infarctus). These experiments clearly demonstrate that in animal's psychosocial stimuli lead to stress and illness.

The question is whether or not such experiments can be interpreted in an analogous manner for human beings. Hamburg (cf. 65, p. 29) showed experimentally in apes and human beins that crowding of individuals in a confined space or increasing contact with unknown individuals provokes aggression both in animals and human beings. Thus, there seems to be a certain interspecies analogy in the physiological reaction to psychosocial stimuli.

Today, there are a great number of studies which prove the impact of psychosocial stressors upon man. Such an impact has been described by Groen (121) and Satin (313) and Cooper and Sylph (62), especially for the incidence of neurotic disorders, and for the incidence of psychotic disorders by Brown et al. (43). Rahe and Lind (288), Rahe et al. (289) and Rahe (352, 355), Theorell described the impact of psychosocial stimuli upon the onset of psychosomatic disorders. They proved that life changes (e.g., marriage, birth, death, changing of jobs) function as psychosocial stimuli or stressors leading to psychosomatic illness in certain subjects. Lucisano (230) reports that they also proved that increasing change, measured in LCUs (i.e., life change units indicating the amount of adaptation to be made) correlates positively with the duration and intensity of psychosomatic disorders. Persons who indicated a yearly life change of 300 or more LCUs suffered from neurotic, depressive, or psychosomatic disorders in 80% of the cases. Of the persons indicating a life change of 150-300 LCU, 53% became ill while, of the persons indicating less than 150 LCUs, only 33% became ill.

As I mentioned elsewhere (cf. 126), the concept of psychosocial stressors is becoming more widely accepted. The quantification of stress, made possible indirectly by the rating scale of Holmes and Rahe (154), has certainly contributed to this concept. These authors selected, on the basis of case reports, a list of 43 life events which function as psychosocial stressors. The event of "marriage" was attributed arbitrarily an amount of 500 LCU. 394 interviewed persons subjectively estimated the number of LCUs for the other 42 life events. This rating scale was successfully used in different investigations and in different cultures.

The effect of psychosocial stressors has been studied under experimental conditions and physiological parameters have been measured. Levi (214) gives an overview of the most important results — psychosocial stressors lead, independently of the duration of their impact, to increased elimination of adrenaline and noradrenaline; to an increase of free fatty acids, triglycerides, and colesterol in the plasma; and to an increase in fibrinolysis and PBI (protein-bound-iodine).

Levi (213) indicates different types of psychosocial stressors. There are, for example, specific and unspecific stressors. Specific stressors are stimuli with a symbolic character for certain individuals and based upon personal experience with these stimuli. Such specific stressors trigger stress only in predisposed individuals who decode the stimulus as being a stressor. Unspecific stressors, however, produce stress in all individuals, although the duration and intensity of the stress process shows certain differences.

Another question (214) is whether or not the psychosocial stressors lead to specific or unspecific illnesses. It seems, generally, that the unspecific reactions prevail. There are, however, positive correlations between psychosocial stressors and specific illnesses (e.g., thyreotoxicosis, peptic ulcer, essential hypertension).

Finally, there is one basic problem — how can we differentiate psychosocial from physical stressors. Mason (cf. 214, p. 14) points out that it is often very difficult to differentiate purely physical stressors (i.e., cold, heat, effort, and trauma) from the psychological importance these events have for a given person. Physical stressors can always function as psychosocial stressors because the individual rarely lives in complete psychosocial isolation.

9.2.1.4 Function of Stress

Every change in the physical, psychological, or social environment provokes a stereotypical and phylogenetically old response. Stress is that response. The function of this stress response is to prepare the organism for flight or fight (213, 214). Levi emphasizes that today this paleolithic response is often inadequate for a given stimulus and, thus, no longer fulfills its original survival maintaining function.

9.2.1.5 Stress and Its Psychological-Physiological Parameters

According to Lazarus (207), stress can only be measured indirectly by the stress response. The indicators of stress are:

- *Disturbed affects and emotions* (e.g., anger, anxiety, culpability, aggression, depression). For a more detailed discussion of these parameters, the reader is referred to the excellent book by Levi (216).
- *Motor behavior* (e.g., tremor, increased muscular tension, speech difficulties).
- *Physiological modifications* in the functions of the neuroendocrine nervous system (e.g., heart-rate, respiration, function of the sweat glands, function of the adrenal gland).

Pflanz (274) indicated that stress can be indirectly measured by the presence of dysfunctional adaptation phenomena or pathological behavior. This statement is suported by my findings (125, 126) that alcoholism and other behavioral disorders correlate with stress and are indirect stress indicators.

There are also biochemical stress indicators which allow an indirect measurement of stress. Selye (323) has already described the way animals under stress eliminate an increased amount of adrenaline and cortisone in the plasma and urine. The existence of a so-called stress axis was observed by Selye (323). Volkow and Rubinstein (cf. 65, p. 27), experimentally proved the existence of such an axis by stimulating for several hours per day over a number of days the so-called defense area in the hypothalamus of rats — the animals developed a fixed hypertension.

According to Levi (213, 214), who systematically discusses the confirmed results of stress research, the stress process in human beings is characterized by:

- An increased activity of the hypothalamo-sympathico-adrenomedullary system,
- An increased activity of the hypophyso-adrenocortical system, and
- A possible increased activity of the thyroidal system.

Whenever stress occurs, the following parameters can be measured: increased production of adrenaline and noradrenaline, increase of cortisone, free fatty acids, triglycerides, cholesterol, and fibrinolysis and PBI in the plasma.

In a longitudinal study, Rahe (cf. 214, p. 40) proved the existence of a positive correlation between the increased number of LCUs and the increased elimination of adrenaline in the urine.

Eventually, stress can also be measured by the presence of changed organic functions. It is generally assumed that stressors induce modifications of physiological functions which, after a certain intensity and duration, may lead to further modifications of the physiological functions. For instance, increased production of noradrenaline may lead to increased blood pressure which, in turn, can become chronic, producing lesions of the myocardium and other body tissues. This last step, however, is still disputed and the definitive formulation of the causal chain leading from the psychosocial stressor to illness has yet to be made.

9.2.1.6 Different Phases of the Stress Process: Concepts and Explanatory Models

Nitsch (265) enumerates a few of the descriptive and explanatory models which try to describe the whole stress mechanism or process. Selye (cf. 265, p. 72) differentiates three phases of the stress process:

- *Alarm:* The organism responds to the stressors by mobilizing the forces of defense. There is an initial shock phase (i.e., vagal phase) in which the resistence of the organismic system is diminished. In the countershock phase (i.e., sympathicotrop-ergotrop phase), the mechanisms of defense for adaptation are activated.

- *Resistence:* A maximal adaptation is reached. Depending upon the quantitative aspects of the shock, an adaptation to a lower level may occur in the area of cognition-perception, as well as in the area of behavior.
- *Exhaustion:* Continuing stress leads to the total consumption of the energy of adaptation and, finally, to exhaustion.

Other authors have developed models of the stress process which represent further variations and refinements of this basic model. Because these variations are of interest for the present study, they will be mentioned briefly.

Mierke (cf. 265, p. 72) described a syndrome of overcharge or overdemand *(Überforderungssyndrom)* which shows three distinct phases:

Aggression: Extreme demands are responded to by a mobilization of the last energy reserves. Primitive behaviors (e.g., disorders of the motor system, attacks) may occur.
Regression: A regression to lower levels of functioning occurs and the psychophysiological balance is restored.
Restitution: Achievement and performance increase on the basis of a recalibration which prescribes new and more adequate goals to pursue.

Using a cybernetic approach, Selbach and Selbach (cf. 265, p. 72 ff) describe the dynamics of organic and psychic crises. These authors characterize the biologic system as a polar-differentiated oscillating system with a variable resonance. The suppression and activation of the performance of this system occurs in the diencephalon, specifically in the modulla oblongata. If a crisis occurs, it proceeds in three stages:

- *Precritical phase of preparation:* Loss of homeostasis leads to a displacement of the vegetative potential in one of the two directions of the polar-differentiated system. If the capacity of recovery is diminished and there is an overdemand in performance, an adrenergic deviation occurs. If there is an overdemand of the restitutional capacity and a suppression of potential activation, a cholinergic deviation of the system occurs.
- *Critical phase:* If a deviation becomes maximal, the system becomes completely unbalanced and the deviation provokes a counterregulation which leads to the relaxation of the system. Depending upon the basic situation, the unbalancing leads to an overcompensatory regulation (i.e., regression or breakdown with archaic vagotroph metabolism) or to an overcompensatory increase of activation (i.e., eruption, aggression) with a sympathotroph metabolism. Primitive and collective reactions are symptomatic of the whole process.
- *Postcritical phase:* Once relaxation has occurred, there is an attenuated oscillation into the premordial or new stable target value situation.

Nitsch (265) comes to a similar formulation. He describes individual and environment as a dyadic communication system in which matter-energy and information are exchanged. Whenever the communication equilibrium is unbalanced, the system is under strain. The degree of the strain depends upon the stimulus input and the coping capacity. The coping capacity depends upon the preceding strain and upon the capacity of the system. A system undergoes critical strain when the following conditions occur:

- The regulation of a disturbance is substantially impeded (e.g., in the case of anticipatory adaptation) or the strain to be expected is unknown or extreme (e.g., reactive adaptation to overstimulation or understimulation).
- A disturbance cannot be compensated by changing the target values (e.g., in the case of extreme exterior constraint, such as social obligations, or extreme inner constraint, such as motivation).

Levi (214, p. 32) proposed a clear and highly interesting model of the stress process (cf. p. 171) which depends upon the degree of stimulation. The more the degree of stimulation leads away from homeostasis, the more stress increases. Understimulation (e.g., sensory or social deprivation) and overstimulation (e.g., exposure to noise) lead to stress which increases exponentially with a linear change of stimulation.

9.2.2 Psychosomatic-Psychoautonomic Reactions

9.2.2.1 The Mind-Body Dichotomy

The concept of the mind-body dichotomy, originating over 2000 years ago with the teaching of Parmenides from Elea and continuing through Aristotle and the scholastics up to Descartes, has created the theoretical dead lock of the so-called psychosomatic problem. As I emphasized elsewhere (cf. 132), because Decartes differentiated between mind *(res cogitans)* and body *(res extensa)* and attributed a different nature and different qualities to each, we are forced to explain how mind and body influence each other. This whole problem increasingly appears to be a problem of a distorted epistemology. Nevertheless, because the concept is so deeply rooted in our thinking that it appears to be nature itself, we have to deal with it.

For Mason (cf. 213, p. 23), the central question is — which functional mechanisms are involved in the psychosomatic illness and how and why are these mechanisms dysfunctional?

Other authors who, like Popper and Eccles (284), take a more philosophic stance, ask how does the conflict move from the soma to the psyche, or vice versa? Further, how are conflicts desymbolized and expressed in a somatic language? Although certain psychoanalysts claim to solve this puzzle, Schneider (318) made clear that this question cannot be answered from a psychoanalytic standpoint which assumes a strict parallelism between soma and psyche. One can only describe with physiological or psychological approaches and methods what goes on on one side of a parallel system. At the same time, Schneider (318) is sceptical about the value of the psychoanalytic approach in the field of psychosomatics and touches on examples of psychoanalytic treatment (i.e., didactic analysis) where the result of the treatment did not include a removal of psychosomatic disturbances. We can assert that, if the pragmatics deduced from a conceptual model are a failure, the value of the concept itself is highly questionable. For a further discussion of this theoretical problem, see Guntern (130).

Strotzka's (345, p. 101) term "psychosomatic" aims at the rejection of a completely organicistic view. Plack (283, p. 199 ff) views the term as obsolete. The term, as he explains, derives from the old mind-body dichotomy which holistic medicine, because it treats organisms and not "minds" or "bodies," has overcome. This is, indeed, the case, though holistic medicine has not yet had enough impact to make the term "psychosomatic" definitively obsolete. In this situation, the term "excitation," because it has a somatic and a psychic aspect, could lead to a holistic organismic concept. This view is held by Grace and Graham (118). As long ago as 1952, they proposed to define emotions in such a way that the definition of the term contained a psychological attitude and a corresponding physiological reaction at the same time. The emotion "anxiety," for instance, would be composed of a feeling of threat or danger and of a physiological reaction of alarm and defense. This view seems to have become generally accepted, as Groen (122, p. 728 ff) and Levi (217, p. 705) report. Nevertheless, it needs further specification and a clearer definition in order to avoid widespread confusion, a problem clearly seen by Brady (38, p. 17 ff).

Despite these new developments, the old thinking still prevails. Many authors are still trying to show how the psychic part of the organism influences the somatic part, and vice versa. In this respect, Luborsky et al. (229), in a systematic analysis of 53 studies concerning the onset of psychosomatic symptoms, found that the premorbid stage was characterized by major psychological symptoms. In particular, they found an increase of frustrations directly before the onset of the psychosomatic symptom and problems of separation which preceded these frustrations.

Within a cybernetic model it is less difficult, as Levi (213) pointed out, to show that excitation flows from the psyche to the soma, although the "how" is not explicable as yet. In 1929, Cannon (cf. 213, p. 15) had already proved experimentally that psychosocial stimuli excite the sympathico-adreno-medullary system. It is also known that psychosocial stimuli increase the production of adrenocortical hormones which influence the metabolism of ions and carbohydrates, thus modifying the contractivity of certain organs and the reaction disposition of certain tissues. Furthermore, although it is known that a viral infection may be accompanied by a reactive depression, the causal links between the two are still unknown.

In my opinion the unresolved problem of the information processing between psyche and soma will be overcome only when the dichotomy concept has been replaced by an organismic concept.

9.2.2.2 Definitions

According to Eastwood and Trevelyan (87), the term "psychosomatic" was originally used by the WHO committee to describe states which were caused by stress. Later, in the framework of the ecological view, the therm was used to describe a general psychophysiological reaction mechanism and, finally, the term has been used for describing physical symptoms without any organic alteration. Groen (122, p. 738) points out that today more and more syndromes are viewed as being psychosomatic. This tendency may increase as more and more researchers adopt the assumption of Wolf (372, p. 619 ff) that psychosomatic mechanisms can be postulated for almost any disease process.

Braeutigam (39) tried to define and separate different psychosomatic reactions and states, differentiating between:

— Illness with organic lesion (e.g., asthma, colitis ulcerosa).
— Physical complaints without organic lesion which are not hysterical symptoms (i.e., not a sexual repression with *libido cathexis* in the functional area).
Such symptoms have a certain signalizing value (e.g., pressure on the chest stands for depressive mood, tachycardia expresses anxiety).
— "Organic neuroses," the functional disturbance of organic systems due to a conflict induced *libido cathexis* (e.g., diarrhea, constipation, cardiospasm).

This differentiation is of limited value. It is made within a narrow and outdated psychoanalytic framework and is not compatible with research based upon more exact contemporary models of thinking.

9.2.2.3 Stress and Psychosomatic Disorders

Levi (214) proposed an interesting theoretical model (cf. p. 169) showing that the combined effect of psychosocial stimuli and the psychobiological program, due to genetic factors and earlier environmental influences, determines the psychological and physiological reactions of an individual. If the intensity and/or duration becomes extreme, then an entire organic system undergoes strain which leads to increasing morbidity and even death.

The model does not propose a one-way process, but rather a cybernetically regulated system, influenced by many variables.

According to Satin (313), there is only one theoretical concept that clearly demonstrates the interconnection of stress and illness. This is the theory of crisis of Lindeman and Caplan, based upon the following assumptions: the individual tries to maintain homeostasis; the homeostasis is determined by demands of the environment and by the coping and adaptation capacity of the individual; and a crisis leads to disturbance, reduced functional capacity, defense, and adaptations of variable efficiency. Efficient adaptation leads to growth and maturation. Inefficient adaptation leads to pathological symptoms (e.g., psychosomatic illness, psychiatric disorders). Groen (121), who holds a similar position, defines illness as behavior of an organism which is coping with stress.

9.2.2.4 Influencing Variables

(1) Genetic Factors. As Hinkle et al. (152) point out, the work of Kallman and other geneticists suggests an influence of genetic factors upon psychosomatic disorders. Hinkle et al. (152) found a family bound increase of certain syndromes (e.g., migraine and allergic rhinitis). It is questionable, however, whether or not these syndromes are due to a transfer of genetic information or a so-called symptom tradition. As suggested by Pflanz (274), they might be due to a certain transactional family style in which a symptom, as demonstrated by Minuchin et al. (255), has a homeostasis maintaining function.

(2) Personality Structure. In all the different stress concepts, it is assumed implicitly or explicitly that the structure of the personality influences the onset, intensity, and duration of the psychosomatic reactions.

Hardyck and Moos (142, p. 171) indicate that, at the beginning of the psychoanalytic era, Dunbar claimed that patients with certain psychosomatic disorders (e.g., ulcus duodeni or migraine) would have specific personality profiles. Later, Alexander (cf. 142) claimed that specific emotional conflict patterns lead to specific psychosomatic reactions. As Grace and Graham (118) mention, there is a still older theory which claims an organ specifity (i.e., the hypothesis that any conflict would lead to a symptom in the "inferior" organ). A statistical study, made by Buck and Hobbs (47), proved this latter hypothesis to be wrong.

As Schneider (318, p. 38 ff) points out, the French authors David, Fain, Marty, and De M'uzan claim to have found a personality structure which is supposed to be specific for psychosomatic patients. However, as Cremerius (64, p. 20 ff) showed, this "psychosomatic personality structure" is an artifact typical for the personality patterns found in the social class from which the French sample of patients was drawn. It would seem, therefore, that, despite the speculations and unsubstantiated claims of an assortment of authors, the psychoanalytic approach has been unsuccessful in its attempts to describe a specific personality structure for psychosomatic patients.

Antonelli and Ancona (12), for instance, claim that the approach of Melanie Klein is very promising. This approach assumes that the psychosomatic person is bothered by an "internalized pregenital mother" who produces psychosomatic symptoms. Here, a reified metaphor resolves the problem of explanation — a hobgoblin or intrapsychic homunculus plays the same *deus ex machina* which once rescued ancient Greek playwrights from the embarrassment into which their wild speculations had maneuvred them. A similarly uncritical position is held by Ammon (cf. 257, p. 33) who accuses, yet again, the early child-mother relationships which produce a "hole in the ego" which the psychosomatic symptom fills up, just as the dentist's filling stuffs the caries-ridden cavity of a tooth. Skinner's (329) criticism that psychoanalysis invented an homunculus in order to explain homo sapiens seems apt. The early mother-child relationship is also accused by Winnicott (cf. 257, p. 34) for producing a pseudoself which is supposed to be the basis for the psychosomatic symptom.

All these speculations have two things in common — they neglect the transactional network in which the child is embedded, a network carefully described by Bateson (17), Jackson (171, 172), Haley (140, 141), Minuchin (253-255), and Wynne et al. (374) and they are also based upon very poor observational data, as Grinker (120, p. 122 ff) made amply clear. By and large, such constructs tell us more about the logical leaps of an author than about the problems he claims to explain.

Aitken (8) criticized that this absence of exact methods, combined with fantastic speculations, is also found outside the psychoanalytic school.

Typical of the unreliable results are the cases where the diagnosis of neurotic disorders in psychosomatic diseases depends mainly upon the diagnostic criteria used. Therefore, Eastwood and Trevelman (87) assume that the coexistence of neurotic and psychosomatic disorders in the same person indicates a general type of psychophysiological instability.

The claim of a specific psychosomatic personality structures is also refuted by the measurement of personality profiles with the help of psychometric tests. Hardyck and Moos (142), using the MMPI-test, investigated individuals who had the same psychosomatic disorders; they distinctly showed different personality profiles.

Approaches which try to demonstrate correlations between certain personality features or attitudes and psychosomatic disorders are more successful. According to Nitsch (265), the way in which a person perceives a given situation as a stressor or nonstressor is important for the susceptibility to become ill. Groen (121) and Levi (214) share similar positions. Levi (214) emphasizes that hypochondriac persons show a tendency to interpret almost any situation as a stressor and, thus, to develop stress and stress indicators.

Hinkle et al. (152) compared groups with a high susceptibility (i.e., high risk group) with persons of low susceptibility (i.e., low risk group) and found significant differences. Patients with high susceptibility were generally altrustic, identified with extraneous goals, and did little to satisfy their own needs. They also showed a general attitude of interpreting an objective situation as challenging, overdemanding, and conflictuous. According to Ackerman (cf. 121), individuals susceptible to illness have a tendency to fail when put into a situation which demands the integration of antithetic roles.

The attitude concept is further substantiated by the observations of Grace and Graham (118). These authors suggest that patients suffering from vasomotoric rhinitis have a general attitude which tends to avoid problems rather than meet the challenge. Patients suffering from asthma are easily frustrated when their coping strategies are blocked. Constipated individuals tend to meet the challenge and hold out even when they are unable to resolve a problem; they tend to "hold without change." Similar findings are reported by Jacobs et al. (174). These authors found that patients with asthma displayed an angry, rebellious attitude whereas patients with hay fever showed a submissive attitude. And. finally, Coddington (59) reports correlations between temperament, behavior, and psychosomatic reactions.

Stanaway (341) experimentally proved that certain personality traits correlate with certain physiological reactions. He found highly significant correlations between "neuroticism" measured according to the personality inventory of Eysenck and the level of blood sugar and lactate.

Especially in the realm of coronary insufficiency, many studies deal with the problem of personality structure of patients. Eastwood and Trevelyan (86) found that persons with a psychoneurotic disorder had a significantly higher incidence of cardiovascular disorders. Hagnell (cf. 86, p. 289) found a significantly higher incidence of psychotic disorders in individual suffering from a cardiovascular disease.

Zohman (379) reports an increase of the neurotic trio (i.e., hypochondria, hysteria, and defensive attitude) in the MMPI of coronary patients. Other authors published similar findings, although their results are often contradictory as Christian and Hahn (56) show. While some psychoanalytic authors do not find neurotic disorders in coronary patients, others do, claiming that a trauma in the "anal" phase is responsible for a personality pattern composed of such traits as overadaptation, tenacity, high achievement motivation, and tendency to dominate.

Similar observations, although not linked to the same explanatory framework, have been made in several epidemiologic studies. Ostfeld, Lebowits, and Shekelle (cf. 379, p. 111) showed in a prospective study that individuals who were tense, mistrusting, and jealous showed a higher frequency of coronary disorders than others. Russek (cf. 379, p. 112) made a study of 12,000 professional individuals and found that general practitioners (i.e., doctors, dentists, and lawers) were especially at risk, having a high achievement motivation and being reactive to a basic passivity. Comparably, Christian and Hahn (56) found that infarction patients were overadapted individuals with a fixation on work and performance and a tendency to lead and dominate. Roseman and Friedman (cf. 56, p. 422), in an interdisciplinary prospective study, describe a behavioral type A which shows the following character traits: intense success motivation, a well-developed tendency to compete, a permanent wish for recognition and success, and a tendency to expect too much of themselves. This behavior type A was especially at risk with regard to myocardium infarctus.

It seems, as Weingarten (366) demonstrates, that good physical training protects against coronary infarctus. Such training, however, depends directly upon motivation which is rooted in a certain personality and also in a field expectation produced by social context. As Nitsch (265) points out, the motivation level is responsible for the readiness to undergo strain of a certain level.

(3) Sociocultural Factors. As I showed in my theory of transactional topology (cf. 129), individuals are embedded in a transactional field which determines their behavior at a given moment and in a given context. A personality is structured in a lifelong process of socialization which, in turn, depends upon the process af acculturation brought about by contact with different human ecosystems. The specific structure of the social organization of a human system determines attitudes and reactions.

According to Pflanz (274, p. 70), sociocultural factors determine whether or not a stimulus is interpreted as a stressor and formulated as a complaint which leads a patient to a doctor. These doctors are also responsible for the organic system in which a disturbance is projected and localized. They decide whether or not complaints are more localized in a specific organ or are more vaguely perceived as fatigue, nervousness, or general uneasiness. They determine how intensely the pain is experienced. These statements are supported by the observations of Cochrane (cf. 274, p. 71) who observed that, in prisoners of war, identical psychosocial stress made Frenchman complain of pain in the liver, Serbs of a belt-like feeling under the chest, Russians of pain in the back, and British of gastric troubles. Satin (313) observed that cultural factors also determine whether or not a patient goes to the doctor with a somatic disorder or a psychological complaint.

The modern industrial society is highly achievement motivated, as McClelland (243) convincingly analyzed. The prevailing achievement ideology determines major areas of our behavior, as Groen (121) states. Boys undergo a different socialization process than girls. In the Western society, boys learn to hide emotions. This makes them susceptible to stressors leading to psychosomatic disorders. The modern mass society is also, as Riesman (297) points out, a producer of lonely crowds in which individuals are isolated. As Groen (121) observes, this isolation leads to a lack of interpersonal security and support within the family and community, thus making the isolated individual even more vulnerable to stress.

Strotzka and Grumiller (347) emphasize the influence of social factors upon psychosomatic disorders and determine their type and frequency. Groen (121) indicates that we find a high frequency of colitis ulcerosa, migraine, impotence, and frigidity in Western culture, possibly due to the suppression of emotions. Eastern cultures have a higher incidence of hysteric disorders because, in these cultures, the acting out of emotional tensions is allowed. In Japan, where aggression is extremely suppressed and well-hidden under the mask of an ever smiling politeness, there is a high incidence of essential hypertension. In other words, the type of social organization determines the type of symptomatic behavior. This fact is corroborated by the sex-specific psychosomatic disorders found in several cultures. Wittcower and Lipowski (cf. 261, p. 240), for instance, attribute the high incidence of gastrointestinal disorders in men in Arab countries to the social organization which demands passive dependency and the higher incidence of disorders of the motor system in Arab women to the socially demanded suppression of aggression.

For this study, it is of special interest to have a look at the impact of acculturation and symptomatic behavior. Theorell and Rahe (352) quote transcultural studies which prove that immigrants take over not only the value patterns and behaviors of the new country, but also the higher frequency of coronary disorders. Wittkower and Dubreuil (371) assumes that social change leads to a higher incidence of psychosomatic disorders when the social change produces anomie (i.e., role confusion, role deprivation, and the coexistence of contradicting value patterns). I demonstrated (cf. 125) that social change increases alcoholism, especially in men.

Since the famous study of Hollingshead and Redlich (153) indicated that correlations exist between a social class and the incidence of psychiatric disorders, this interconnection has attracted the interest of several investigators. Braeutigam (39), Groen (121), Hinkle et al. (152), and Theorell and Rahe (352) published data which corroborate this interconnection. Hinkle et al. (152) showed that there is a correlation between a low level of education and coronary disorders when individuals of the same occupational group are compared. Groen (121) described class-specific stressors. In the upper social class, emotional deprivation, lack of support, and isolation with, at the same time, inhibition of motor and verbal acting out are the stressors leading to stress and neurotic and psychosomatic disorders. The lower social class suffers from stressors such as overcrowding and material deprivation, but, since emotional acting out is permitted, social deviance and aggressive behavior are the consequences. Pflanz (274, p. 265) indicates that hypertension; ulcus pepticum, and ventriculi, vegetative exhaustion, coronary disorders, and neurosis with somatic complaints have a high incidence rate in the lower social classes. In the upper classes, asthma, hay fever, and colitis ulcerosa are frequent.

That social change increases the incidence of psychosomatic disorders is a well-established fact, especially since Holmes and Rahe (154) introduced a rating scale for the quantification of change. Interestingly enough, this concept had already been stressed years ago by Meyer (cf. 264, p. 465), who postulated that each patient should have a so-called life chart in which life events could be registered. As Zwaga (382) reports, even small events (e.g., problem resolution in an experimental setting) can lead to stress. More dramatic events produce more dramatic consequences. Fritz and Marks (cf. 79, p. 167) observed, after a tornado had swept through Arkansas, that 90% of the population showed some kind of symptoms — 49% showed nervousness, irritability, and hypersensitivity; and 46% exhibited sleeping troubles.

There are also positive correlations between life events and psychosomatic symptoms, as Hinkle et al. (152) and Grace and Graham (118) report. Dohrenwend (78), after a review of the international literature, concludes that the concept of "life event" or "life change" subsumes two concepts — the concept of change and the concept of desirability of change. According to Dohrenwend (78), change in itself is more important than its subjective interpretation. This view has been experimentally confirmed by Levi (214) who measured physiological reactions using film demonstrations which induced stress.

The already mentioned LCU concept of Holmes and Rahe (154) instigated a great number of studies, especially since Coddington (59) and Ruch and Holmes (305) proved that the same rating scale can be used for children and adults. The validity of the rating scale was tested in a transcultural study done by Harmon et al. (144) concerning a comparative study in Japan and the United States using a study done in Italy by Lucisano (230). The latter author proposed a minor modification of the scale in Italy. There are now a great number of studies which prove the correlation between psychosomatic disorders and life change, such as the studies of Brown et al. (43), Cooper and Sylph (62), Holmes and Holmes (155), Nelson et al. (264), Rahe and Lind (287), Rahe et al. (288, 289), and Uhlenhuth and Paykel (60).

A positive correlation between a high number of LCUs and the frequency of onset, sometimes leading to death, has been particularly well demomstrated in the case of coronary disorders. Theorell and Rahe (352) found, in a study of 3000 individuals, a positive correlation between high LCUs and coronary infarctus. The same authors (353), investigating 30 outpatients treated after a myocardium infarctus, report that the number of LCUs increased two times in the 18 months preceding the infarctus. Syme et al. (cf. 352, p. 25) found the incidence of coronary disorders to be two to three times higher in individuals who had changed jobs, and four or more times higher for individuals who had changed their domicile two or more times. Rahe and Lind (287) took a sample of 39 patients who died of coronary infarctus and followed their life changes in their last few years, comparing the number of LCUs at different times. They found that all showed a significant increase in the number of LCUs in the 6 months preceding the coronary infarctus. In accordance with these findings, Rahe et al. (289) compared the life history of 279 patients surviving coronary infarctus with 226 patients who died following coronary infarctus. They found that the latter group had a significantly higher number of LCUs within the last 6 months preceding the infarctus.

(4) Age. It is generally assumed that younger individuals have a higher incidence of psychological symptoms, whereas older individuals indicate psychophysiological symptoms.

According to Uhlenhuth and Paykel (360), younger patients are more often anxious, whereas older patients are more often depressive. Leighton et al. (cf. 360, p. 747) report a higher frequency of psychophysiological disorders and a higher frequency of neurotic symptoms (e.g., anxiety) in younger patients. These findings support the concept of the life cycle analyzed by Erikson (92, p. 155 ff) who describes the adolescent as entering a critical phase of life where he risks identity diffusion and breakdown when exposed to a high number of stressors. Even children of 6 or 7 years old can be exposed to a high number of LCUs leading to psychological symptoms, as Coddington (60) reports. According to Pflanz (274, p. 227 ff), it is very difficult, methodologically, to differentiate age-specific biological, psychosocial, and sociological factors. Investigating patients of a medical policlinic, he found a higher incidence of the symptoms of constipation and insomnia in older patients, while all the other symptoms were more frequent in younger patients.

(5) Sex. It is difficult to differentiate between biologically linked and socioculturally linked sex-specific incidences of different psychosomatic symptoms and disorders.

I mentioned before that Musaph (261) reported studies which showed the sex linked difference in psychosomatic disorders in Arab countries. Schaefer and Blohmke (cf. 228, p. 321) claim that women adapt better to environment than men. Holmes and Holmes (155) assume that women, more frequently than men, react with pathological symptoms upon short term intrusions into the daily life routine. Roghman and Haggerty (300) emphasize that women, especially mothers, visit health care facilities less frequently than men when under stress. Fischer (101) points out that the different sex-specific labeling process is responsible for women ending up more frequently in health care facilities. This view is diametrically opposed to the view of Roghman and Haggerty (ibid.). Obviously, it is difficult to get a coherent picture of the sex linked frequency of psychosomatic disorders. In my opinion, the differences are probably due to the cultural differences of the observed samples.

Generally, it is assumed that women express emotions more easily than men. This view is held by Fischer (Esquisse d'une sociologie de la psychologie de la femme, unpublished manuscript), Groen (121), and Pflanz (274). Uhlenhuth and Paykel (360) reports that women express stress by means of depressive symptoms while men express stress by becoming obsessional and irritable.

Pflanz (274) indicates that the sex-specific differences decrease as women increasingly occupy the same economic and occupational roles as men. Although women tend to be absent from work more frequently than men, they are not more susceptible to illness, but often have jobs which allow for brief absences. According to Pflanz (274, p. 224), there are certain psychosomatic disorders with a clearly sex-specific difference in the rate of incidence: ulcus ventriculi and duodeni are more frequent in men and hypertension, hyperthyreosis, and functional cholecystopathia are more frequent in women.

(6) Occupational Roles. The type of occupational role and number of workhours are well-known stressors. The same holds true for the interpersonal conditions of occupational settings, the so-called working climate.

Erickson et al. (91) points out that status congruency (e.g., work time, wage, age, marital status) between individuals and peer groups are a significant indicator for the predictability of stress.

Zohman (379) studied 100 young coronary patients. He found that 25% had two occupational roles at the same time and 46% worked 60 or more hours per week. Russek (cf. 379, p. 112), in a study which included 12,000 professionals from 14 professional categories, found that long work hours combined with high intensity were important stressors for coronary patients.

Jones and Doll (cf. 121, p. 202), investigating a sample of ulcus duodeni patients, demonstrated a positive correlation between occupational roles and social function, on the one hand, and psychosomatic illness, on the other. Glatzel (cf. 274, p. 286) sees the following set of factors as responsible for the high frequency of ulcers in blue collar workers — their capacities for further development are blocked, the quality of their job performance is not valued, and they are not respected as individuals.

A similar correlation is described by Musaph (261) and Satin (313). Heady et al. (cf. 8, p. 286) found differences of incidence between workers of apparently the same occupation. English bus drivers, for example, have a higher incidence of myocardium infarctus than the ticket collectors of the bus. It is not clear, as Aitken (8) writes, whether or not this difference can be explained simply by the fact that the ticket collectors move more than the drivers.

According to Pflanz (274, p. 287 ff), employees of the bureaucracy are exposed to social change and, consequently, to stress. They, for example, have a higher frequency of coronary disorders and constipation. Pflanz (274, p. 287 ff) claims that this is an indicator of a certain occupational ideology because the same symptoms could also be found in the wives of these employees.

9.2.2.5 Frequency of Psychoautonomic and Psychosomatic Symptoms

(1) Headache. It is extremely difficult to specify the factors responsible for headaches. The cause of a headache, whether or not the complaint is indicated in a question-

naire or in an interview with a doctor, cannot be specified. There are many possible causes. To name only a few, a headache may be an expression of psychic conflict, of an endogeneous depression, hypertension, infection, or a degenerative or proliferative process. Furthermore, Pflanz (274, p. 70) emphasizes the format of the questionnaire which does not permit a clear diagnostic separation between organic and purely functional complaints.

Pflanz (274, p. 75) mentioned that women complained about headaches more frequently than men. Approximately 50% of the women, 30-39 years old, complained about frequent and severe headaches. The peak of the distribution curve was found in the 39-year-old age group.

Other authors, quoted by Pflanz (274, p. 76 ff), report the following frequencies of headaches. Essen-Moeller found 13% in the total population of southern Sweden. Koos, studying the rural population of the United States, found variations within the different social classes; 80% in the upper class, 56% in the middle class, and 22% in the lower class. Lilienfeld reported, for the total population of the United States, a frequency of 42.5% in nonsmokers and 46.1% in smokers. Grandjean, comparing male and female postal employees in Switzerland, found the symptom in 28% of the males and 33% of the females. DUC, investigating Swiss couples with marital conflicts, found headaches in 21% of the men and 44% of the women. Birkmayer showed that individuals under stress complained more often about headaches than individuals without stress and that 60% of the patients with vegetative exhaustion indicated the symptom.

These studies, reported by Pflanz (274), will be quoted subsequently without further description of the sample. The reader is referred to the above description.

(2) Vertigo. Pflanz (274, p. 80) reported the following investigations of the incidence of the symptom vertigo: (Lilienfeld) 40.1% nonsmokers and 47.1% smokers; (Essen-Moeller) 10%; and (Birkenmayer) 62% in patients with vegetative exhaustion. Pflanz (274, p. 79) found the symptom most frequently in miners, in recently married patients, and especially in social climbers (up to 62%). The peak of the distribution curve was between 50 and 59 years for both sexes.

(3) Palpitations of the Heart. According to Pflanz (274, p. 81 ff) there is little indication of the frequency of this symptom in the international literature. It oscillates between 10% and 50%. In his own sample, Pflanz (274, p. 81 ff) found 40% of the women and 22% of the men indicating the symptom. The peak of the distribution curve was between 50 and 59 years.

(4) Precordialgia. According to Pflanz (274, p. 82 ff), the following data are reported: (Duc) 96% men and 42% women; (Birkmayer) 52%; (Pflanz) 20% men and 40% women. The peak of the distribution curve was between 50 and 65 years.

(5) Restlessness. Restlessness subsumes nervousness, irritability, excitation, anxiety, tension, and so forth.

According to Pflanz (274, p. 85) the following data are found: (Essen-Moeller) 4.5%; (Lilienfeld) 59.9% nonsmokers and 70.3% smokers; (Grandjean) 26% men and 58% women; (Birkmayer) 41%; (Pflanz) 25% men and 42% women. Young women do not complain about the symptom very frequently. This is, according to Pflanz (274, p. 85), an indicator of the protective function of marriage. The peak of the distribution curve was between 30 and 59 years.

(6) Fatigue. Fatigue is the general feeling of psychophysiological exhaustion which cannot be localized. Fatigue is a symptom that accompanies different syndromes and disorders. It is an ubiquitous phenomenon. According to Pflanz (274, p. 89 ff), the following data are reported in the international literature: (Koos) 80% in the upper class, 53% in the middle class, and 19% in the lower class; (Grandjean) 32% men and 52% women; (Birkmayer) 92%; (Pflanz) 40% men and 52% women. The peak of the distribution curve was between 50 and 59 years for men. There was no clear peak for women.

(7) Insomnia. Pflanz (274, p. 97 ff) reports the following data: (Essen-Moeller) 8% men and 10% women; (Duc) 24% men and 35% women; (Lilienfeld) 37.1% nonsmokers and 42.6% smokers; (Birkmayer) 28%; (Pflanz) up to 35%, slightly more frequent in women. The peak of the distribution curve was between 49 and 59 years. In contrast to other symptoms, the frequency of insomnia does not diminish after 50.

(8) Constipation. Constipation is essentially a functional symptom which is often regarded as a signal in interhuman communication. Several authors claim that constipation represents a "not willing to give" attitude.

Pflanz (274, p. 97 ff) indicates the following data: (Birkmayer) 24%; (Pflanz) 33%, more frequently in women than men. The peak of the age distribution curve was at 30 for women with a slow increase towards 70. Men showed a continuously increasing frequency up to 70.

(9) Abdominal Complaints. According to Pflanz (274, p. 93 ff) there are only a few indications in the literature: (Duc) 36% men and 38% women.

9.3 Methods of Data Collection

I used the questionnaire, discussed above (cf. p. 36), to interview a representative sample of the population.

The sample was instructed to indicate only those complaints and symptoms they were suffering from on a continuous basis. A "continuous" symptom was defined as a symptom bothering the individual at least once or twice a week. There is one exception to this definition; "menstruational difficulty" was considered a continuous symptom when the complaints occurred monthly. The symptoms were described in everyday language. When a professional term was used, it was explained to every individual.

9.3.1 Symptoms

Table 14 gives the indicated symptoms according to their frequency. The total number of subjects was 120.

9.3.2 Syndromes

As expected, most of the subjects indicated several symptoms and complaints. Because certain symptom clusters seemed to be repetitive and more frequent than others, Fischer

196

Table 14. *Overall distribution of symptoms*

	n	%
Chronic fatigue	29	24
Muscular fasciculation	25	21
Precordialgias	23	19
Lumgalgias	22	18
Palpitations of the heart	21	17
Vertigo	20	17
Finger tremor	16	13
Constipation	15	12.5
Arthralgias	13	11
Profuse sweating	13	11
Lack of appetite	12	10
Menstrual complaints	10	8
Hypertension	9	7.5
Respiratory difficulties	9	7.5
Ear ringing	8	7
Hypotension	8	7
Abdominal pain	8	7
Meteorism	7	6
Diarrhea	6	5
Bladder troubles	5	4
Globus hystericus	5	4
Frigidity	5	4	(8% of all the women)
Impotence	4	3	(6% of all the men)
Suicidal ideas	2	2

Table 15. *Types of syndromes*

Psychic syndromes
    Chronic fatigue
    Insomnia
    Irritability

Neurocardiovascular syndromes
    Precordialgias
    Palpitations of the heart
    Profuse sweating
    Hypertension
    Hypotension
    Vertigo
    Headache
    Ear ringing

Motoric syndrome
    Arthralgias
    Muscular fasciculations
    Finger tremor
    Lumbalgias

Digestive syndrome
    Abdominal pain
    Lack of appetite
    Constipation
    Diarrhea
    Meteorism

(cf. p. 197) constructed several clearly defined syndromes, using the configuration-frequency analysis of Lienert (225). These syndromes are different from the classical nosological entities. We constructed them for the purpose of a comparison during the different stages (i.e., cross-sectional studies) of the followup study.

A syndrome was defined as a constellation of at least two symptoms or, in the case of the neurocardiovascular syndrome, of three symptoms in the above defined frequency. The syndromes were as shown in Table 15.

The definition of these syndromes was checked with the configuration-frequency analysis of Lienert (225) which makes it possible to identify so-called configural types or syndromes in a number of t alternative symptoms. The analysis compared the frequency f of the 2^t symptom clusters with the expected frequency e. It was based upon the zero hypothesis that the t symptoms are totally independent. A symptom configuration is a type if the chi-square component $(f\text{-}e)^2/e$ transcends a defined threshold.

The picture of the configuration-frequency analysis of the symptom cluster is as shown in table 16.

Table 16. *The configuration-frequency analysis of the symptoms*

Number of symptoms per component										
2 S1	3 S2	2 S3	2 S4	f_{ijk}	$f1$	$f2$	$f3$	$f4/n^2 = e_{ijk}$	e_{ijk}	$x^2_{ijk} = (f\text{-}e)^2/e$
+	+	+	+	2	40.	20.	21.	$7/99^2$	0.12	29.5
+	+	+	-	22	40.	20.	21.	$92/99^2$	1.58	0.11
+	+	−	+	0	40.	20.	78.	$7/99^2$	0.45	0.45
+	−	+	+	0	40.	79.	21.	$7/99^2$	0.47	0.47
−	+	+	+	1	59.	20.	21.	$7/99^2$	0.18	3.74
+	+	−	−	8	40.	20.	78.	$92/99^2$	5.86	0.78
−	+	+	−	4	58.	20.	21.	$92/99^2$	2.33	1.20
−	−	+	+	2	59.	79.	21.	$7/99^2$	0.70	2.41
+	−	+	−	2	40.	79.	21.	$92/99^2$	6.22	2.86
+	−	−	+	2	40.	79.	78.	$7/99^2$	1.76	0.03
−	+	−	+	0	59.	20.	78.	$7/99^2$	0.66	0.66
+	−	−	−	24	40.	79.	78.	$92/99^2$	23.13	20.03
−	+	−	−	3	59.	20.	78.	$92/99^2$	9.66	4.59
−	−	+	−	8	59.	79.	21.	$92/99^2$	9.19	0.15
−	−	−	+	0	59.	79.	78.	$7/99^2$	2.60	2.60
−	−	−	−	41	59.	79.	78.	$92/99^2$	34.13	1.38
				n = 99					99.04	$\chi^2 = 50.96$
										$p = < 0.001$

The following abbreviations are used in the above table:

n = number of probands indicating symptoms
S1 = psychic syndrome (with two or more symptoms)
S2 = neurocardiovascular syndrome (with three and more symptoms)
S3 = motoric syndrome (with two and more symptoms)
S4 = digestive syndrome (with two or more symptoms)

There are 16 possible configurations which are indicated at the beginning of the above figure. f_{ijk} indicates the n-distribution and e_{ijk} indicates the theoretical frequency. χ^2_{ijk} indicates the chi-square calculations. The global chi-square gives a highly significant value ($\chi^2 = 50.96, p = < .001$) (i.e., the four syndromes or configurational types are clearly distinguished).

A methodological problem arose in the evaluation of the symptom headache which was indicated by 32 subjects, i.e., 27% of the sample (Table 17). Only 9 subjects, (i.e., 7.5% of the sample) indicated this symptom as the only one they suffered from. The symptom was frequently indicated in conjunction with the neurocardiovascular symptom or other symptom configurations found outside the four main syndromes. We, therefore, indicate the symptom headache as S5 in the following figure and headache in combination with other symptom clusters outside the four basic syndromes as S5+. Finally, we indicate a combination of several symptoms which are not found in the four basic syndromes as S6. So stands for the subjects who indicated no syndrome at all.

Table 17. *Frequency of syndromes*

Syndrome	n	%
S0	21	17.5
S1	15	12.5
S2	29	24
S3	21	17.5
S4	12	10
S5	9	7.5
S6	13	11
Total	120	100
S5+	32	25

The following chapters discuss only the four main syndromes which have the following order of frequency: neurocardiovascular syndrome (24%), motoric syndrome (17.5%), psychic syndrome (12.5%), and digestive syndrome (10%).

Even though the number of chronic symptoms and syndromes seemed to be high, 80% of the sample indicated that they were in "good health" at the time of the interview. To have a chronic complaint or symptom is obviously not identical with labeling it as pathological and, therefore, with feeling ill and behaving like a patient. Indeed, I found more symptomatic people in the survey than my observations in the general practice led me to expect.

Based upon the daily experience in the medical practice, I had formulated some working hypotheses on the correlations between symptoms and the following factors: age, sex, marital status, work time, subjective interpretation of the season, evaluation of the importance of tourism for the financial situation, evaluation of a possible economic crisis, symptoms during early childhood and adolescence, vertical social mobility, state of health at the time of the interview, consumption of alcohol, occupation, number of occupational roles, and income.

Three of the hypotheses are omitted because the number of the subjects who answered the questions was too small to permit statements of any significance.

9.4 Symptoms and Working Hypotheses

9.4.1 Chronic Fatigue

Working Hypothesis. The symptom "chronic fatigue" is more frequent in women than in men. Its frequency increases with increasing worktime (i.e., hours per day). It is more frequent in the middle age groups and in subjects who experience subjectively the strain of the season as an intolerable stressor.

Results. There is no significant correlation between sex and frequency of the symptom. There is no statistically significant correlation between the symptom and the number of work hours per day, although there is a tendency ($p = <0.10, >0.5$) for the frequency to increase with an increasing number of workhours. There is a statistically significant correlation ($p = <0.02, >0.01$) between the frequency of the symptom and the various age groups. Table 18 shows that it is found most frequently (55%) in age group 3 (definition of groups cf. p. 44 ff) and least frequently (10%) in the oldest group.

Table 18. *The age-specific distribution of the symptom "chronic fatigue"*

	Indication of symptom (%)			
	Yes	No	%	n
Group 1	10	90	16.7	20
Group 2	25	75	16.7	20
Group 3	55	45	16.7	20
Group 4	10	90	16.7	20
Group 5	20	80	16.7	20
Group 6	25	75	16.7	20
Total	24	76	100	120
	$x^2 = 14.960$	$p = <0.02,$	>0.01	

Moreover, there is a highly significant correlation ($p = <0.001$) between this symptom and the subjective evaluation of the season. Probands who experience the season

as an intolerable stressor indicate the symptom more frequently (50%) than probands
who experience it as being a tolerable stressor (14%) (Table 19).
N.B. Since the number of figures for this book is restricted, I made a selection. The
main part of the results is presented in the text, including the significance of the correlations.

Table 19. *The evaluation-specific distribution of the symptom "chronic fatigue"*

| | Indication of symptom (%) | | % | n |
	Yes	No		
Tolerable stressor	14	86	71	85
Intolerable stressor	50	50	27	33
Total	24	75	98	118
	$x^2 = 20.112$	$p = < 0.001$		

9.4.2 Insomnia

Working Hypothesis. The symptom is more frequent in men than in women; its frequency increases with age and the number of work hours; and it is more frequent in probands
who experience the strain of the season as an intolerable stressor than in those who experience it as a tolerable stressor.

Results. There is no significant correlation between indications of the symptom and
sex or the way in which the season is experienced. There is no significant correlation
between the symptom and the number of work hours. Interestingly enough, however,
42% of the probands who work 10-12 hours per day indicate the symptom, but only
24% of the probands who work 12-15 hours per day indicated it. There is no statistically significant correlation between age and indication of the symptom, although there is
a slight tendency for older age groups to indicate the symptom more frequently.

9.4.3 Irritability

Working Hypothesis. The symptom is more frequent in women than in men; its frequency increases with the increasing number of daily working hours; and it is more frequent
in the middle aged groups and in probands who experience the season as an intolerable
stressor.

Results. There is a highly significant correlation ($p = < 0.01, > 0.001$) between sex
and indication of the symptom (Table 20).

There is no significant correlation between the symptom and the number of daily
workhours, although there is a slight tendency for the symptom to increase with the
number of hours. There is no significant correlation between age groups and symptom,
although there is a tendency for it to decrease with increasing age. While only 25% of
the oldest group indicate the symptom, it is indicated by 45-65% of the three youngest
groups. There is a highly significant correlation ($p = < 0.02, > 0.01$) between the frequency of the symptom and the subjective valuation of the season (Table 21).

Table 20. *Sex-specific distribution of the symptom "irritability"*

| | Indication of symptom (%) | | % | n |
	Yes	No		
Men	32	68	50	60
Women	57	43	50	60
Total	44	56	100	120
	$x^2 = 7.603$ $p = < 0.01, > 0.001$			

Table 21. *Evaluation-specific distribution of the symptom "irritability"*

| | Indication of symptom (%) | | % | n |
	Yes	No		
Tolerable stressor	36.5	63.5	71	85
Intolerable stressor	66	34	27	33
Total	44	46	98	118
	$x^2 = 10.863$ $p = < 0.02, > 0.01$			

9.4.4 Vertigo

Working hypothesis. The symptom is more frequent in women than in men; its frequency increases with age and with the number of work hours; and it is more frequently indicated by probands who experience the season as an intolerable stress than by others.

Results. The symptom is significantly ($p = 0.05$) more frequently indicated by women than by men. While only 10% of the men indicate the symptom, 23% of the women do. There are no significant correlations between symptom and age, symptom and number of work hours, and symptom and the way in which the season is experienced.

9.4.5 Headache

Working Hypothesis. The symptom is more frequent in women than in men; it is more frequently in middle age groups than in others; it increases with the number of daily work hours; and it is more frequent in probands who experience the season as an intolerable stressor.

Results. There is a highly significant correlation ($p = < 0.001$) between sex and the indication of the symptom, as shown in Table 22.

There is no significant correlation between the symptom and work hours, the symptom and age, or the symptom and the way in which the season is experienced.

Table 22. *Sex-specific distribution of the symptom "headache"*

| | Indication of symptom (%) | | % | n |
	Yes	No		
Men	12	88	50	60
Women	42	58	50	60
Total	27	73	100	120
	$\chi^2 = 13.807$	$p = < 0.001$		

9.4.6 Palpitation of the Heart

Working Hypothesis. The symptom is more frequent in women than in men; its frequency increases with age and with increasing number of daily workhours; and it is more frequent in subjects who experience the season as an intolerable stressor.

Results. There are no significant correlations between symptom and sex, symptom and age, symptom and the number of daily work hours, or symptom and the way in which the season is experienced.

9.4.7 Arthralgias

Working Hypothesis. The symptom is more frequent in women than in men; its frequency increases with increasing age and increasing number of work hours; and it is more frequent in subjects who experience the season as an intolerable stressor.

Results. There is a significant correlation ($p = < 0.01, > 0.001$) between sex and symptom; 2% of the men and 20% of the women indicate the symptom. There is no significant correlation between the symptom and the number of work hours. There is no significant correlation between the symptom and age, but there is a tendency for the older groups to indicate the symptom more frequently and for the youngest group not to indicate it at all. There is a statistically significant correlation ($p = < 0.01, > 0.001$) between the symptom and the evaluation of the season; only 7% of the subjects who experience the season as a tolerable stressor indicate the symptom, while it is indicated by 19% of the subjects who experience it as an intolerable stressor.

9.4.8 Profuse Sweating

Working Hypothesis. The symptom is more frequent in women than in men; its frequency increases with the increasing number of work hours; it is more frequent in the middle age groups; and it is more frequent in probands who experience the season as an intolerable stressor.

Results. There is no significant correlation between symptom and sex, symptom and age, symptom and the number of work hours, or symptom and the way in which the season is experienced.

9.4.9 Muscular Fasciculations

Working Hypothesis. The symptom is more frequent in men than in women; its frequency increases with the increasing number of work hours; it is more frequent in the middle age groups; and it is more frequent in probands who experience the season as an intolerable stressor.

Results. There is no significant correlation ($p = > 0.10$) between symptom and sex, and symptom and the number of workhours, although no proband who works the minimum (5-8 hours per day) indicates the symptom. There is a significant correlation ($p = < 0.02, > 0.01$) between symptom and age; 45% of group 4 indicate the symptom, while it decreases symmetrically in the older and younger groups; none of the probands of the oldest age group indicates the symptom. There is a significant correlation ($p = < 0.05, > 0.02$) between the symptom and the way the season is experienced; only 14% of the probands who experienced it as a tolerable stressor indicate the symptom, while it is indicated by 37.5% of the probands who experience it as an intolerable stressor.

9.4.10 Precordialgias

Working Hypothesis. The symptom is more frequent in women than in men; its frequency increases with the age and with the number of daily workhours; and it is more frequent in probands who experience the season as an intolerable stressor.

Results. There is a significant correlation ($p\ 2 < 0.05, > 0.02$) between symptom and sex; only 12% of the men, as compared to 27% of the women, indicate the symptom. There is no significant correlation between the symptom and the number of work hours. There is a significant correlation ($p = < 0.05, > 0.02$) between symptom and age; 35% of the subjects of age group 3 and 4 indicate the symptom and its frequency decreases in the older and younger age groups. There is a highly significant correlation ($p = < 0.001$) between the symptom and the way the season is experienced; only 12% of the probands who experienced the season as a tolerable stressor indicate the symptom, while it is indicated by 37.5% of the probands who experience it as an intolerable stressor.

9.4.11 Lumbalgias

Working Hypothesis. The symptom is more frequent in women than in men; it is more frequent in middle age groups than in others; its frequency increases with the increasing number of work hours; and it is indicated more often by subjects who experience the season as an intolerable stressor.

Results. There is a highly significant correlation ($p = < 0.01$) between symptom and sex; only 7% of the men as compared to 30% of the women, indicate the symptom. There are no significant correlations between symptom and age, symptom and number of work hours, and symptom and the way in which the season is experienced.

9.4.12 Constipation

Working Hypothesis. The symptom is more frequent in women than in men; its frequency increases with increasing age and increasing number of workhours; and it is more frequent in probands who experience the season as an intolerable stressor.

Results. There is a highly significant correlation ($p = < 0.001$) between symptom and sex; 2% of the men and 23% of the women indicate the symptom. There is no significant correlation ($p = > 0.10$) between the symptom and the number of workhours, symptom and age, or symptom and the way in which the season is experienced.

9.4.13 Finger Tremor

Working Hypothesis. The symptom is more frequent in men than in women; its frequency increases with the increasing number of work hours and increasing age; and it is more frequent in probands who experience the season as an intolerable stressor.

Results. There is no significant correlation between symptom and sex, symptom and the number of work hours, or symptom and the way the season is experienced. There is no significant correlation between symptom and age, although no proband of the oldest group indicates the symptom and 25% of the two youngest age groups do.

9.4.14 Menstrual Complaints

Working Hypothesis. The symptom is more frequent in women with a high number of workhours; it is more frequent in women of the middle age groups; and it is more frequent in women who experience the season as an intolerable stressor.

Results. There is no significant correlation between the symptom and the number of workhours, between the way in which the season is experienced, or the symptom and age. This latter result has to be critically examined. One of the women of the oldest and four women of the second oldest age group indicate menstrual problems, yet, these women are between 55 and 75 years old. According to Pschyrembel (286, p. 523) menopause occurs in 75% of the cases between 45 and 55 years of age. According to a statistical study od Doehring (cf. 286, p. 523), the average age of menopause in 1959 was 49.3 years. Considering these findings, we can assume that the older women indicated climacteric complaints, thus, there appears to be a clear tendency for the symptom to decrease with age; 50% of group 6 (the youngest), 30% of group 5, 10% of group 4, and 10% of group 3 indicate the symptom.

9.5 Working Hypotheses for Syndrome Distribution

9.5.1 Sex

Working Hypothesis. All syndromes are more frequent in women than in men.

Results. Globally, there is a highly significant correlation ($p = < 0.01, > 0.001$) between the indication of the syndromes and sex (Table 23).

Table 23. *Sex-specific distribution of the syndromes*

	Sex-specific frequency of syndromes (%)		%	n	p
	Men	Women			
S0	86	14	100	21	< 0.001
S1	53	47	100	15	> 0.05
S2	34.5	65.5	100	29	< 0.05, > 0.02
S3	33	67	100	21	< 0.05, > 0.02
S4	50	50	100	12	> 0.05
S5	33	67	100	9	> 0.05
S6	61	39	100	13	> 0.05
Total	50	50	100	120	
S5+	20	80	100	32	< 0.001
	$x^2 = 19.02$	$p = < 0.01, > 0.001$			

Within the single syndromes, there are significant correlations between sex and S0, S2, S3, and S5+. Women more frequently indicate the neurocardiovascular syndrome (S2), the motoric syndrome (S3), and the combined headache syndrome (S5+); 86% of the probands without a syndrome are men.

9.5.2 Age

Working Hypothesis. The psychic syndrome (S1) is most frequent in the youngest age group. All the other syndromes are most frequent in the middle age groups.

Results. Globally, there is no significant correlation between age and the syndromes. There is, however, a slight tendency ($p = > 0.05$) for the psychic syndrome (S1) to be more frequent in the younger age groups. Only 27% of the two oldest and the two middle age groups indicate the syndrome while it is indicated by 46% of the two youngest age groups. The two middle age groups have a sightly higher frequency (58%) in the digestive syndrome (S4) than the two oldest (17%) and the two youngest (25%) age groups.

9.5.3 Marital Status

Working Hypothesis. The psychic syndrome (S1) is more frequent in single subjects than in others. For the frequency of the other syndromes, the marital status is not important.

Results. Globally, there is no significant correlation between marital status and frequency of syndromes. There is a significant correlation, however, between the psychic syndrome (S1) and the marital status; 47% of the single subjects indicate the psychic syndrome as compared to 20% of the total distribution.

9.5.4 Number of Work Hours

Working Hypothesis. All the syndromes are more frequent in subjects who work a high number of hours daily.

Results. Globally, there are no significant correlations between the syndromes and the number of work hours. The combined headache syndrome (S5+), however, is more frequently indicated by subjects with a high number of workhours. There is a significant correlation (p = < 0.05, > 0.2) between the subjects who indicate no syndrome (S0) and the number of workhours; 57% of the subjects with less than 10 hours per day, 29% with 10-12 hours, and only 14% with more than 12 hours indicate no syndrome.

9.5.5 Subjective Evaluation of the Season

Working Hypothesis. All the syndromes are more frequent in subjects who experience the tourist season as a tolerable stressor.

Results. Globally, there are significant correlations (p = < 0.05, > 0.05) between the way the season is experienced and the syndromes (Table 24).

Table 24. *Evaluation-specific distribution of syndromes*

	Evaluation-specific frequency of syndromes (%)		%	n	p
	Tolerable stressor	Intolerable stressor			
S0	25	5	100	21	< 0.02, > 0.01
S1	67	33	100	15	> 0.05
S2	62	38	100	29	> 0.05
S3	67	33	100	21	> 0.05
S4	42	58	100	12	< 0.02, > 0.01
S5	78	22	100	9	> 0.05
S6	85	15	100	13	> 0.05
Total	71	29	100	120	
S5+	63	37	100	32	> 0.05
	x^2 = 13.60	p = < 0.05, > 0.02			

Within single syndromes, there are significant correlations (p = < .02 > .01) only for the digestive syndrome (S4) and for no syndrome S0; 95% of the subjects who experience the season as a tolerable stressor indicate no syndrome (S0).

9.5.6 Attitude Towards a Possible Economic Crisis

Working Hypothesis. Subjects who indicate great anxiety about a possible economic crisis indicate the psychic syndrome (S1) and the digestive syndrome (S4) more frequently. There are no correlations between the attitude towards a possible economic crisis and the syndromes.

Results. Globally, there are no significant correlations between the attitude and the syndromes. There is a significant correlation ($p = <0.05, >0.02$), however, for the digestive syndrome (S4); 67% indicate great anxiety vis-à-vis a possible economic crisis while only 8% think that the economic crisis would be a bearable damage.

9.5.7 Vertical Social Mobility

Working Hypothesis. Vertical social mobility correlates positively with all the syndromes; social climbers and/or descenders indicate all syndromes more frequently, especially the psychological syndrome (S1).

Results. There are no significant correlations between syndromes and vertical social mobility.

9.5.8 Number of Occupations

Working Hypothesis. Probands with two or more occupations indicate all the syndromes more frequently than probands with only one occupation.

Results. There is no significant correlation between the number of occupations and the syndromes.

9.5.9 Early Childhood Developmental Problems

Working Hypothesis. All the syndromes are more frequent in probands who had two or more developmental difficulties or disturbances.

Results. There is no significant correlation between syndromes and the number of developmental disturbances. Obviously, this fact questions some basic psychoanalytic assumptions about neurotic problems of early childhood, personality structure, and psychosomatic disorders.

9.5.10 Health Status

Working Hypothesis. Probands who feel ill at the time of the interview indicate syndromes more frequently than probands who feel well.

Results. There are no significant correlations between the health status at the moment of the interview and the frequence of syndromes.

9.5.11 Daily Alcohol Consumption

Working Hypothesis. Increased alcohol consumption correlates positively with increased frequency of syndromes.

Results. There is no significant correlation between daily alcohol consumption and the frequency of syndromes.

9.5.12 Monthly Income

Working Hypothesis. Probands with a low income have a higher frequency of the psychic (S1) and the neurocardiovascular (S2) syndromes.

Results. Globally, there is no significant correlation between syndromes and monthly income. There are, however, significant correlations ($p = < 0.05$) between the psychic (S1) and the motoric syndrome (S3) and income; subjects with the psychic syndrome (S1) belong in 73% to the lower income class (less than 2000 Swiss francs monthly) and subjects with the motoric syndrome (S3) belong in 62% to the higher income class (more than 2000 Swiss francs monthly).

9.6 Discussion of Results

There is no doubt that, in 1970, the villagers were exposed to a great number of stressors and had been for some time prior to that date. All of these stressors produced both stress and stress indicators. Psychosomatic symptoms and syndromes, quantified in the questionnaire, are only one type of stress indicators. Because stress is the organism's response to any demand made upon it and stress could not be measured by physiological parameters in this study, I measured it indirectly by the observable stressors and stress indicators. Stressors and stress indicators and their importance and relationship with the data reported in international literature will now be discussed briefly.

9.6.1 Stressors

The existence of stress may be predicted with some probability from the existence of stressors.

The village, in 1951, underwent a major social change. This change created a great number of stressors, defined by Dohrenwend (78) and Groen (121) as factors which demand adaptational efforts from individuals, families, and the system as a whole.

One of the major stressors was the fact that the season lasted almost 10 months and demanded a 7 day workweek with long workhours each day. Of the subjects between the age of 15 and 75, 42.5% worked more than 10 hours daily. Even if we take into account that the intensity of work varied during the day, this constituted a considerable strain.

Women worked more than men (cf. p. 142). This asymmetry was due to the systemic contradictions, these being the contradictions of the social organization with its uneven distribution of responsibilities and role expectations, and were a stressor of a new sort. An important consequence of the woman's longer workhours was the loss of time for sleep. As the worktime lengthened, therefore, the time meeded to recover from work, through sleep, was shortened.

With the exception of the oldest age group, there was an equal distribution of workhours across the different age groups. As could be expected, the middle age groups worked hardest, a fact which was responsible for the high number of stress indicators they reported.

Beside the social change in the different subsystems and the daily stress of worktime and work rhythm, there were other, less conspicuous, stressors due to the goal oriented social organization. On the basis of the life change concept of Holmes and Rahe (154), it is quite clear that the inhabitants of the village had to make a number of adaptations every day. Almost everyone in the tourist industry and, thus, each person was constantly exposed to a high number of social interactions with tourists he did not know and whose language he did not speak. The guests had many expectations and the villagers were supposed to fulfill them. Their education had prepared the villagers for a tenacious fight with nature, but not for smooth functioning in multiple social interactions. Social interactions, thus, were a constant source of stressors. Women were especially exposed to the wear and tear of tourism because they had more and less glamorous roles than men. Guests usually stayed in the village from 1 to several weeks. They then left and new guests arrived. Departures and arrivals unbalanced the transitory homeostasis of the guest-villager system and increased the daily stress. Moreover, there were problems with employees and one's own family. All these factors led to a general overstimulation and an increase in the number and intensity of stressors and, therefore, to stress.

The construction of tourist facilities put everyone into debt. The rebalancing of the financial situation depended, to a great extent, on the international political and economic situation. This constituted an additional source of stressors leading to anticipatory stress, as analyzed by Lazarus (208).

The questionnaires show how important such stressors were. More than three-quarters indicated that they would be hurt and felt threatened by a possible economic crisis. More than one-third indicated that they experienced great anxiety when thinking of a possible economic crisis.

Levi's (213) differentiation between specific and nonspecific stressors in an experimental situation was not possible with my approach. Moreover, its usefulness is questionable in a field study if we consider the observation of Dohrenwend (78) that change in itself is a stressor rather than the subjective meaning of change. Still, considering the correlation of many symptoms with the way the season is experienced rather than with the number of work hours per day, it seems that the subjective interpretation of a stressor is important for the amount of stress produced by an event.

Also, it seems to me, that it is impossible to differentiate physical from psychological stressors. A physical stressor (e.g., the number of daily workhours) may or may not, according to the framework of a personal or familial value system, be experienced as a stressor. It is the personal epistemology which makes the physical stressor a psychological one. It is the conceptual grid put upon events which qualifies the semantics of reality.

Finally, the social and sensorial deprivation, experienced in the "dead season" (i.e., in the interseason and partly in the afterseason) also constitutes a source of stressors leading to stress. This observation fits the explanatory model of Levi (cf. p. 171), showing that understimulation and overstimulation are stressors. Interseason and part of the afterseason moved the village into a recreational phase which corresponds to the regression phase of Mierke (cf. p. 184). During this time, the stimulus input was diminished and the coping capacity of individuals, families, and the village as a whole was recovering. There was a gradual adaptation to the understimulation, after which the oscillation capacity of the village increased again. Gradually, there occurred a postcritical recalibration towards new target values (Nitsch, Selbach and Selbach, cf. p. 183 f.).

During the preseason, an anticipatory adaptation began and, with it, a slow ergotrop reorientation of the system. The village moved into the precritical preparation phase and the individuals were gradually becoming activated. The communicative balance now slowly shifted to the positive side; in the direction of an increasing stimulation. The boundaries between different subsystems inside and outside the village became more and more permeable and there was an increased exchange of matter-energy and information. The bureaucratic subsystem started to awaken and take up its habitual functions. The tourist facilities were getting ready to receive, feed, and entertain the many thousands of guests. As a field observer, I was intensely aware of the general increase of activity and tension in the whole population as the village process gained momentum.

During the season, the whole community was under intense strain. Individuals were clearly overstimulated. The defense and coping mechanisms were mobilized. The human system was in a maximal critical phase of strain. It gradually led to a disturbance or loss of homeostasis which could not be rebalanced by a change in the target values (i.e., by giving up the tourist industry). Outer constraint (e.g., epidemical onset of Christmas tourism) and inner constraint (e.g., extreme achievement motivation) forced the system onto a course of maximum performance to the point of exhaustion.

In the afterseason, there was a final activity spurt to close down the tourist facilities. After this, the system shifted into a cholinergic metabolism and the village began to show patterns of exhaustion and regression.

9.6.2 Stress Indicators

Pflanz (274) points out that stress is indirectly measurable by the number of dysfunctional adaptations and pathological behaviors. My observations are congruent with those made by Lazarus (207) and Pflanz (274) —pathological behaviors, disturbed affects, disturbed motoric behavior, and physiological change in the function of the autonomous and vegetative-nervous system are expressions of stress.

The frequency of symptoms in the village is indicated on page 196. The list is headed by psychic symptoms such as irritability (44%), insomnia (32%), and chronic fatigue (24%). They are followed by symptoms of the musculoskeleton system such as muscular fasciculations (21%), lumbalgias (18%), and finger tremor (13%). Clinical experience teaches that lumbalgias are usually a general fatigue with a nonspecific localization due to an increased use of the paravertebral-lumbal muscles.

The third place is taken by neurocardiovascular symptoms, such as precordialgias (19%), palpitations of the heart (17%), and vertigo (17%). Constipation (12.5%) is indicated rather frequently. Sexual disorders are very rarely indicated. They are not even mentioned by probands who were in treatment for the disorders. This, again, illustrates the limits of a questionnaire which does not take into account the fact that people of a rural Catholic area might not want to disclose their sexual performance outside the doctor-patient setting.

Suicidality was low. Only two out of 120 subjects indicated frequent (i.e., once or twice a week) suicidal thoughts. In the 19 years from the construction of the road to my investigation, there was only one case of suicide reported – a villager hospitalized for endogenous depression committed suicide during hospitalization.

The catalogue of symptoms is impressive, especially the quantitative limit of threshold which indicates a symptom. Compared to the quantification of "very frequent," "frequent," "occasional," and "rare" used by Pflanz (274), I assume that my quantification is situated between "very frequent" and "frequent." Keeping this difference in mind and also the fact that the samples are chosen according to different criteria, I will compare my results with those reported by Pflanz (cf. p. 194 f).

9.6.2.1 Symptoms

(1) Irritability. The frequency of irritability (44%) of my sample is much higher than the results by Essen-Moeller (4.5%), but it corresponds with the findings of Birkmayer who indicates 41% in cases of vegetative exhaustion.

The sex distribution of the symptom (32% men and 57% women) corresponds with the findings of Grandjean and Pflanz.

The peak of the age distribution is between 25 and 45 years in 65% of the cases, thus, it is different from the findings of Pflanz (274).

(2) Insomnia. Insomnia is indicated by 32% of my sample. It corresponds with the results of Pflanz (274). Essen-Moeller and Birkmayer report a lower frequency.

The sex distribution of the symptom (27% men and 39% women) corresponds with the findings of Essen-Moeller, Duc, and Pflanz.

The peak of the age distribution is between 45 and 75 years, thus, it is different from the findings of Pflanz (274).

(3) Headache. Headache is indicated by 24% of my sample. All the other authors indicate a higher frequency.

The sex distribution (27% men and 22% women) corresponds with the data of Pflanz (274). Grandjean reports an inverse sex distribution.

The age peak between 45 and 55 years corresponds with the findings of Pflanz (274).

(4) Precordialgias. Precordialgias are indicated by 19% of my sample. All the other authors report a higher frequency.

The sex distribution (12% men and 27% women) corresponds with the findings of Duc and Pflanz.

The peak of the age distribution is between 35 and 55 years. Pflanz (274) indicates an earlier peak.

(5) Palpitations of the Heart. Palpitations are indicated by 17% of my sample. Pflanz reports differences in the international literature, ranging from 10% to 50%.

The sex distribution (13% men and 22% women) corresponds with the findings of Pflanz (274).

The peak of the age distribution, corresponding with the findings of Pflanz (274), is between 45 and 55 years.

(6) Vertigo. Vertigo is indicated by 17% of my sample. This is higher than the findings by Essen-Moeller and lower than the findings of all the other authors.

The sex distribution (10% men and 23% women) cannot be compared because Pflanz (274) does not indicate it.

The age peak, corresponding with the findings of Pflanz, is between 55 and 65 years.

(7) Constipation. Constipation is indicated by 12.5% of my sample. This is lower than the findings of all the other authors.

The sex distribution (2% men and 23% women) corresponds with the findings of Pflanz (274).

The age peak is between 55 and 65 years. The oldest group (65–75) does not indicate the symptom at all. Thus, the findings are different from those of Pflanz (274) who indicates a regular increase up to the age of 70.

(8) Other Symptoms. The frequency of sex and age distribution of other symptoms is not discussed because it is too low to permit statistically significant statements.

9.6.2.2 Syndromes

Most of the subjects indicated several symptoms. Therefore, we constructed symptom clusters or syndromes (cf. p. 197 ff). The frequency of these syndromes is the following: no syndrome (S0) = 17.5%, neurocardiovascular syndrome (S2) = 24%, motoric syndrome (S3) = 17.5%, psychic syndrome (S1) = 12.5%, mixed syndrome (S6) = 11%, and digestive syndrome (S4) = 10%. The headache syndrome (S5+), also contained in other syndromes, has a frequency of 25%.

The frequency of these syndromes demonstrates to what extent the population of Saas-Fee was under stress. The kind of expression of stress was influenced by many variables, as discussed before, and was also dependent on the physical training of the individuals. According to Weingarten (366), physical training is a protective factor against stress and the physical training of the villagers was relatively high.

Some of the influencing variables are discussed briefly.

9.6.2.3 Variables Influencing Symptoms and Syndromes

(1) Age. There is a maximal frequency of certain symptoms in the youngest age group (15-25 years) which indicates that the youngest group experiences a special stress. Irritability (45%), tremor (25%), menstruational troubles (50%), psychic syndrome (46%), and mixed syndrome (46%) are found most frequently in this group.

This age group is generally in the process of leaving the nuclear family, establishing heterosexual relationships, finding jobs, and participating special teaching programs. The findings emphasize the importance of the definitions of the psychosocial self, as described by Erikson (92). This period of transition increases the number of the above mentioned symptoms and syndromes, a fact also observed by Leighton et al. (cf. 360).

Certain symptoms, however, are not indicated at all by the youngest group – palpitations of the heart, arthralgias, and profuse sweating. Other symptoms (e.g., headache, precordialgias, insomnia) have the lowest frequency in the youngest group. It is probable that biological reasons mainly are responsible for this fact, although psychosocial factors may sometimes play a major role. Moreover, certain persons at certain stages of their life process have different ways of expressing stress.

The middle age groups (35-55 years) indicate a maximal frequency in almost all the symptoms. It is very probable that the role accumulation and, consequently, the number of responsibilities, work hours, and work intensity are responsible for this accumulation of symptoms.

The oldest age group (65-75 years) indicate insomnia (45%) with a maximal frequency. Other symptoms (e.g., muscular fasciculations, constipation, finger tremor) are not indicated by this group. Based on clinical observation, I would have expected that especially constipation and finger tremor would be frequent in this group; however, it seems probable that many probands were used to the symptoms and no longer found them disturbing or worth reporting.

Of the probands who did not indicate any syndrome, 52% belong to the oldest age group. Of the probands indicating neurocardiovascular symptoms, 40% belong to the two oldest groups (55-75 years). This corresponds with clinical experience. Moreover, the two oldest groups indicate the lowest frequency in the psychic, digestive, and motoric syndromes.

(2) Sex. All the symptoms, with the exception of chronic fatigue, are more frequent in women. In a few symptoms, sex-specific differences are slight. In others, the differences are important. For instance, arthralgias are indicated by 2% of the men and 20% of the women. Constipation is indicated by 20% of the men and 23% of the women.

I agree with Fischer (Esquisse d'une Sociologie de la psychopathologie de la femme, unpublished manuscript), Groen (121), and Pflanz (274) that such differences are not likely to be due to biological variables. It is more probable that women more readily express complaints and emotions because the sex-specific difference in the socialization process has taught them to do so. Men, however, have been taught to "clench their teeth," which is a different strategy for expressing stress. However, consumption of alcohol permits the men to regress as well as act out in a ritualized way, as will be discussed in the next chapter.

Obviously, the higher number of daily work hours (cf. p. 142) plays a determinant role for the higher frequency of psychosomatic symptoms in women, although this is only one of many influencing variables. I agree with Pflanz (274) that women who integrate more and more in the economic process, taking over more and more roles and responsibilities, are increasingly exposed to a wide field of stressors. They, therefore, increasingly develop stress indicators.

Amazingly enough, chronic fatigue is a symptom more frequent in men (27%) than women (22%). Considering the sex-specific distribution of workhours, sleeping hours, and work rhythm, this finding is surprising. In my view, there are various possible reasons for it; men officially own the tourist facilities, they are officially responsible for the debts, they often feel guilty about not working enough. They have a work pattern which is defined by excentric dispersion (cf. p. 142) and they drink a fair amount of alcohol, a cerebral depressant that makes them more tired. Often they are bored and understimulated in routine jobs.

Men indicate the psychic and the mixed syndrome more frequently. All the other syndromes are more frequently indicated by women.

(3) Personality and Sociocultural Factors. Our methodological approach does not permit direct statements about the personality structure of the subjects who indicate psychosomatic symptoms.

For the correlations between the type of developmental disturbances and the number and type of syndromes, the number of subjects was too small to yield statistically significant statements. The correlations were not significant.

There are indirect hints that personality or character structure influences the way in which the seasonal strain is experienced. In all the symptoms, with the exception of lumbalgias and finger tremor, the percentage of those probands prevails who experience the season as an intolerable stressor. I am aware of the fact that there is only a statistical correlation between indication of symptoms and the way the season is experienced. As to the causal relationship between the two phenomena, it is impossible to make statements supported by facts. Once again, we have to give up monocausal and unidirectional models of thinking (cf. 123) and adopt circular models which replace the straight cause-effect line by a cybernetic loop in which cause and effect are inseparable.

As far as the syndromes (cf. p. 204 f.) are concerned, only in the digestive syndrome does the number of probands prevail who experience the season as an intolerable stressor. On the other hand, only 5% of the probands who indicate no syndrome also experience the season as an intolerable stressor. For the digestive syndrome, comparable results are found for the way in which subjects confront a possible economic crisis (cf. p. 207).

Social mobility, number of occupational roles, and consumption of alcohol are also factors which would allow an indirect evaluation of the personality structure, but the results are not significant (cf. p. 207).

My results correspond, however, to the findings of Groen (121), Hinkle et al. (152), Levi (214), and Nitsch (265) who attribute the major importance to the way in which a person interprets a given situation. The high frequency of the neurocardiovascular syndrome (cf. p. 198) is congruent with the fact that personality type A, described by Roseman and Friedman (cf. 56, p. 422), is probably the prevailing character type of the village.

Although the number of the symptoms and syndromes reported is rather high, only 20% of the subjects indicated feeling ill at the time of the interview. As discussed, the reason for this seeming contradiction might be protective sociocultural factors which inhibit the social labeling process which would turn symptomatic individuals into patients. The coherence of families and the community as a whole was still strong enough to protect individuals and guarantee caring and mutual support.

Thus, the solitude characteristic of industrial societies (297, 121) was not very important. The interseason, despite its general understimulation, permitted a relatively intense social exchange among family members and villagers. For most of the year, however, the high number of business-like interactions with employees and guests did not permit enough intimate relationships with family and villagers.

Vertical mobility (cf. p. 207) did not lead to increased morbidity. On the one hand, the definition of a clear and unambiguous social stratification was very difficult within the village and, on the other hand, the village as a whole had become upwardly mobile. According to the principle of relativity, the specific move of one individual and one family is less stress inducing when their mobility is embedded in a general village process.

I found statistically significant correlations between the monthly income and the frequency of syndromes (cf. p. 208). The psychic and motor syndromes were strongly associated with the higher income classes — the psychic in 73% of the cases and the motor in 62%. Although an interpretation of this finding is difficult, it is probable that these individuals strove harder than others for economic success and the price they paid was the symptom.

(4) Marital Status. The standard distribution of single probands was 20%, yet, 47% of those indicating the psychic syndrome (S1) were single (cf. p. 205). This fact, however, may be explained more by the age of the probands than the circumstance of being unmarried. Adolescents go through a period of difficult recalibration and this stress produces stress indicators of mainly a psychological type.

(5) Occupations and Work Hours. There were no statistically significant correlations between the type of occupation and the psychosomatic symptoms and syndromes. The number of types was too great and the number of probands per type too small to allow significant statements. The correlations between the number of occupations held at the same time and the distribution of the symptoms were also statistically insignificant. Compared to the standard distribution, however, a tendency does appear for the neuro-cardiovascular and headache syndromes to be more frequent in probands who indicate two or more occupations.

There are no statistically significant correlations between the daily workhours and the distribution of particular symptoms. Again, there is a tendency with regard to certain symptoms [e.g., chronic fatigue, arthralgias, profuse sweating, muscular fasciculations, finger tremor (i.e., motor symptoms)] for the frequency to increase proportionally to the increasing number of daily work hours. However, vertigo and palpitations of the heart tend to have an increasing frequency with the increasing number of daily work hours.

For probands who indicate no syndrome, there are significant correlations with the daily workhours (cf. p. 206): 57% of these probands work less than 10 hours; 29% work 10-12 hours; and only 14% work more than 12 hours. Therefore, my results are not in accordance with the findings of Zohman (379), although many of my probands indicate a maximal work time. It is possible that the status congruency (92) plays a protective role. Most of the probands had a work time congruent with the performance of the majority of the same age group.

9.7 Answers to Four Basic Questions

9.7.1 Variation in Frequency Distribution

Generally, the distribution of the frequency of symptoms corresponds to the frequency observed in the medical practice. There are, however, some exceptions.

On the one hand, I rarely treated patients with the symptoms "headache," "irritability," or "insomnia." These patients probably treated themselves with the analgesics and tranquillizers available in pharmacies and drugstores.

On the other hand, I treated patients with precordialgias and hypotension or hypertension relatively often. These symptoms probably provoke anxiety which pushes people to seek medical help. These symptoms are not treated either with grandmother's home remedies or modern tranquillizers, although home visits taught me that most of the families had a substantial stock of analgesics and tranquillizers.

I treated fewer women with menstrual problems than indicated in the questionnaire. Due to the specific history of the practice (cf. p. 178), women generally preferred to consult gynecologists outside the valley. I often treated patients with symptoms of the musculoskeleton system, mainly due to sport accidents. Moreover, chronic fatigue and stress often lead to muscular tensions and dysfunctional distortions of joints and muscles. The resulting pain brings the patient to the practitioner.

Sexual disorders are less frequently reported than found in the medical consultations. The reasons for this fact have been discussed before.

9.7.2 Variation in Sex-Specific Distribution

The sex-specific distribution of symptoms and syndromes found in the medical practice corresponds, more or less, to the results of the inquiry. Woman indicated psychosomatic symptoms more frequently, although the symptom "chronic fatigue," the psychic syndrome, and the mixed syndrome were exceptions to this rule. I also treated more women than men for psychosomatic problems. While men offered mainly somatic complaints, often covering psychosomatic problems, men had other means (e.g., drinking) for the expression of stress.

9.7.3 Work Hours and Subjective Attitude Towards Tourism: Correspondence to Symptoms

There are no statistically significant correlations between daily work hours and the frequency of symptoms and syndromes; however, of the probands indicating no syndrome, 57% work less than 10 hours per day.

Corresponding to my expectations, there are statistically significant correlations between all the symptoms, except lumbalgias and finger tremor, and the way the season is experienced. The same correlation is found for the digestive syndrome — 95% of the probands indicating no syndrome evaluate the season as a tolerable strain.

There is, therefore, a correlation between attitude to the season and tourism and the frequency of symptoms. The subjective interpretation of reality seems to be more important for the genesis of stress than the objective reality. This finding seems to question Dohrenwend's (78) claim that life change in itself is a stressor and not its subjective interpretation. I have used the phrase "seems to question" advisedly, of course, because the relationship found between the subjective experience of the season and the indication of symptoms is based on statistical correlations, not on causality. Moreover, Dohrenwend (78) speaks of life change while my probands evaluated their changing life situation.

9.7.4 Pathogenic or Pathoplastic Function of Social Change

It was the conviction of the key persons and the probands interviewed that their psychosomatic disorders had increased since the construction of the road in 1951.

Such statements, however, have to be interpreted with caution. It is well-known that older people tend to cling to the myths of the good old times, when everything was so much better. Moreover, people have a tendency to use unilinear, monocausal, and reductionist models of explanation for all kinds of phenomena. Still, it is obvious that the construction of the road is a timemarker. It coincides with the beginning of a rapid social change and, therefore, with the production of a field of stressors leading to stress and stress indicators.

Only the further results of the follow-up study will give clearer answers concerning the correlations between social change and its pathogenic and pathoplastic functions. For the time being, there are strong arguments for the fact that the social change created a great number of stressors. At this point, I can only describe the space-time pattern of the structures changed and the statistical correlations between the symptoms found and the village structure of 1970. For a clear proof of a strictly causal interconnection, we would need a before-after study or a number of comparative studies which would corroborate my hypothesis. A before-after study could not be made in Saas-Fee since I arrived only after about 2 decades of intensive change which had started with the construction of the road. A study combined with specific interventions inducing change into the field of observation would also prove a causal relationship between change, stress, and stress indicators; however, interventions of this kind are precluded for ethical reasons.

9.8 Final Remarks

In comparing the results of this investigation with the results reported in the international literature, I have come to some conclusions and considerations which have to be taken into account for the next cross-sectional study in 1980. It would be interesting to construct, in accordance with the social readjustment rating scale of Holmes and Rahe (154), a rating scale which allows the quantification of adjustment demanded daily or weekly (e.g., arrival and departure of guests, beginning and end of season, conflicts with employees, changes in the international political and economic situation). The studies of Holmes and Rahe (154) and many other authors (43, 59, 60, 62, 144, 155, 264, 287-289, 352, 353, 360) are a promising approach which could be used in the framework of this followup study.

It would be interesting to include in each of the questionnaires a psychometric test (e.g., MMPI test) in order to have some quantifiable psychometric data about the personality structure of the individuals interviewed.

It would be desirable to investigate individually, whether or not there are somatic findings behind the indication of psychosomatic complaints. Such an endeavor would demand the collaboration of all the general practitioners inside and outside the valley and a thorough checkup of all the probands.

Finally, it seems imperative that the next cross-sectional study be made with an interdisciplinary team. Although Fischer, a sociologist, collaborated in this study and, in fact, was completely responsible for the statistical elaboration of the results of the questionnaire, a future interdisciplinary collaboration will have to be both more intensive and more extensive. An optimal team would include at least one psychiatrist, one psychologist, one sociologist, and one epidemiologist or another scientist with experience in statistical methods.

10. Consumption of Alcohol

10.1 Introduction

Alcohol consumption in the village was high, as well as conspicuous. Drinking was the outstanding phenomenon I observed in 1968. In fact, the present study grew out of the initial intention to investigate the alcohol consumption of the village. Once started, it soon became clear that heavy drinking was only one indicator of the vast field of stressors and stress indicators to be investigated.

At first glance it seemed that alcohol consumption was sanctioned positively by a permissive value pattern and that drinking fulfilled a communicative-integrative and utilitarian function. I was interested in investigation this problem further because few studies exist that are concerned with alcohol consumption in rural areas. The interested reader is referred to the separate study (cf. 125) on stress and alcohol consumption which includes many detailed figures and tables. The findings of the latter publication have been integrated into the present larger conceptual framework.

10.2 Stress and the Consumption of Alcohol: Brief Overview of International Literature

Keller (185) points out that the definition of an alcoholic has been marked by "insecurity, conflicts, and ambiguity" for a long time, nor has there been any recent improvement. Each of the following definitions is unsatisfactory in some measure.

10.2.1 Definition of an Alcoholic and of Alcoholism

According to Lundquist (232), Bleuler, in 1969, offered the following definition: "the person who clearly damages himself and his family by the consumption of alcohol without being able to take advice or without having the will or the force to improve, must be considered an alcoholic." This definition contains moral and ethical aspects. Furthermore, it is useless for epidemiologic purposes because it cannot be quantified in any way.

Similar objections can be applied to the following definition of alcoholism of the World Health Organization (WHO), quoted by Chafetz (54): "alcoholism is a chronic behavioral disorder manifested by repeated drinking of alcoholic beverages in excess of the dietary and social uses of the community and to an extent that interferes with the drinker's health or his social or economic function." As Chafetz (54) points out, this definition is descriptive, symptomatic, and neglects etiologic considerations. It lends itself to quantification of a moralist kind because it outlines the aspect of social deviance more than individual discomfort. Different observers, according to their own value patterns, will make the diagnosis of a clear functional disorders at different stages of the process of drinking, but it is virtually impossible to decide whether or not relationship problems and social functioning are due to alcohol consumption or whether or not they precipitated the alcohol consumption.

More operational definitions were proposed by Berner (27) and Keller (185). Berner (27) defines an alcoholic as a person who is drunk at least 4 times a week without necessarily showing signs of excessive drinking. Keller (185) proposes a definition explicitly formulated for epidemiologic purposes — drinking must be described in terms of chronicity, repetition, and undesirable characteristics concerning quality, frequency, and drinking pattern; drinking is implicative (i.e., provoking suspicion) or manifest; it must be described with respect to the pathogenous effects upon the drinker, the social and interpersonal dimensions, and, finally, the economic situation (e.g., behavior at work, changing jobs, neglect of property).

Even these definitions are not satisfactory for epidemiologic purposes. Again, it depends upon the observer and his explicit or implicit value patterns, his training, and his prevalent conceptual grid whom he declares as being "drunk" or as "being disturbed in his interpersonal dimensions by drinking." On the other hand, I have no better definition to offer. We do not know enough about drinking and social interactions, drinking and family structure, quantitative aspects of drinking, and physical disorders to propose a satisfactory definition.

Given this situation, I adopted the following policy: when consumption of alcohol is concerned, I indicate the amount of daily drinking; and when alcoholism is concerned, as in the direct field work, I use the definition of the WHO. Although its reliability is questionable, at least it has the advantage of being widely accepted.

10.2.2 Variables Correlating With Type and Quantity of Drinking

(1) Age. Age plays a major role in correlation with the onset of drinking, the time of manifestation of clinical symptoms, and the long term prognosis.

Warder and Ross (362) report the results of studies investigating the correlations between age at the beginning of drinking and the consumption of alcohol. Foulds and Hassal (cf. 362) found a significant correlation between the early onset of drinking and the gravity of alcoholism. Foulds proposes, therefore, that age at the beginning of drinking should be used as a criterion for the classification of different types of alcoholism. Hassal (cf. 362) notes that the beginning of drinking tends to gradually shift to earlier ages. The onset age he reports is 15.5 years, fully 2 years younger than the age reported in comparable studies. Rosenberg (cf. 362) compared groups of alcoholics who were over and under the age of 30; the younger group shows the more extreme disorders.

Obviously, the onset of drinking is influenced by many variables (e.g., heredity, family structure, socialization. sociocultural value patterns, economic status).

The period of risk for the manifestation of clinical symptoms and hospitalization lies mostly between 40 and 50 years, as reported by several investigators [Rubington

(304), Warder and Ross (362), Wieser and Kunad (369)]. This corresponds to an average drinking career of 25 to 35 years of regular alcohol consumption.

The above findings are supported by an extensive and methodologically exact catamnestic study of Ciompi (57). He shows that the life expectancy of alcoholics, especially of alcoholics with an organic brain syndrome, is significantly shortened. On the other hand, the age at the beginning of drinking does not necessarily play a decisive role in the long term prognosis of alcoholics. He emphasizes that the actual physical and psychosocial situation of the drinker plays a destructive or, when optimal, a protective role for the evolution of the old drinker and alcoholic.

(2) Sex. Many authors [Bales (14), Becker (20), Dollard (80), Field (98), Guntern (125), Heath (148), Jackson (173), Jessor et al. (180), Lemert (209), Maddox (233), Simmons (328), and Stacey and Davies (340)] show that men drink more than women. What Adler (2, p. 120) calls "the obligation to virility" seems to be prescriptive for the behavior of adolescents in all western cultures. To drink is often an expression of manhood, a communication of virility, and a status indicator. In my view, drinking is a sex-role-specific strategy of men for dealing with life stresses.

As many observes emphasize, among them Mead (247, p. 127), sex roles are in the process of change. Drinking becomes a signal which marks a change in status, as indicated by Jessor et al. (180). Dollard (80) reports that women drink more as they enter higher social classes, a finding which is also emphasized by Falk (96). He shows that status in the economic sector correlates with the drinking pattern (i.e., the number of female drinkers increases proportionally to the women's rising status in the economic world). The same observation is made by Becker (20) who explains this fact by the existence of a hidden matriarchy caused by their double function as housewives-mothers and wage earners.

According to Becker (20), the proportion of male to female drinkers was 10 to 1 before World War II, 3 to 1 during World War II, 7 to 1 just after the war, and reached 3 to 1 again in 1956 — clear evidence for the trend towards an increase in female drinking and alcoholism. Drinking becomes a strategy for coping with stress shared by men and women, to the extent that occupational roles and economic status are shared by both sexes.

(3) Civil Status. Wieser and Kunad (369, p. 416 ff) quote the findings of Bacon, Rosenblatt, Rosenbaum, Straus, Baily, and Malzberg which show the correlations between drinking and civil status — the percentage of single, separated, divorced, and widowed alcoholics is high. There are, however, as Straus and Bacon emphasize, sex-specific differences in the distribution of frequency of drinking. Malzberg (cf. 369, p. 416 ff) indicates a high percentage of married alcoholics in the upper social class.

(4) Occupational Roles. The clearer (i.e., the better defined) the role prescription and role expectation within occupational roles and the corresponding professional training, the less an occupational role becomes a stressor. This is a fact which can be generally observed and also indirectly deduced from the discussion of Daheim (66, p. 364) concerning professionalization.

On the other hand, there is no doubt that the position in the economic process is linked to the degree of "alienation," as observed long ago by Marx (cf. 111, p. 57). Increasing frustration in lower socioeconomic classes, job insecurity, low gratification level, and low status or status insecurity, for instance, in top management where one can be hired and fired at will are certainly factors which induce men and women to drink.

The occupational roles linked with the production, distribution, and sale of alcohol (e.g., wine producer, wine merchant, waitress, barman, innkeeper) are especially at risk. At the same time, these are the preferred jobs for people who like to drink.

Wieser and Kunad (369), investigating the occupational roles of drinkers, found the following rank order: the greatest number of drinkers is in trade and commerce; followed by skilled laborers, farmers, and construction workers. Becker (20), in an inquiry made in West Germany, reports that the female drinkers prevail in the middle level positions. They had the following distribution of occupational roles: 39% housewives, 35% employees (partly in high positions), and 20% unskilled workers. By contrast, male drinkers were found mostly in the lower classes with lower prestige jobs. These results might be linked to the economic and sociocultural situation of West Germany.

(5) Religion. Although the influence of religion on drinking behavior is emphasized by Fouquet (99), it is denied by Stacey and Davies (340), a contradiction probably due to the different ethnic-cultural samples investigated by these authors.

Fouquet (99) was studying the drinking behavior in France where he found that religion and religiosity were significant influences. Irgens-Jensen (170), investigating drinking behaviors in Norway, reports that individuals who indicate religious activity drink less than others. Skolnick (330) found, in a comparative transcultural study, that religion strongly influences individual drinking patterns and value patterns. He argues that such inhibiting influence is important in Jews, Episcopalians, and Methodists whereas in Irish and Italian Catholics, the national background seems to be a more significant determinant of drinking patterns than religion.

(6) Birth Order. Generally speaking, findings concerning birth order and position within the siblings are contradictory and comprehensive studies in the field of psychiatry have never adequately proven that birth order shows a significant correlation with pathological behavior.

Nevertheless, Barry and Blane (15) found that male alcoholics in the last birth position (i.e., youngest of the siblings) are overrepresented; Navratil (263) holds that the fact of being the last child plays an important pathoplastic function in alcoholism; and Barry and Blane (15) indicate that this overrepresentation becomes more obvious the greater the number of siblings and it is more significant in men than women.

(7) Social Mobility. According to Dollard (80), social climbers show a high frequency of so-called problem drinking. On the other hand, Wieser and Kunad (369) emphasize that downward vertical mobility can be an indicator of social desintegration, a consequence, rather than a cause, of drinking.

(8) Genetic Factors. Reviewing the literature, Lundquist (232) concludes that the studies of Kaij (1960), Partanen, Bruun, and Markanen (1966), investigating the drinking behavior of monocygotic twins, clearly proved the importance of genetic factors. This view is shared by Schuckit (320).

The basic question, however, is – how do the genetic factors determine the drinking behavior? Lundquist (232) emphasizes the importance of genetically determined biochemical factors (e.g., the NAD/NADH-quotion). He quotes a study of Amark who shows a correlation between a genetically determined personality structure and drinking. According to Amark, psychopaths are very frequently found among alcoholics. Rubington (304), studying skidrow drinkers, points to the important factor of marginal personalities who are most often found among this severe type of alcoholism. Such studies, I should like to emphasize, do not differentiate between the personality as cause or effect of the drinking and they certainly neglect the systemic approach in which personality and drinking patterns interact in multiple feedback processes governed by certain rules.

Barry and Blane (15) quote a study of Ross who compared 36 children with at least one alcoholic parent with 25 children of nonalcoholic parents. Both groups were reared by foster parents. At the age of 30, there were no significant differences in the drinking behavior of the two groups; none of the children had become an alcoholic and only "very few" were drinkers.

(9) Personality Structure. Whereas sociologists have a tendency to neglect the importance of personality structure, it is very much emphasized in studies made by psychiatrists. Obviously, different training leads to different tendencies of focusing upon one or the other aspect of the field of investigation.

Jellinek (179) emphasizes that it is methodologically difficult to differentiate between prealcoholic and postalcoholic personality traits when the alcoholic is the object of study. Only prospective studies, even when made a posteriori, as in the work of McCord and McCord (244), are able to make this differentiation. This study will be discussed later.

In a syngenetic view, we must conceive of personality structure as the result of a network of factors which determine all behavior. Logically, therefore, the personality structure influences the drinking behavior. The process of socialization may be controlled by a deferred gratification pattern. This pattern will have a prohibitive function upon drinking. On the other hand, a deferred gratification pattern is already the expression and result of prohibitive-restrictive value patterns. During adolescence, individuals undergo an identity crisis, a process well described by Erikson (92, p. 140). This is also the time when drinking begins in the Western societies. Alcohol, a depressant for the central nervous system and an anxiolytic drug, is consumed by persons who rebel against a prohibitive value pattern or by persons who have a syngenetic program with permissive value patterns. Alcohol is a "helper," a strategic tool which, in the short range, cures and, in the long range, often destroys.

Immediate gratification (e.g., by drinking) sews the seeds of future self-destruction, as claimed by Plack (283, p. 220). This mechanism has been carefully described by Reich (292, p. 192) in the case of addictive mountain climbing, which is especially interesting in the context of my study. The more an individual exposes himself to a real physical threat *(Realangst),* the more this exposure decreases via generalizing the neurotic anxiety, which can be due to the socially controlled repression of "drives" and needs. With time, this mechanism becomes self-perpetuating.

Moreover, as Bateson (17, p. 309 ff) suggests, drinking is a coping strategy which makes the alcoholic more normal in terms of his own epistemology, whereas he becomes abnormal in the eyes of the environment. Haley (140) stresses the communicative aspect of the drinking behavior. In a systemic view, drinking can be a strategy to cope with an unbearable situation, maintain a threatened family homeostasis, or control the environment by means of a "one down" position. Obviously, there are individuals who successfully maintain, at least in the short run, their identity and integration by drinking.

Although these considerations are convincing, a prevailing reductionism poses the danger of explaining complex phenomena with one-dimensional concepts. Horton (163) warns against a psychological reductionism in the explanation of drinking behaviors, a warning which is especially needed in psychoanalytic circles. Here, wild speculations have flourished for a long while. For instance, drinkers and alcoholics are considered as latent homosexuals, a term indicating everything and nothing. Gibbins and Walters (115) investigated the hypothesis of latent homosexuality with a series of experiments. They concluded that there was not the slightest evidence in favor of it. Nonetheless, it is still held by certain authors.

In order to avoid reductionism, authors such as Jessor et al. (180) and Robins et al. (298) stress the psychosocial factors more than the individual psychological factors influencing drinking behavior. Many authors, however, such as Connor (61), Navratil (263), Stacey and Davies (340), Schuckit (320), Walton (361), and Warder and Ross (362), postulate a clear correlation between personality structure, drinking, and alcoholism. Essentially, these authors try to prove that there is a connection between the way in which individials cope with impulses and emotions and the tendency to drink.

The most interesting study in this context was made by McCord and McCord (244). They investigated the probands of Talbot's followup study (Cambridge-Somerville Youth Study), started in 1953, in which personality profiles of boys had been recorded. McCord and McCord (244) proved that all the boys who later became alcoholics showed a similar personality pattern. The characteristic features were strong self-confidence, no abnormal anxieties, indifference towards mother and siblings, uncontrolled and aggressive behavior, sadism, sexual fears, and a high level of activity. In other words, these boys showed all the character traits which are typically masculine in Western societies. Obviously, they were overadapted to the prevalent sex-specific value patterns. Why, then, did they become alcoholics? The authors give the following explanation: the boys became alcoholics when they entered puberty. They now had to repress definitely the already repressed needs for support and dependence. The more society demanded altruistic roles, the more the neurotic equilibrium was pushed to the brink of decompensation. In this crisis, alcohol consumption seemed to be an optimal solution. It satisfied the needs for dependence and, at the same time, it was an expression of virility which permitted acting out and was in accord with the sex-specific value pattern. Thus, for the time being, the social integration of the drinker was guaranteed.

(10) Family. The works of Bateson (17), Jackson (172), Bowen (36, 37), Haley (140, 141), Minuchin (253), Minuchin et al. (254, 255), Wynne et al. (374), and many other family investigators have made it amply clear that alcoholism, like any other behavior, has to be viewed and interpreted in a systemic way. A symptom helps to maintain the threatened homeostasis of a human system. Erikson (92) and Koenig (196, p. 254 ff), although using different conceptual frameworks, share similar views. The role of the "broken home" has become a generally accepted factor in the genesis of all kinds of pathological or dysfunctional behavior.

There are several studies which substantiate the claim of an interrelation between family structure and drinking. Schuckit (320) indicates a family-specific increase of the frequency of alcoholism. Park (268) stresses the importance of the family process for the socialization of the drinking behavior. This view is shared by Haes (137), who holds that family and groups of friends are responsible for the drinking behavior and the norms governing drinking. According to Lundquist (232) and Stacey and Davies (340), the first drinking occurs within the family. The family can have a protective role, as described by Evreux (97), or a destructive role, as described by Jackson (173) and Wardner and Ross (362).

(11) Group. At present, in complex industrialized society, the peer group has an increasing impact in socialization, while parental influence seems to be gradually declining. This fact is stressed by Bruun (46), Lemert (211), Maddox (233), and Stacey and Davies (340). Jessor et al. (180) claim that the influence of the small group is a basic criterion for the type of drinking behavior, while Haes (137) stresses that the group influences especially the drinking behavior of men. This, in turn, influences the drinking behavior of their female partners.

(12) Socialization. As mentioned before, socialization is a learning process in which the individual is trained in the value patterns and behaviors a given society considers appropriate. Socialization builds up the syngenetic program which governs human transactions. Maddox (233) stresses that drinking is usually a social act. It is the social expectations and rituals which determine who drinks and when, where, with whom, and how much.

As Guntern (123) has shown, an increasing number of studies indicate that the learning processes during the phase of socialization shape drinking behavior. Among the many authors studying this interconnection, only a few are mentioned here: Horton (163), Jackson (173), Jellinek (178, 179), Lawrence and Maxwell (206), Lemert (209, 211), Park (268), Pittman (280), Simmons (328), Snyder (332), and Zucchi (380).

Pittman (280), however, argues for caution. According to him, the reliable data to prove such a claim in a quantitative way do not yet exist. He advices waiting for more exact studies to substantiate the thesis that drinking behavior is influenced by socialization.

Today, the mass media increasingly take over socialization. In the United States, in 1978, an average child watches TV more hours per day than he attends school. Quite obviously, his socialization is considerably influenced by TV. Considering this influence, Falk (96) and Stacey and Davies (340) especially stress the socializing influence of the TV idols with which the advertizing industry floods individuals and families.

(13) Sociocultural Factors. All the above discussed factors and elements operate in the context of a certain culture and they are, therefore, shaped by it. As Habermas (133, p. 177) makes clear, a society has a certain tendency to project or displace systemic conflicts onto the individual in order to treat the ensuing dysfunctional behaviors as technically and bureaucratically resolvable problems. As Fromm (110) stresses, such a tendency becomes clearest when the distribution of work and the form of organization of a society lead to an increasing alienation of the individual. Wyss (375) discusses the anthropology of Freud and Marx who hold that individual of the industrialized society,

who is degraded to an object, becomes neurotic and, thus, the socially determined conflict is twisted into an intrapersonal one. Drinking permits the individual to revoke, at least temporarily, such alienation. This is stressed by Bateson (17, p. 309 ff) and exemplified in the study of McCord and McCord (244). From a psychoanalytic standpoint (cf. 67, 227, Mendel 250), the question arises as to how social factors interact with "drive" factors in order to generate intrapersonal problems leading to drinking.

The influence of sociocultural factors upon drinking behavior is best studied in the transcultural work edited by Pittman and Snyder (281). The general impression deduced from these comparative studies indicates that drinking is least pathologic when it is socially well integrated, thus corresponding to the prevailing cultural value patterns.

The influence of sociocultural factors in so-called primitive cultures was investigated by Bunzel (48), Field (98), Heath (148), Horton (163), and Sangree (312). Drinking behavior in complex societies has been studied by Becker (20), Berner (27), Gabriel (113), Irgens-Jensen (170), Pichler (279), and Solms (333). The influence of sociocultural factors in Europe and the United States has been studied by Jellinek (179-180), Lemert (210-212) and Solms (333).

To what extent sociocultural factors influence the drinking behavior of certain social classes and subcultures is studied by Bales (14), Bruun (46), Dollard (80), Rubington (304), and Snyder (332). It is interesting to note that Rubington (304) describes the social organization and the drinking behavior of seemingly disorganized and anomic skidrow drinkers as highly structured and organized. Snyder (332) suggests that the rigidly ritualized and institutionalized drinking behavior of ethnic minorities (e.g., American Jews) are responsible for the fact that they are rarely alcoholics sensu strictu, although their consumption of alcohol is high. It seems that their well developed ingroup-out-group consciousness is responsible for the high social cohesion which inhibits the dropping out of drinkers.

Pittman (280) differentiates four value patterns which govern the drinking behavior of cultures all over the world. These value patterns are responsible for four types of drinking cultures:

Abstinent cultures. The prevailing value patterns governing drinking are negative and prohibitive (e.g., in the cultures belonging to Islam).
Ambivalent cultures. Contradictory value patterns coexist (e.g., in the United States).
Permissive cultures. Drinking is permitted, but drunkenness and deviant behavior is prohibited (e.g., in Spain).
Permissive-dysfunctional cultures. Drinking, drunkenness, and deviant behavior while being drunk are allowed. This attitude is found in certain primitive societies and in complex societies undergoing rapid social change (e.g., the Cambas tribe in Bolivia; Japan; and, to some extent, France).

(14) Economic Factors. Economic factors influence the drinking behavior, although not in a monocausal way since wine producing countries with similar economics (e.g., Italy, France) have totally different drinking patterns.

According to Solms (333), the general alcoholization in France is an integral element of life, lifestyle, and nutrition. The number of inns (i.e., 1 per 97 inhabitants) indicates how many people are economically interested in the production, distribution, and sale of alcohol. In a country that produces as much wine as France, the nation easily identifies with the needs of the wine producers, as Jellinek (178) states. This identification influences the value patterns and makes drinking a highly desirable and socially demanded behavior. These value patterns also inhibit the social desintegration of drinkers because the culture accepts alcoholism as a pattern of normal life style.

(15) Function of Drinking. Pittman (280) presents two different typologies for the function of drinking. One stems from functionalist sociology which considers drinking as integrative for society and the individual; anxiety reducing, especially for the individual; or disintegrative for society and the individual. The other stems from Bales who differentiates between the following functions:

- Religious (e.g., in the context of the holy communion in the Catholic Church).
- Ceremonial-ritual [e.g., in the *rites de passage* from birth to death (e.g., marriage, birthday, Irish Wakes)].
- Hedonistic-convivial (e.g., in the context of hospitality, toasts, "to get high" in order to lose inhibiting behavior, to become more "social").
- Utilitarian (e.g., in the context of satisfying personal needs, anxiety reduction, the manipulation of others for a specific goal).

There are several studies which show that all of these functions have some impact upon the drinking patterns in different cultures. The integrative function of drinking in primitive societies has been illustrated by Bunzel (48), Fields (98), Heath (148), and Simmons (328). The integrative function of drinking in complex societies has been observed by Bacon (13) who stresses that drinking integrates aggressive and competitive tendencies and supports the need for an optimal interpersonal functioning. Dollard (80), Pittman (280), Stacey and Davies (348), and Stone (344) come to similar conclusions, as does Rubington (304) who shows that even skidrow drinkers are socially integrated by certain drinking rituals and behavior patterns.

The communicative aspect of drinking, enhancing *Gemütlichkeit*, and pleasurable interaction is described by Bales (14), Bruun (46), and Clinard (58). Maddox (233) stresses the first drinking as a ritual of initiation into the world of grownups and Snyder (332) shows the ethnocentric integration of drinkers in Jewish subcultures.

Several authors focus upon the anxiety reducing function of drinking. In his often quoted cross-cultural study, Horton (163) integrates psychoanalytic and behavioral concepts. He comes to the conclusion that drinking, in all societies, primarily serves for the reduction of anxiety produced by wars, catastrophes, and acculturation, and creating contradictory situations and consequent anxiety. Simmons's (328) hypothesis that alcohol serves primarily for the reduction of expectation anxiety in social interactions goes in the same direction, as does Bacon's (13) study which stresses that modern societies, with the hierarchically organized gradient of responsibility and the status specific prestige thinking, produces more anxiety than primitive cultures.

Irgens-Jensen (170) did not confirm Horton's hypothesis in a study of rural Norway. Field (98), however, confirms Horton's hypothesis, although somewhat modifying it. He shows that acculturation can reduce anxiety by creating better life conditions.

The disintegrative function of drinking in a primitive society (e.g., Peruvian community) is described by Simmons (328). Bruun (46) and Dollard (80) describe the same function in modern societies. Although Lemert (211) assumes that drinking and alcoholism have only a disintegrative function, this view is contradicted by Stacey and Davies (340). They reject a strict correlation between heavy drinking and deviant social behavior. The latter view is questioned by the report of Wieser and Kunad (369) who emphasize that drinking can lead to total social disintegration and anomie. It seems to me that such contradictory views are due, on the one hand, to the fact that different samples were investigated and, on the other hand, to the fact that the authors do not effectively differentiate between the function of drinking (i.e., motivation) and the consequences of drinking. However, on a more general level, the cybernetic model of explanation makes linear cause-effect thinking impossible. Carefully planned cross-cultural followup studies would be very helpful in clarifying these issues.

The religious function of drinking is stressed by Fouquet (99). The ceremonial-ritual function is emphasized by Heath (148) and Snyder (332). Heath (ibid.) describes the rigorously ritualized drinking pattern of the Cambas tribe in Bolivia, which seems to be responsible for the fact that even highly concentrated alcohol does not lead to pathological behavior. Similarly, Snyder (332) shows that orthodox Jews, although having an early onset of drinking, do not have an alcoholism problem in the strict sense.

The hedonistic-convivial function of drinking for primitive cultures was stressed by Bunzel (48) and Heath (148). Bales (14) describes the convivial function of drinking among Irish Catholics, pointing out its communicative and solidarizing function. The hedonistic aspect is reported by Snyder (332) and Adler (2, p. 235) who show that alcohol diminishes the culturally determined inhibitions which block the expression of fun and pleasure. Similarly, Solms (333) points to the *chaleur communicative* which arises whenever people drink together.

In primitive cultures, the utilitarian function of drinking, in the framework of magical practices, is often preponderant. Heath (149) reports that Bolivian Cambas think that drinking "kills parasites, stomach troubles, and liver sickness." As Sangree (312) indicates, certain tribes use alcohol in order to exorcise witches.

The utilitarian function of drinking in modern society is reported by many investigators, such as Bacon (13), Globetti and Pomery (116), Horton (163), Lemert (211), Pichler (279), and Pittman (280). These authors indicate that alcohol serves as food. It is supposed to help digestion and sleep and protect against cold and fatigue. It is also taken as a medicine for the production of blood or the reduction of tensions and anxiety.

(16) Causes of Drinking. Some authors seem to favor monocausal explanations for such a complex behavior. Horton (163) holds that anxiety and Schuckit (320) that heredity is the determinant of drinking. Fields (98) critizises Horton's approach as reducing complex social phenomena to the monocausal level of emotions or "drive." According to Field (98), alcoholism in primitive society is not due to anxiety, but, rather, to the level of disorganization of social structures. Especially the lack of kinship structures, which are stabilizing, permanent, and integrating because of their clear structure and function, is a factor responsible for drinking.

In earlier publications, I stressed (cf. 123-125) that monocausal models of thinking are insufficient. I instead postulated multifactorial models of explanations for drinking and alcoholism. My views are shared by Gabriel (113), Solms (335), and especially Lundquist (232) who differentiates between genetic factors; quantity, quality and frequency of drinking; time and duration of drinking; type of drinking pattern; behavior and attitudes of the environment with respect to drinking; and occasional factors (e.g., conflicts, hard work, anxiety, depressive moods) which function as stressors triggering drinking. To this list can be added the structure of the social organization of the human system (e.g., couple, family, kinship, community, state, culture) in which drinking occurs.

10.2.3 Types of Alcoholism

Practically all the types of alcoholism referred to in international literature are based upon Jellinek (179). He differentiates between loss of control drinkers (i.e., alcohol addicts) and habitual symptomatic excessive drinkers without loss of control. Loss of control means that the drinker cannot stop drinking once he has started. For Jellinek (179), both groups are ill, although the second type drinks mostly in order to cope with individual stress. He thinks that the excessive drinker can drink even more than the alcohol addict, but that loss of control often occurs only after 30-40 years of controlled drinking. In some cases, actual loss of control does not occur at all.

Jellinek (178) also describes culturally determined subtypes of alcoholism, (e.g., the *alcoolisme sans ivresse* in France). This type presupposes the consumption of great quantities daily, but it is evenly distributed over the whole day. In contrast to this type, a drinker in the United States usually does not drink during workhours, but in the evening he drinks large quantities of highly concentrated alcohol within a short time. The typical Swiss drinker is characterized by Jellinek (178) as a "primitive hedonist" who has a rather limited field of interests. He is not interested in social interaction and drinks mostly alone. Solms (333) shows that in Switzerland there is a new type of alcoholism which has developed under the influence of the alcoholism treatment programs — it is a hidden alcoholism with rare drunkenness and difficult to observe.

Based on Jellinek's typology, Walton (361) differentiates between a "loss of control drinker" and an "inability to abstain drinker." The former, also called compulsive or gamma drinker, is addicted. He drinks in increasing cycles until physical impairment occurs. He drinks until he is totally helpless and all the available alcohol is consumed. He often displays alcohol intoxication and disorganized public behavior. The latter type, also called inveterate or delta drinker, cannot live without alcohol, but he does not need to drink excessively. Drunkenness and social disintegration do not occur. He often lives in a milieu in which regular drinking is tolerated or required. He develops a syndrome of abstinence when without alcohol.

A more complex typology, based on Jellinek and Fouquet, is proposed by Solms (333). In this typology, the degree of importance of the sociocultural influences is indicated by three, two, or one asterisks, as follows:

- Continual habitual alcohol consumption with alcoholic disorders and symptoms. It is not yet an addiction. It is typical for wine producing areas. Sociocultural influence***.
- Irregular conflict drinking of primarily abnormal personalities leading to excessive drinking or to secondary impairment due to intoxication. It is not an addiction. Typical in the United States and northern Europe. Sociocultural influence*.
- Heavy irregular drinking with frequent and, often, abnormal drunkenness, psychosocial disintegration, somatic impairment, and loss of control. It is an addiction. Typical for the United States and northern Europe. Sociocultural influence*.
- Heavy continuous drinking with few states of drunkenness. Psychosocial disintegration. Inability to abstain. Somatic impairment. It is an addiction typical for wine producing areas. Sociocultural influence**.

10.2.4 Consequences of Drinking and Alcoholism

Generally, in the international literature, psychological, somatic, social, and economic consequences of drinking are discussed. In this study, I am interested primarily in the psychosocial consequences of drinking.

As Heath (148) makes clear, extensive and repetitive drinking does not necessarily lead to manifest disorders. The tribe of the Cambas drink large amounts of highly concentrated alcohol in a rigourously ritualized way. Hangovers, hallucinations, and pathological symptoms do not occur.

To what extent the drinking patterns determine the outcome of drinking and alcoholism is also shown by Simmons (328) and Bruun (46). The latter stresses the status position of the drinker within a group as a determinant. When the prevailing drinking pattern is prohibitive, the consequences of alcoholism are more pathological, as Solms (333) observed in the United States and Stacey and Davies (340) observed in adolescents. If adolescents grow up in a prohibitive environment, they become problem drinkers more frequently than if they grow up in a permissive culture.

As Bacon (13) describes, the economic consequences of drinking and alcoholism are especially high where work distribution and work rhythm require exact timing, sensitivity, prudence, and efficiency (i.e., in industrialized areas). The same fact is stressed by Trice and Wahl (359) and Lemert (211). Lemert (211) points out the interdependence between economic productivity, high transactional speed, and a health oriented social organization which cannot tolerate alcoholism without high economic and psychosocial losses.

Finally, alcoholism may lead to deviant behavior, as pointed out by Palola et al. (267), Park (268), Pittman and Wayne (282), and Wieser and Kunard (369). Wieser and Kunard (369) differentiate between two possible criminological types — the "early" criminal for whom alcoholism is only a concomittant phenomenon and the "late" criminal for whom alcoholism plays a causal role.

10.2.5 Alcoholism in Rural Areas

Although Lemert (209) and Maddox (233) argue that the urban lifestyle produces more alcoholism than the rural, other authors point out that we do not know enough about alcoholism in rural areas. Berner (27) and Guntern (124-127) emphasize that rapid social change with industrialization and urbanization promote drinking and can lead to intensive alcoholism in rural areas.

Irgens-Jensen (170), investigating drinking in rural Norway, finds few alcoholics, but Evreux (95) reports that, in rural Britain, 63% of the adolescents are habitual cider drinkers. Berner (27) quotes a study made in rural Canton Wallis where 6.4% of the population are alcoholics. An indicator of increasing rural alcoholism is the increasing number of patients hospitalized for alcoholism, as reported by Haes (151) in rural Yemen and by Wieser and Kunad (369) in rural Germany.

The most comprehensive study concerning this question, to my knowledge, was made by Amsler (10). In interviews with 795 French general practitioners in rural areas, he found that alcoholic symptoms played a major role in 75%. Asked whether or not alcoholism in rural areas of France was increasing 50% indicated that it was stationary, 35% that it tended to increase, and 11% that it decreased.

10.3 Methods of Data Collection

The methods of data collection correspond to the general methods discussed erarlier.

The construction of the questionnaire concerning drinking and the organization of the direct field observation followed the methodological indications given by Campbell and Katona (50), Cannel and Kahn (51), and Katz (182). The direct field observation was aimed at the observation of drinking patterns and of alcoholism in situ. The questionnaire focussed on the subjective aspects, the information about age at the onset of drinking, the quantity (i.e., probands were asked how much beer, wine, and highly concentrated alcohol they drank per day), drinking customs, motives and causes, emotional reactions following drunkenness, and the evaluation of alcohol consumption of the proband, his or her partner, his or her father, and the villagers.

I simplified the quantification of alcohol because the number of probands was 120. Many of the probands were nondrinkers and most of the drinkers drank wine. For operational reasons, I defined "one glass of alcohol" as one unit. This was epidemiologically useful and could also be indicated easily by the probands. This simplification is also justifiable since the volume of alcohol in a glass of beer, wine, or hard liquor and its concentration are indirectly proportional (i.e., all three contain approximately the same amount of alcohol).

10.4 Working Hypotheses About Drinking and Results

Based upon my experience in the medical practice, the direct field observation, and the interviews with key persons, I formulated 22 working hypotheses. A few of the working hypotheses will be mentioned only briefly. Because the number of probands was too small, they did not yield significant results. The main working hypotheses posited correlations between onset, patterns, and amount of drinking.

There were 120 probands, of these, 91 indicated that they drank alcohol daily. The onset of drinking and the daily amount of alcohol consumed by the 91 regular alcohol consumers is presented in Fig. 38 and 39.

10.4.1 Value Patterns

Working Hypothesis. The villagers assume a permissive-dysfunctional attitude towards drinking (Table 25).

Results. The permissive attitude allows drinking as healthy, tolerable, and normal. The nonpermissive attitude considers it to be harmful and a sign of illness. The dysfunctional attitude holds that drinking is an unavoidable evil; it is healthy and at the same time an unavoidable evil; is normal and at the same time an unavoidable evil; or is impairing and at the same time an unavoidable evil.

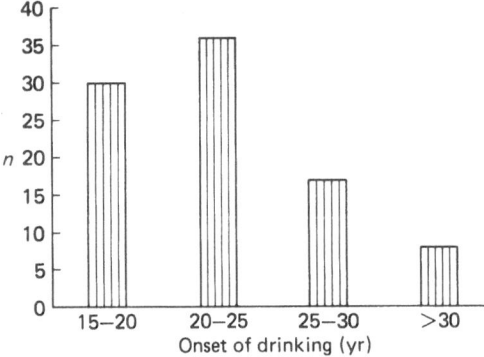

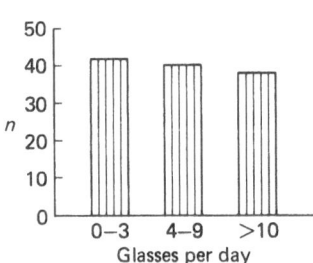

Fig. 38. The overall distribution of the onset of drinking of the regular alcohol consumers

Fig. 39. The overall distribution of the daily amount of alcohol consumed

Table 25. *Percentage distribution of the different attitudes*

Evaluation of drinking	Permissive (%)	Nonperm. (%)	Dysfunct. (%)	Nondrinker (%)	No response (%)	Total (%)	n
Own	79	6	8	7	-	100	120
Partner	60	9	7	5	19	100	94
Father	61	15	8	3	13	100	120
Villagers	20	42	35	-	3	100	120
Total	56	18	15	4	8	100	
	$x^2 = 134.10$		$p = < 0.001$				

The different categories show statistically significant differences ($p = < 0.001$). Probands have a very permissive attitude (79%) toward their own drinking. They are less permissive when the drinking of their partner or father (60-61%) is concerned. Only 20% have a permissive attitude toward the drinking of the villagers in general, 42% are nonpermissive toward the drinking of nonfamily members, and 35% describe the drinking of nonfamily members as dysfunctional.

The findings support the working hypothesis.

If we distinguish the different categories "healthy," "normal," and "tolerable," on the one hand, and "harmful" or "sick" on the other hand, we again find significant differences ($p = < 0.01$) (Table 26).

In both figures there is a continuous split between attitudes towards in-clan drinking and out-clan drinking. Social distance and the tendency to describe the other's behavior as pathological are directly proportional to each other.

Table 26. *Percentage distribution of permissive and nonpermissive attitude*

| | Permissive | | | Nonpermissive | |
| | Health | Norm. | Tol. | Harm-ful | Sick |
	(%)	(%)	(%)	(%)	
Own	19	28	32	6	-
Partner	15	23	23	5	4
Father	13	28	20	11	4
Villagers	-	4	16	27	15
	$\chi^2 = 19.29$		$p = < 0.01$		

10.4.2 Age and Value Patterns

Working Hypothesis. Younger age groups have a more permissive attitude than older age groups.

Results. There is a highly significant correlation ($p = < 0.001$) between the different categories of value patterns and the age groups (Table 27).

Table 27. *Percentage distribution of the value patterns per age group*

	Permissive (%)	Non-perm. (%)	Dysfunctional (%)	%	n
Older	30	2	4	36	43
Younger	37	1	2	40	48
	$\chi^2 = 18.71$		$p = < 0.001$		

The older group has twice as many nondrinkers (8%) than the younger group (4%). The permissive attitude in the younger age groups is higher, while the nonpermissive and dysfunctional attitudes show an inversed pattern.

The findings support our working hypothesis.

N.B. The number of nonresponses and nondrinkers is indicated only if they highlight a point.

10.4.3 Value Patterns and Amount

Working Hypothesis. The consumption of alcohol is high when the value pattern is permissive, and vice versa.

Results. There were no significant correlations between early onset of drinking and value pattern. The drinking pattern, however, changes with the value pattern. Whereas

234

only 4% of the probands with a permissive value pattern drink alone, 14% of the probands with a nonpermissive value pattern drink alone.

The correlation between permissive-nonpermissive value patterns and the amount of daily alcohol consumption is given in Table 28.

Table 28. *The distribution of the daily amount of drinking in relation to the value patterns*

Evaluation	Drinking quantity (glasses/day)	%	n
Healthy	4- 5	16	19
Normal	5- 6	23	28
Tolerable custom	6- 7	25	30
Harmful	15-16	4	5
Total	6- 7	68	82
	$\rho = 0.98$ $p = < 0.001$		

The result falsifies the working hypothesis. People with a permissive attitude drink less than people with a nonpermissive attitude. The results fit, however, with certain field observations – the more a person is convinced of the utilitarian function of drinking, the more he drinks in a regular and highly controlled way; the more a person drinks in an uncontrolled way, the more he is convinced that drinking is harmful, but unavoidable.

10.4.4 Age of Female Alcohol Consumers

Working Hypothesis. The daily alcohol consumption of younger female drinkers (15-45 years old) is higher than the daily consumption of older female drinkers (45-75 years old).

Results. There are highly significant correlations ($p = < 0.001$) between age and drinking, as shown in Table 29.

Table 29. *Distribution of the daily consumption of alcohol in the two female age groups*

	Drinking quantity (glasses/day)				%	n
	1-6	7-12	13-15	Average		
Older group	81	19	-	2-3	15	17
Younger Group	52	44	4	5	17	19
Total	65	33	2	4-5	32	36
	$t = 7.84$		$p = < 0.001$			

The working hypothesis is supported by the results.

10.4.5 Early Childhood Environment

Working Hypothesis. Probands from disturbed early childhood environment drink more than others.

Results. There is a highly significant correlation ($p = < 0.001$) between early childhood milieu and drinking, as shown in Table 30.

Table 30. *Distribution of the daily consumption of alcohol in relation to the early childhood environment*

Environment	Drinking quantity (glasses/day)	%	n
Undisturbed	5-6	66	79
Disturbed	6-9	10	12
Total	6-7	76	91
	$\rho = 0.96$	$p = < 0.001$	

Probands with an undisturbed early childhood (i.e., both parents alive and together) drink lower quantities than probands from a disturbed childhood environment.

There is also a highly significant correlation ($p = < 0.001$) between the quality of the marriage of the parents of the probands and their own alcohol consumption. Probands who indicate that their parents' marriage was "good" drink 5-6 glasses per day, probands who indicate that it was "unconspicuous" drink 6-7 glasses per day, and probands who indicate that it was "troubled" drink 9-10 glasses per day.

The findings support the working hypothesis.

10.4.6 Developmental Problems and Amount

Working Hypothesis. There is a positive correlation between developmental problems of childhood and the daily amount of drinking.

Results. There are significant correlations ($p = < 0.001$) between the number of developmental problems (e.g., enuresis, nail biting, encopresis, pavor nocturnus, stuttering, temper tantrums, isolation, educational problems, stealing) of the probands and their daily consumption of alcohol. Probands who indicate none of the above problems drink 5-6 glasses per day, probands who indicate one of the above problems drink 7 glasses per day, and probands who indicate 2 or more of the above problems drink 7-8 glasses per day.

The findings support the working hypothesis.

10.4.7 Early Onset of Drinking and Amount

Working Hypothesis. Early onset of drinking correlates positively with the daily amount of drinking. The earlier a proband begins to drink the more he drinks.

Results. There is a highly significant correlation ($p = < 0.001$). Probands who started to drink at the ages of 15-20 drink 8 glasses per day and probands who started to drink between the age of 25-30 drink 4-5 glasses per day.

The findings support the working hypothesis.

10.4.8 Age of Wife and Amount of Husband's Drinking

Working Hypothesis. Men married to an older partner drink more than men married to a younger partner.

Results. There is no significant correlation between the age of female partner and the daily amount of drinking.

The working hypothesis is not supported by the findings.

10.4.9 Sex

Working Hypothesis. Men drink much more than women.

Results. There is a highly significant correlation ($p = < 0.001$). On the average, men drink 8 glasses of alcohol per day while women drink 4-5 glasses per day.

10.4.10 Living Conditions

Working Hypothesis. There is a correlation between living condition and drinking; the better a proband lives the less he drinks.

Results. There is a highly significant correlation ($p = < 0.001$) between number of available rooms and daily amount of drinking. The more rooms a proband has the more he drinks. This correlation is difficult to interpret and is probably purely accidental.

There is no significant correlation between the type of apartment, own house, own business, or rented house and drinking. And there is no significant correlation between whether or not probands are satisfied or dissatisfied with their dwellings and their daily amount of drinking.

The working hypothesis is falsified.

10.4.11 Parental Social Status

Working Hypothesis. Parental social status of a proband and his daily alcohol consumption are indirectly proportial.

Results. There is a significant correlation ($p = < 0.05$) between the social status of the parents and the daily alcohol consumption of probands. Probands who indicate that their parents social level is above average drink 6 glasses per day, probands who indicate that it is average drink 6-7 glasses per day; and probands who indicate that it is below average drink 8-9 glasses per day.

The findings support the working hypothesis.

10.4.12 Economic Change

Working Hypothesis. Probands who have undergone an economic change since 1951 drink more than others.

Results. There is no significant correlation between the daily alcohol consumption and economic change, although a trend supports the working hypothesis. Probands who had an economic improvement before 1951 drink 4-5 glasses per day, whereas probands with an economic improvement after 1951 drink 6-7 glasses per day.

10.4.13 Functional Competence

Working Hypothesis. A gap between the educational level and the level of required performance is a stressor which increases the daily alcohol consumption.

Results. There is a highly significant correlation ($p = <0.001$). Probands who indicate a "good" education drink 7 glasses per day, while probands who indicate a satisfactory or nonsatisfactory education drink only 5 glasses per day.

The result falsifies the working hypothesis. It also contradicts the findings of the field observation. It is possible that younger drinkers who drink both in more quantity and more often and have a good education are responsible for this result.

10.4.14 Work Conditions

Working Hypothesis. Role accumulation and unsatisfying work conditions increase the amount of drinking.

Results. There is no significant correlation; however, there is a tendency for the consumption of alcohol to increase when the number of jobs increases. Probands with one job drink 5 glasses per day, probands with two jobs drink 7 glasses, and probands with 3 jobs drink 7-8 glasses per day.

There is, however, a highly significant correlation ($p = <0.001$) between the type of occupation and the daily drinking. Probands who are strictly housewives or housewives with one additional job drink 4 glasses per day; probands who are merchants, artisans, workers, ski instructors, or hotel managers drink 7-8 glasses per day; and probands who are farmers, mountain guides, innkeepers, or hotel managers plus one additional job (e.g., mountain guide, artisan, or ski instructor) drink 10 glasses per day.

The results confirm the working hypothesis.

10.4.15 Drinking Patterns

Working Hypothesis. Integrated drinking patterns decrease drinking, while disintegrated drinking patterns increase drinking.

Results. There is a highly significant correlation ($p = <0.001$) between the number of combined drinking patterns (e.g., drinking alone, while eating, with work collegues, with drinking buddies, with guests) and the daily consumption of alcohol. Probands who indicate one drinking pattern drink 2 glasses per day, probands who indicate 2 drinking patterns drink 5 glasses per day, and probands who indicate 3-4 drinking pattern drink 8-9 glasses per day.

There is also a significant correlation ($p = < 0.05$) between the type of drinking pattern and the daily amount of drinking. Probands who have a tendency to drink alone drink maximal quantities (i.e., 8 glasses per day), probands who drink mostly while eating drink the lowest quantity (i.e., 5 glasses per day), and probands who drink with collegues and guests or with collegues and guest and alone drink average quantities (i.e., 7-8 glasses per day).

The results support the working hypothesis.

10.4.16 Emotional Reactions After Drunkenness

Working Hypothesis. The smaller the number of indicated emotional reactions after drunkenness, the greater the amount of drinking.

Results. There is a highly significant correlation ($p = < 0.001$) between emotional reactions and drinking. Probands who indicate no emotional reactions drink 5 glasses per day, probands who indicate 1-2 emotional reactions (e.g., religiously motivated feelings of culpability, concern for health, culpability vis-à-vis partner or other persons) drink 7-8 glasses per day, and probands who indicate 3-4 of the above reactions drink 9 glasses per day.

The working hypothesis is falsified. Although these results contradict my field observation, they fit with a general clinical experience, namely that drinkers find themselves in a vicious circle of emotional reactions, self-accusations, and drinking.

10.4.17 Motivations

Working Hypothesis. The smaller the number and the more socially accepted the type of motivation for drinking, the smaller the amount of daily alcohol consumption.

Results. There is no significant correlation ($p = > 0.10$) between the number of certain motivations (i.e., anxiety, anger, inhibition, isolation, boredom, habitude, opportunity) and the daily amount of drinking.

There is a significant correlation ($p = < 0.05, > 0.02$) between the number of certain motivations (e.g., longing for togetherness, desire to be anesthesized, wish to be drunk, increase of performance, solution for sexual inhibitions, relief of aggressivity, display of virility) and the daily amount of drinking. Probands who indicate 2 or more of these motivations drink 9-10 glasses.

There is also a significant correlation ($p = < 0.05, \geq 0.02$) between the type of motivation and the daily consumption of alcohol. Probands who indicate the motivations "anger in work or marriage" and "wish for stupefaction" drink 5-6 glasses per day; probands who indicate the motivations "resolution of aggressiveness," "isolation," "opportunity," "increase of performance," and "longing for solidarity and togetherness" drink 7 glasses per day, probands who indicate "opportunity," "anxiety," "display of virility," and "resolution of sexual tensions" drink 8-9 glasses per day; and probands who indicate "anger in business," "desire for stupefaction," "inhibition," and "boredom" drink 10 glasses per day.

The findings falsify the working hypothesis as far as the number of motivations is concerned. They partly support the working hypothesis as far as the type of motivations is concerned.

10.4.18 Nonelaborated Working Hypotheses

Five of 22 working hypotheses could not be elaborated. For two, a sufficient control sample was lacking. The correlation between social mobility or work order and drinking yielded no significant results. The correlation between sexual behavior and drinking could not be elaborated because the majority of the probands did not answer the questions on this issue.

10.4.19 Results of the Direct Field Observation

Some field observations modify or complement the results of the questionnaire:

— In many cases, the amount of drinking indicated was lower than the actual consumption observed by the partner, another family member, or by myself. There is a general, conscious or unconscious, tendency of dissimulation. We can assume that the daily amount of alcohol is between one-fifth and one-third higher than the proband indicated.
— The type of drinking observed in the village corresponds to the type of *"alcoolisme sans ivresse"* described by Jellinek (178) (i.e., to drink small amounts during the whole day). Many villagers are continuously slightly drunk and a few are heavily drunk in the evening.
— I observed three different types of female drinkers. One group, between 18-25 years old, visited a number of bars, inns, and dancehalls, where they drunk and sometimes got drunk. Some villagers critizised these women and others showed resignation vis-à-vis a new and seemingly unavoidable trend. The second group was composed of married women who usually went to only one or two specific bars where they drank and sometimes got drunk. The third group was composed of married women who accompanied their husbands to bars, inns, and dancehalls. They all drank and sometimes got drunk. All three groups were composed of from two to five individuals. In general, the drinking behavior of the women was more controlled than the drinking behavior of the men. Since the women's behavior was conspicuous, it was noticed. This should be emphasized to put the facts into the right perspective. The three groups indicated more of a tendency than a serious problem.
— According to the direct field observation, in 1970, there were 45 men (i.e., 5.6% of the population) and 3 women (i.e., 0.3% of the population) considered alcoholics, according to the WHO definition.

10.4.20 Interviews of Key Persons

The key informants yielded results which usually corresponded with the results of the questionnaire and the direct field observation.

All key informants agreed on several basic questions — that the drinking began after 1951, the villagers drink too much, the tendency to drink increases every year, the younger generations drink more than the older, and women drink increasingly more and increasingly more women drink.

10.5 Discussion of Results

The overall results confirm the first field impression of 1968 – there is a considerable and measurably high consumption of alcohol in the village.

More than half of the sample who indicates drinking alcohol (cf. p. 232) drink approximately three-quarters liter per day. In fact, the actual alcohol consumption is one-fifth to one-third higher than indicated by the probands. This fact is confirmed by yet another observation – among the 12% of the probands who do not indicate drinking, there are some well-known alcoholics. Thus, in 1970, the factual amount of drinking is above average.

Some of these partial results shall be discussed more extensively below in the process of comparing them to the findings of the international literature.

10.5.1 Permissive-Dysfunctional Attitude Toward Drinking

According to Pittman (280) the paradoxical permissive-dysfunctional attitude about drinking is found most frequently in modern industrialized societies which have experienced social change. Saas-Fee has experienced a major social change since 1951 and has, in 1970, a permissive-dysfunctional attitude towards drinking and drunkenness.

Approximately 80% of the probands have a permissive attitude towards their own drinking; however, it is accompanied by a nonpermissive attitude towards the drinking of fathers, partners, or, especially, outclan villagers. It appears that drinking behavior is measured with different parameters. Possibly, the accusations about the behavior of other villagers serves as an outlet for aggressiveness.

Approximately 35% of the probands have a dysfunctional attitude towards the drinking of the villagers. They describe it as a sign of illness or as physically and psychologically harmful. At the same time, they assume that it is an unavoidable evil. In practice, this means that drinking and drunkenness are simultaneously condemned and excused; accepted at a behavioral level and rejected at a verbal level. The drinker is seen as a victim of unfortunate circumstances. His behavior is not considered deviant from the norm and, therefore, is not sanctioned.

The divergence of the different parameters of judgment (cf. p. 233) fits with similar observations of Globetti and Pomery (116), who show that different towns in the same American district had different attitudes and value patterns towards drinking. Saas-Fee shows different value patterns not only within the village but also within the same individual, depending on whose behavior is being judged; a pattern which is as old as human kind. In fact, it is already reported in the Bible.

It seems obvious that this coexistence of different value patterns and the prevalence of the permissive-dysfunctional attitude is due to rapid social change. The key informants indicate that there was a nonpermissive attitude before 1951, a claim substantiated by the old chronicles. In 1970, this nonpermissive attitude is found especially in older women (cf. p. 233). Younger persons drink more than older persons. Younger women drink larger amounts than older women. Younger women have fewer nondrinkers than older women. Younger women, as well as younger men, have a tendency to drink increasingly highly concentrated liquors (e.g., whisky, cognac, gin) instead of wine, the preferred drink of the older generations.

All these changes and contradictions in the value patterns are interdependent with social change and, especially, with acculturation. After 1951, the number of stressors increased and heavy drinking developed into a strategy for coping with stress. Such a goal, of course, influences tha value patterns and makes them more permissive. Still, the syngenetic program of most of the villagers in 1970 is composed of an agglomerate of integrated and nonintegrated value patterns. As long as this patchwork exists, the set of rules governing behavior in general and drinking in particular will be contradictory, as will be the behavior itself. This assumption is substantiated by the result (cf. p. 234) which shows that probands with high permissiveness drink the least, while probands with nonpermissiveness drink maximal quantities.

Contradictions and value patterns are generators of stressors inducing stress. Since drinking is a strategy for coping with stress, the vicious circle will continue until the social contradictions are resolved or other major sources of stressor production are eliminated. This can become reality as soon as the village has adapted sufficiently to its new structural roles.

10.5.2 Influence of Early Childhood Environment and Socioeconomic Level

10.5.2.1 Birth Order and Drinking

The claim that there is a correlation between drinking and birth order, as reported by Barry and Blane (15) and Navratil (263), is not substantiated by my findings.

10.5.2.2 Family Structure and Drinking

The role of the "broken home" or the disorganized family structure, stressed by Jackson (173), Park (268), Schuckit (320), and Warder and Ross (362), is corroborated by my findings; however, there was no divorced or separated couple in the village. On the other hand, the overorganized family, mentioned by Koenig (196), and families whose personality inventory was changed by death were found to influence the drinking behavior. Probands whose parents died before they were 15 drank more than those who lost one or both parents after this age.

Probands who described the marriage of their parents as good drank less (cf. p. 235). Another finding shows (cf. p. 235) that the number of neurotic symptoms or developmental problems which are clearly related to the family structure increase the consumption of alcohol in a linear way.

The direct field observation showed that the alcoholics came from a family whose structure had a redundant process pattern and was distinctly dysfunctional. The typical family background of the male alcoholic involved an indulged childhood, the early onset of drinking, and a conflictful parental marriage. The marital conflict blocked the parents from taking a joint, firm, and unequivocal stand against the son's drinking. Once becoming an adult, the male alcoholic married a woman from outside the village — invariably an active and energetic person who dominated the household and their tourist business. The more she took over, the more her husband could regress and drink. The more he regressed and drank, the more she was motivated to take over. Finally, the husband was maneuvred, and maneuvred himself, into a marginal position. From this position, he would sometimes noisily interfere, but most of the time he would remain gloomily apart and mutter about "lack of respect." This lack of respect was displayed in disguised ways by his wife who had, in the meantime, accumulated responsibilities, functions, and decisionmaking powers and, more directly, by his children who tended to refer to him as a "poor devil."

He drowned his own lack of self-esteem in alcohol, but his drunken behavior triggered responses from the environment which further decreased his low self-esteem. From time to time, he would pathetically announce a "total change." The family, however, would be skeptical about his motivation and his ability to overcome the drinking. Their attitude made him angry and irritable. Soon, both he and the family wished he would drink again. Thus, he found himself in a whirlpool of self-defeating currents, a labyrinth of self-constructed and family-constructed traps, and, eventually, he would give up and return to drinking. As soon as this happened, the stress of the family decreased. Mother would function smoothly in the economic sector, the children would avoid "the poor devil," and he would avoid the family. Thus, the family homeostasis was maintained, though in a dysfunctional way. A similar process of social schizmogenesis in the Jatmul tribe in New Guinea was observed by Bateson (16, p. 171 ff).

Once again, we are faced with a paradoxical reality which is partly due to the syngenetic approach. There is both a intrafamilial acceptance and rejection and there is both an extrafamilial acceptance and rejection of the drinker. According to the adopted vantage point, one of the complementary aspects seems to be all important while the other fades out.

10.5.2.3 Dwelling Conditions

The dwelling conditions in the village correlate with the drinking behavior. Probands who live in a rented apartment (cf. p. 236) drink more than those who live in their own house. Mostly, probands in a rented apartment belong to the lower economic class and, therefore, they have to cope with a greater number of stressors. As discussed before, it is difficult to interpret the fact (cf. p. 236) that probands in apartments with many rooms drink more than probands in apartments with fewer rooms. The finding might be a pure statistical coincidence or might be dependent upon unknown variables.

There is a tendency (cf. p. 236) for probands who evaluate their dwelling conditions as nonoptimal to drink more than others. Actually, there are no major differences in the dwelling conditions of the villagers. Thus, their behavior can be little affected by the generally satisfying dwelling situation.

10.5.2.4 Socioeconomic Level

Although it is difficult to differentiate social levels in the village, I constructed three socioeconomic groups according to these criteria — income, prestige, status, education, and actual occupational role. I found the following correlations: probands of the lower socioeconomic level drink most and probands of the upper socioeconomic level drink least (cf. p. 236).

The socioeconomic level of the parents (cf. p. 236) correlates with the drinking behavior — probands whose parents belong to the upper social level drink least and probands whose parents belong to the lower social level drink most.

There is no direct correlation between drinking and social mobility. Such a correlation, discussed by Dollard (80), is, however, indirectly confirmed by my findings (cf. p. 237). There is a tendency for probands who have experienced a socioeconomic amelioration after 1951 to drink more than others. Since most of the people have experienced an economic takeoff after 1951, accumulating debts at the same time, it is difficult to judge to what extent someone has bettered or worsened his economic position. Moreover, all experienced the same social change and the same stressors, but not all drank. This illustrates that the economic situation is only one factor in a web of interconnected factors which have a determining influence upon drinking.

10.5.3 Age, Sex, and Drinking

Figure 38 (cf. p. 232) shows that the majority of the drinkers had started drinking by the age of 15-20. Drinkers with an early onset (cf. p. 236) drink twice as much as drinkers with an onset after 25. This finding corroborates similar findings by Foulds and Hassal (cf. 362) about the negative influence of early onset. Early onset in the village is increasingly stimulated by the general availability of alcohol; the high number of inns, bars, and restaurants; and the paradoxical value patterns of villagers, guests, and employees.

The alcohol consumption of men is much higher than that of women (cf. p. 236). The female population has five times more nondrinkers and the drinking quantity of men to women is 1.8 to 1. Younger women drink more than older women (cf. p. 234) and they increasingly drink highly concentrated alcohol. This points to an increasing number of female alcoholics in the future.

Using the WHO definition, the village has 45 men and 3 women alcoholics. The difference (i.e., 15 to 1) is an indicator of the women's abstinence in earlier times, since it takes 15-20 or more years until the manifestations of alcoholism become easily observable.

I agree with Falk (96) that female alcohol consumption increases proportionally to the extent to which women are integrated into the economic process. The correlation between the hidden matriarchy in the village and female alcoholism, also observed in another context by Becker (20), is obvious. A glass of alcohol is a "medicine" against arising problems, available in every house and tourist business. Women and men function more fluently in multiple interactions when slightly inebriated. The operant conditioning provided by drinking, positive feedback of guests, and relaxation leads to a vicious circle. This vicious circle might, however, be interrupted by, as yet, unknown factors with a counterimpact.

10.5.4 Work Conditions and Drinking

Contrary to my expectations, there was no significant correlation between the accumulation of jobs and drinking (cf. p. 237); however, the direct field observation made it clear that the number of indicated jobs does not necessarily correlate with the intensity of work. Many an innkeeper is an occasional ski instructor, mountain guide, or laborer. When he indicates several professions or jobs, he does not necessarily indicate the accumulation of functions and intensity of work, although it may be assumed.

There is a highly significant correlation between the type of job or occupation and drinking (cf. p. 237). Women who are only housewives drink the least. Merchants, artisans, laborers, ski instructors, and hotel managers drink slightly above average quantity.

The highest alcohol consumption is found among farmers, mountain guides, innkeepers, and hoteliers; the latter with an additional profession. Farmers drink more than artisans. This result is in contrast to the results of Wieser and Kunad (369). The difference might be related to the different samples investigated — Wieser and Kunad (369) studied alcoholics while I investigated a normal population.

It is easy to understand why innkeepers and hoteliers with an additional job drink maximal quantities. It is less obvious why farmers and mountain guides drink maximal quantities. My explanations for this phenomenon (cf. 124, 125) are briefly outlined:

- Hard physical work creates thirst. Thirsty men in a wine culture — the Canton Wallis is famous for its wine production — drink wine.
- Agriculture is in a crisis and so are those few farmers (i.e., 1% in 1970) who did not adapt to social change by moving into the service sector.

Berner (27) observed that social change in rural areas is a factor of risk which can induce farmers to drink. Some farmers, by selling land, became rich. To become rich overnight can unbalance the homeostasis of a person or family. The traditional character of the farmer, bred over centuries, did not easily permit him to socialize with strangers invading the village and, thus, the leap into the new era was not always possible. Alcoholism and drinking are simultaneously indicators and results of the farmers' dysfunctional adaptation.

It is, however, astonishing that mountain guides drink maximal quantities. They belong to a profession traditionally looked upon as requiring sober individuals full of strength and self-control. Why then do they drink?

The several explanations for this phenomenon are complementary. In 1970, the mountain guides were in a crisis. In 1952, the village had 61 mountain guides of a total population of approximately 520 (i.e., one-eight of all the Swiss mountain guides). In 1959, although the population had increased there was only half the number of mountain guides left and, by 1970, this number had further decreased. Why did this happen?

The classical time for mountain climbing was coming to an end. Ambitious climbers now attacked mountains in the Himalayas. The Alps did not offer enough challenge any more. Moreover, Switzerland had developed a great number of climbing schools which taught the younger generations the technical skills. Once trained, they did not need guides. The repercussions of this process produced a disillusioned group of guides who rarely went on an interesting expedition any more. Most of them were busy heaving overweight people up the run-of-the-mill peak, the Allalinhorn, which an average person can easily climb alone. Such tours, sometimes repeated daily, became boring which, in itself, is a factor of risk leading to drinking, as much as the professional crisis does.

- Mountain climbing is dependent on weather. Rainy days force the guides to wait in a mountain cabin or in the village. They lose guests and income temporarily and they become demoralized.
- Among the drinkers who identified themselves as mountain guides were a few who had given up mountain climbing long ago. Since these former guides often drank maximal quantities, they artificially increased the amount of drinking of the actual mountain guides.
- Mountain guides tend to have a schizoid personality or a high unconscious anxiety level. Reich (292) convincingly demonstrated that exposure to physical danger diminishes the existential

danger; the inner anxiety. Mountain guides are rather withdrawn and timid. When put into social contexts, the drink to "loosen up." Alcohol successfully reduces their general and anticipatory anxiety (i.e., anxiety in anticipation of impending social interaction), as discussed by Bacon (13), Horton (163), and Simmons (328).
- Mountain guides work during the summer. In winter, they are laid off or take up another job, a fact which can create dissatisfaction. Job dissatisfaction is a factor of risk for drinking.
- McCord and McCord (244) suggest the most convincing hypothesis. They found that boys, overadapted to the virility ideal of a society, are most likely to become alcoholics.

Up to the time of the construction of the road, the profession of a mountain guide was considered to be the most virile occupation. Men, complying with the virility ideal of the village, chose this profession. They had to repress the character traits which did not conform to the expected role pattern. In doing so, they built up a dysfunctional homeostasis which had to be kept in equilibrium by any means available. When decompensation of the dysfunctional homeostasis threatened, drinking seemed to resolve the problems. Drinking permitted regression and the display of "feminine" behavior. They could display emotions and, at the same time, "drink like a man." Thus, accepted and repressed character traits could be expressed at the same time. Drinking became a possible strategy to deal with an impossible situation, a double bind (cf. 18) in which there was no way to win.

10.5.5 Drinking Patterns and Function of Drinking

As expected, the indicated drinking patterns influenced drinking both quantitatively and qualitatively. The most striking drinking pattern of the village is the "paying a round," as discussed earlier.

The more drinking pattern a proband indicates (cf. p. 237), the higher is his consumption of alcohol. A proband who drinks alone (cf. p. 237) drinks maximal quantities. A proband who drinks in an integrated way (e.g., during meals), drinks the smallest quantity. These findings correspond to similar findings reported by Maddox (233) and Pittman and Snyder (281).

The function of drinking can be deduced from the direct field observation of from the number and pattern of motivations indicated in the questionnaire. The consumption of alcohol increases with the number of indicated motivations (cf. p. 238). The quality of the motivations also plays a determining role. Probands who drink because they are angry, they wish to get drunk, or they are inhibited or bored, drink maximal quantities. Anger in business is a daily experience during the season, as is boredom during the interseason. Both, the overstimulation and the understimulation foster the wish to "get high" or "drunk" in order to escape.

Bacon (13) points out that the integrative function of alcohol is very important in modern industrialized societies. Alcohol consumption in the village, plays a major role in the integration of aggressive competition. Its centrifugal forces have to be socially bound so that the Pearl of the Alps can maintain its Arcadian image, undisturbed by the cracks of social conflict. Drinking, then, and especially drinking together, becomes a strategy and a ritual of social survival, although a dysfunctional one. These considerations support the discussions by Bacon (13), Bales (14), Bruun (46), Clinard (58), Dollard (80), and Pittman (280).

The communicative-solidarizing function of convivial drinking, described by Bales (14), plays a major role in the contact with the guests. Drinking helps to overcome interactional inhibitions. Inhibition, as we have seen, is indicated by the probands as a major motivation for drinking.

The anxiety reducing function of alcohol, described especially by Horton (163), plays a major role in the village, although it is not frequently indicated. Since anxiety is usually unconscious, it cannot be elicited by a questionnaire. Indeed, as I observed, the level of anxiety in the village was high, and there is reason enough for it. The cultural lag (i.e., individuals living in a world with many contradictory beliefs, ideas, and value patterns) is a threatening situation. Financial indebtedness and the economic dependence on the political and economic situation of Europe, and the entire western world, makes the village vulnerable and induces anxiety. Almost 90% of the sample indicated that an economic crisis would harm or even ruin them.

Simmons (328) emphasizes that alcohol reduces the anxiety of expected social interaction. This seems to be an important reason for the villagers to drink so much. Their generally insufficient education, their lack of speaking foreign languages, and their traditional character traits of mountain dwellers does not function in favor of easy talk and smooth social functioning. They mistrust the urban *Gruezini* (linguistically derived from *gruezi,* a Swiss German word for "hello," a label coined for extracantonal Swiss citizens). In the late afternoons, when the tourists come back from their mountain trips, the villagers "grease up" in order to glide more easily out of the paralyzing grip of inhibitions.

Drinking, in summary, fulfills anxiety reducing, integrative, hedonistic, convivial, communicative-solidarizing, and utilitaristic functions at the same time. The overall function, however, is to enable themselves to reach the goals of every tourist resort — to satisfy the guests in order to make good business and survive.

10.6 Alcoholism

10.6.1 Quantitative Aspects

Given the high alcohol consumption, one can expect that alcoholism, as defined by the WHO, is very high. The direct field observation yielded the following: 45 men (i.e., 5.6% of the population) and 3 women (i.e., 0.3% of the population) are alcoholics. Since I applied the WHO definition in a very restricted sense, these data are probably at the lower limit of reality.

According to offical data, in 1970, 2% of the Swiss population were alcoholics. The village had an alcoholism rate three times higher than the whole of Switzerland. This is a significant difference, but, compared to the amount of drinking, even these 5.0% seem to be a low number. How can this fact be explained?
- Heath (148) showed, in a highly interesting study, that extreme and repetitive drinking and drunkenness do not lead, eo ipso, to pathological consequences, given that the drinking occurs in a ritualized and socially integrated manner. In the village, people drink mainly while eating, in a highly ritualized form with guests, in the "pay a round" ritual, and with villagers during the festivities and events organized by clubs,

associations, and political parties. Such integration protects against a depraved career of alcoholics which would lead to social ostracism.

— Berner (27), Gabriel (113), Pichler (270), Solms (333), and Pittman and Snyder (281) stress that drinking, if it corresponds to the prevailing value patterns of a society, is less pathological than if it contradicts the value patterns. I have described before the villagers' permissive-dysfunctional attitude (cf. p. 240) toward drinking. A drinker in the village is not expelled from society, but is, instead, accepted or even pitied. This value pattern protects him from getting into the ever escalating spiral of drinking-shame-culpability and more drinking.

— Another reason why the village has a great number of heavy drinkers, but relatively few alcoholics, lies in an economic stituation which tends to protect drinkers. The work situation is such that most of the jobs can be done while slightly drunk and, thus, the consequences of drinking at work are not immediately apparent or punished. A few jobs (e.g., technicians) demand exact timing, high precision, and differentiated coordination. In these jobs, the drinker is quickly fired when his performance declines. Most of the villagers, however, have jobs like innkeeper, ski instructor, or merchant. It does not matter if they are slightly inebriated. When the men who hold these jobs are utterly drunk, their wives or somebody from the kinship network takes over. Moreover, they do not risk being fired because most of the villagers own the facilities they work in.

— As Warder and Ross (362) and Wieser and Kunad (369) stress, the disturbing manifestations and heavy consequences of alcoholism often become apparent only after 20-30 years of drinking.

Heavy drinking in the village started in 1951 and my field observation took place 19 years after this event. Thus, the next cross-sectional study, in 1980, will probably reveal many more alcoholics. This supposition is justified by the development shown in Tab. 34 (cf. p. 284), which indicates that the number of hospitalizations for alcoholism is increasing.

10.6.2 Types of Alcoholism

The types of alcoholism in the village corresponds to the *alcoolisme sans ivresse* (i.e., drinking without drunkenness), described by Jellinek (178). People drink smaller or greater quantities, mor or less evenly distributed over the day, getting increasingly inebriated as the day proceeds. This type does not correspond, however, to the "primitive-hedonist" type, described by Jellinek (178), and supposed to be typical for Switzerland. As we have seen, drinking and alcoholism fulfill a complex set of functions in the village. Contrary to the drinker with loss of control, described by Jellinek (179), the drinker with control is prevalent in the village. Most of the villagers are able to abstain from alcohol when major negotiations are in view.

The comparison with the typology of Solms (cf. p. 239) is more difficult. The village has no wine production, but it is part of the Canton Wallis which is well-known for its wine. To drink in a region whose economy is based, in part, on the production of alcohol is virtually a patriotic duty.

The drinker of Saas-Fee best resembles the habitual drinker with alcohol intoxication typical for a wine producing area. He is heavily influenced by socioeconomic factors.

10.7 Final Remarks

The village has a severe alcohol problem. It shares this problem with many tourist resorts in the area. The reasons for alcoholism are manifold. Some might decrease and others increase in the future. The next cross-sectional study will falsify or support my assumption that alcoholism in Saas-Fee will increase in general, but especially in young people and women, at least until the cultural lag decreases.

Alcoholism, in 1970, seems to be mainly a sex-specific coping strategy for men. Like many other strategies, it helps for the immediate relief of distress, but becomes self-defeating in the long run.

Once the village has successfully adapted to social change, either because its speed slows down or because, in the meantime, several generations will have learned to adapt to social change, the consumption of alcohol will decrease. This, at least, is what one could expect. Life teaches us, however, that coping strategies are often maintained beyond the point where the purpose is reached.

11. Consumption of Drugs

11.1 Introduction

The experience in the general practice and the direct field observation suggested that drug consumption constituted only a minor health problem in the village.

However, it is well-known that drug consumers have a tendency to dissimulate their consumption, if strictly prohibitive value patterns govern drug consumption. The dissimulation tendency is important in the contact with the doctor because he usually warns, or is expected to warn, the patient against drug abuse. In the function of the village doctor, it is quite possible that I did not fully perceive the extent to which the drug consumption was a problem.

The dissimulation tendency was less severe where tranquillizers were concerned, because the patients had to ask for a prescription. I knew, however, that many villagers illegally got tranquillizers in different pharmacies. The attitude towards tranquillizer consumption was permissive. The publicity of pharmaceutical industries created the impression that there was no danger of addiction. Tranquillizers were mostly consumed by overworked women who did not drink.

In one case, a mother reported that she put tranquillizers into the milk of her baby to quiet him "since the guests hated his screaming." This might have been an exceptional case or the indicator of a more frequent hidden habit.

The flood of modern drugs (e.g., cannabis, hallucinogens, opiates), which reached Switzerland towards the end of the 1960s, had not yet reached the village in 1970. The geographic distance from the urban drug scene, the relatively strong religious bonds, the conservative value patterns, and the low consumption of medical drugs by the older generations were protective factors blocking the influx of illegal drugs. A few years later, this hypothesis was gradually disproven by events. Tourist resorts became the places for drug dealing. The modern drugs came via seaports into the major cities and then up onto the mountains, into the tourist resorts, and only from there did they flow back to the cities. Thus, in the light of the later developments, the situation in 1970 depicted here has to interpreted cautiously.

11.2 International Literature

I briefly will discuss the literature relevant for our purpose. Pharmacodynamic aspects of drug consumption and different types of drugs will not be discussed.

11.2.1 Definitions

According to Kielholz and Ladewig (186, p. 11), a drug is defined as a substance which is able to change one or more functions within an organism. Psychoactive drugs have a special influence upon the central nervous system.

According to the definition of WHO (cf. 186, p. 12), drug dependence is a state of psychological or psychic and physical dependence on a substance which influences the central nervous system and which is taken temporarily or continuously.

Drug abuse (186, p. 13) is the consumption of a drug without medical indication or in an excessive way.

11.2.2 Types of Drug Dependence

Kielholz et al. (187, p. 499) points out that pharmacological viewpoints permit a differentiation of seven types of drug — morphine, barbiturate-alcohol, cocaine, cannabis, amphetamine, khat, and hallucinogens. All seven types create a psychic dependence and, some of them (e.g., morphine), also a somatic dependence.

11.2.3 Causes of Drug Dependence

The main motivations for drug consumption are pleasure, increasing performance, avoidance of disagreable states or pain, and "expanding the mind."

There are three main groups of factors which influence the pursuit of the above goals via drug consumption.

(1) Socioeconomic Factors. Kielholz et al. (187, p. 498) points out that the following socioeconomic factors influence drug consumption and drug dependence: familial environment, occupational roles, economic stituation, social status, social mobility, laws, religion, value patterns, the advertising industry, fashion, and general customs of consumption.

Economic factors play a major role. As Somerhausen (336) claims, we are today in the process of creating a "pill culture." He emphasizes that modern business and industry aim at maximizing profit rates by elaborating and ameliorating the means of production and distribution. They also, via advertising, promise happiness for everybody.

To what extent economic interests may foster future drug consumption and dependence can be indirectly deduced from the data which Zacune et al. (376, p. 55) collected in Great Britain:

- In 1959, the industry sold drugs for 153 million pounds; in 1968 the sale grossed 292 million pounds.
- Between 1961 and 1968, the number of prescriptions for barbiturate-free sleeping pills rose from 3.4 to 5.8 million.
- Between 1961 and 1968, the number of prescriptions for barbiturate-containing drugs was constantly over 15 million.
- From 1961 to 1968, the number of prescriptions for tranquillizers rose from 6.2 to 16 million, while the number of prescriptions for amphetamine drugs sank from 6 to 3.9 million.

According to Schmidbauer and Vom Scheidt (317, p. 185), in 1968, 30 million prescriptions for barbiturates, 1.6 million for amphetamine, and 50 million for tranquillizers were registered in Germany.

These data, of course, concern only the drugs sold by prescriptions and supplied by the pharmaceutical industry. There is, however, an illegal market for certain drugs which has its own network of production and distribution and which yields large profits.

According to Zacune et al. (377, p. 123), in 1954, there were 57 officially known heroin addicts in Great Britain; in 1968 there were already 2,240. In 1963, there were 296 white and 367 black cannabis consumers; in 1967 there were already 1,737 white and 656 black cannabis consumers.

The advertising industry plays an important role both in creating new drug markets and in maintaining the traditional ones. Thomas (355, p. 42) speaks of "brain washing" which has become so important and ubiquitous that nobody can escape it. It is based on an arsenal of techniques from different scientific sources — behaviorism, ethology, psychoanalysis, and the theory of communication. Thomas (355, p. 42) reports that Packard calculated that the United States, in 1957, spent about one billion dollars on advertising which produced a gross sale of 3,000 billion dollars. Certain specialists in the field of advertising, for instance Kutter (205), rather understate the impact of advertising; however, most of the industries seem to believe in it or they would not invest so much money. Thomas (355, p. 43) reports that some agencies feel no moral restrictions in the choice of their means of persuasion. For example, the visual combination of the product with religious pictures of the Holy Virgin or other saints successfully increased the sale of Aspirin to Indians.

According to Hordern (158), social change and the consequent insecurity concerning value patterns and behavior produce a high level of anxiety which encourages drug consumption. Taking drugs becomes an attempt at self-healing. According to the same author, the Protestant ethic has been replaced in certain countries by a leisure ethic which creates a vacuum [i.e., a general meaninglessness — well analyzed in many of its implications by Frankl (100)] which stimulates drug consumption, as well as the consumption of music and sex.

Social change and the problem of competition demands adaptations and produces frustrations which, as Solms (334, p. 43) stresses, also foster the need for regression. In such a situation, drugs promise quick regression and a pharmaco-happiness.

Kielholz and Ladewig (186), and Kielholz et al. (187) make clear that the "broken home" and, with it, the family structure has a major influence on drug consumption. Kielholz and Ladewig (186, p. 20) quote a Canadian study which shows that adolescents from families where the parents use tranquillizers and psychostimulantia are more frequently drug consumers than adolescents from families with prohibitive value patterns.

As to be expected, the value patterns of a global population and its attitude toward drug consumption plays a determining role. Kielholz et al. (187, p. 514) reports that in Norway, where the population has a very prohibitive attitude towards LSD, the consumption of psychotrop drugs is much lower than in nearby Sweden, where the prevailing value pattern is more permissive.

Kielholz and Ladewig (186, p. 34 ff) stress that the consumption of drugs is also influenced by the work situation and occupational roles. Men seem to consume drugs mostly for professional reasons (e.g., lack of education, overdemanding work, rivalry), while women take drugs for mainly emotional reasons. Women seem to be more susceptible to the family homeostasis. Tensions in marriage or family (e.g., problems with children or partner, lack of love and support, sexual dissatisfaction) instigate their drug consumption.

(2) The Drugs. Kielholz et al. (187, p. 512) suggest that the choice of drugs depends on the availability of drugs, on the normative pattern of the custom of consumption of a given society, and, finally, on the expected or desired effect.

Solms (334, p. 35) emphasizes, however, that the choice of drugs depends upon psychological motivations or the goal to be reached. To avoid disagreable states, gain pleasure, or "expand the mind" instigate the specific choice of the drug.

(3) Personality. Certain types of personality and character structure are overrepresented among drug dependent individuals. As Kielholz and Ladewig (186), and Kielholz et al. (187) report, 60% of the drug dependent individuals come from families where toxicomania, tentamen, suicide, and alcoholism are frequent. The prevailing premorbid character shows the following: anxiety, reserve, sensitivity, vulnerability, and a leptosome-asthenic constitution. They are very often conscientious, ambitious, and perfectionist. They maneuvre themselves into chronic feelings of insufficiency which favor drug consumption.

The same authors (186, 187) report that the earyl childhood environment plays a role in determining personality structure and drug consumption. Hoff (cf. 187, p. 512) points out that 83% of a sample of drug addicts came from broken homes. According to Kielholz et al. (187, p. 511), 72% of the juvenile polytoxicomanic patients indicate a negative relationship with father and 32% a negative relationsships with mother. These indications might be an expression of the often accused "fatherless society," or, as Somerhausen (336) suggests, they might be due to a type of reaction specific for adolescents. In their struggle to gain autonomy and define their identity, they often respond to conflict by passive rebellion. If it fails to provoke the desired response, the adolescents escalate in their means of rebellion by consuming drugs. On the other hand, it is probable that drug consumption deteriorates the relationships with parents. There is a general cause and effect problem that most of the epidemiologic studies do not take into account.

11.2.4 Consequences of Drug Consumption

The consequences of drug consumption (186, 187, 350, 355) are well-known and do not need further discussion in this context. Mainly, they consist of psychic or physical dependence. The latter, especially, leads to an increase of tolerance and, therefore, to an increase of the dosage consumed. Dependence creates the basis for chronic drug consumption which, according to the type of the drug, leads to physical or psychological destruction, with its individual and social consequences.

11.2.5 Epidemiologic Data

Kielholz and Ladewig (186, p. 16) report that there are a few general trends discernable:

- Increasingly younger people become drug consumers.
- New drugs and new ways of consumption connected with the cultural change, fashion, and new motivations spread into all social classes.
- The 30-40-years-olds increasingly consume hypnotics and antipyretic analgesics, "uppers" (i.e., brain activating drugs), and tranquillizers.
- Polytoxicomania increases.

(1) Age. A general survey (187, p. 505). made in Germany in 1961, shows that 9% of the population regularly consume somnifera, psychostimulantia, tonics, or some kind of medication against nervousness; 39% of the women and 19% of the men regularly use pain relievers against headache. By contrast (187, p. 505), only 0.1% of the Swiss population are drug dependent.

The consumption of certain drugs has become particularly popular. Kielholz et al. (187, p. 505) report that 0.5% of the population of Stockholm are amphetamine dependent and the tranquillizer consumption in the United States increased from 7%, in 1957, to 27%, in 1967; 80% of the drug patients in the United States (188, p. 507) are under 40 years old, while Europe has two major groups of drug dependents: 16-22-years-olds and 30-45-years-olds.

The drug consumption of adolescents is especially well studied. As Somerhausen (336, p. 186) reports, a survey by Bättig of 307 college students in Zurich revealed that 81.4% consumed alcohol, 43.6% pain relievers, 18.6% cannabis, 16.6% tranquillizers, 12.4% amphetamins, and 4.9% somnifera. Angst et al. (11, p. 12) mentions a study, by Gnirrs in 1969, which indicates that 10.3% of a sample of 881 adolescents are drug consumers. Angst et al. (11) made a survey of 6.315 male students and 1,381 female students – 24% of the males and 16.1% of the females indicated the consumption of one or several drugs, one or several times. Taeschner (349, p. 2276) reports the findings of comparable studies in Germany where the consumption varied between a frequency of 21.7% and 34%.

In a pilot study with 81 recruits, Battegay and Muehlemann (19) come to the following results: 16% consume cannabis, 6.2% LSD, and 9.9% amphetamines or psychostimulantia and 4.9% indicate an excessive consumption of prescribed drugs. No one indicates consumption of opiates or cocaine.

There seem to be important differences in the frequency of drug consumption between rural and urban youth. In a Swedish survey (cf. 187, p. 506), made in 1967, 18.9% of the adolescents of Stockholm had experience with psychoactive drugs, while only 1.5% of the total Swedish youth had had such an experience.

(2) Sex. All the authors seem to agree that the drug consumption of women is less significant than the drug consumption of men. The sex-specific distribution of drug consumption depends upon age, type of drug, and sociocultural factors. If these determinants change, the sex-specific distribution changes. As Kielholz et al. (187, p. 507) reports, amphetamines were originally consumed by men to increase their performance and achievement, while it is now used increasingly by women to lose weight.

Hypnotics and analgesics are more frequently consumed by women (cf. 187, p. 507) than by men in the proportion of 3 to 1. In adolescents, the number of male consumers is higher than that of female consumers, as Angst et al. (11) point out.

(3) Marital Status. Most of the authors emphasize that drug addicts have disturbed interpersonal relationships and that they have an increased number of separations and divorces.

(4) Occupational Roles. According to Ball (cf. 187, p. 508), only 32.1% of the narcotic addicts practice a legitimate profession. In a study of 2,000 drug dependents in Switzerland, Kielholz et al. (187) found that antipyretic analgesics are mainly consumed by artisans and housewives, while hypnotics are mainly consumed by employees of the middle or upper hierarchical level.

(5) Social Class. Field studies and the elaboration of data collected in clinics show that lower social classes consume cannabis, hallucinogenics, and amphetamines more frequently than middle or upper classes.

Before the modern drug wave arrived in Europe, opiates were consumed mostly by individuals in medical professions. Today, juvenile consumers prevail. In the United States, different studies come to different conclusions. Zacune et al. (377, p. 128) point out that some authors find differences between social classes and an overrepresentation of professional workers, employees, and managers. Other authors claim that no such differences exist. The discrepancy in the results is probably due to the differences in the samples studied.

11.2.6 Polytoxicomania

It is well-known that there is a general increase in polytoxicomania. Habituation and increase in tolerance and undesired side effects of certain drugs induce an increasing number of drug consumers to try out different drugs. Sleeping problems after amphetamine consumption are treated with hypnotics, while the protracted effect of barbiturates is corrected by amphetamines and other "uppers." Sometimes, the nonavailability of a certain drug on the illegal market induces a drug dependent individual to shift to other drugs.

Zacune et al. (377, p. 135 ff) report that adolescent drug consumers in Great Britain are consuming an increasing range of different drugs. The same individuals often consume nicotine, alcohol, and drugs. The same fact is also emphasized by Glatt (cf. 377, p. 137), who found 41.5% of female alcoholics were, at the same time, dependent on barbiturates.

The overall impression is that the mechanistic epistemology and the general manipulation of modern man pushes him more to manipulate his moods with drugs. The mechanistic view of man in the technological society makes him treat his body as a machine, neglecting its alarm signals, and overcome natural reactions with "uppers" and "downers."

11.3 Methods of Data Collection

The methods correspond to the general method of data collection used so far. Ten questions deal with drug consumption. These covered the type and amount of consumption and the attitude the probands had towards their own drug consumption. Because of the low number of drug consumers expected, the questionnaire did not ask about motivations leading to drug consumption. After seeing the results, however, it was apparent that this would have been desirable.

I define as "habitual" or "regular drug consumption" a consumption at least two times per week.

11.4 Working Hypotheses About Drug Consumption and Results

11.4.1 Age

Working Hypothesis I. Drugs of the morphine type are consumed mainly by middle and older age groups.

Results. There is no significant correlation between age and consumption. There are only 3 probands (2 of the oldest and 1 of the second oldest age group) who regularly consume drugs containing morphine or codeine.

Working Hypothesis II. Barbiturate are consumed mainly by the middle age groups.

Results. There is no significant correlation between age and consumption. The number of regular consumer ($n = 3$) is too small to allow any significant statements.

Working Hypothesis III. Tranquillizers are consumed mainly by probands who are 25-45 years old.

Results. There is no significant correlation between age and consumption. Of the 15 probands indicating regular consumption of tranquillizers, 9 belong to the older group (45-65) and 4 belong to the younger group (25-45).

Working Hypothesis IV. Amphetamines are consumed mainly by probands who are 35-55 years old.

Results. There is a highly significant correlation ($p = < 0.01, > 0.001$) between age and consumption (Table 31).

Table 31. *Age-specific distribution of amphetamine consumption*

	NR	Yes	No	%	n
G 1	3	-	17	100	20
G 2	-	-	20	100	20
G 3	1	4	15	100	20
G 4	2	-	18	100	20
G 5	1	-	19	100	20
G 6	1	-	19	100	20
Total	8	4	108	100	120

$x^2 = 24.889$ $p = < 0.01, > 0.001$

All 4 probands indicating regular consumption of amphetamines belong to the 25-45-years-olds. This is the only finding which supports the working hypothesis on age and type of drug consumed.

11.4.2 Age and Evaluation of One's Own Drug Consumption

Working Hypothesis. The two middle age groups (34-55) tend to evaluate their drug consumption as harmful or pathological.

Results. There are no significant correlations between the possible categories of evaluation (i.e., normal, harmful, and pathological) and the age of the consumers.

One-third of the probands ($n = 41$) do not indicate any evaluation; most being non-consumers. Half the probands ($n = 61$) indicate that their consumption is normal. 15 indicate that their consumption is harmful (10 of them belong to the 35-55-years-olds) and only 3 probands consider their consumption as pathological (2 of them belong to the youngest age group).

11.4.3 Sex

Working Hypothesis I. Men consume drugs of the morphine type more frequently than women.

Results. There are no significant correlations between sex and consumption. The number of probands ($n = 3$) is too small to make relevant statements.

Working Hypothesis II. Women consume barbiturates more frequently than men.

Results. There are no significant correlations between sex and consumption of barbiturates. 2 women and 1 man indicate being regular consumers of barbiturates, but the number of probands ($n = 3$) is too small to permit any relevant statements.

Working Hypothesis III. Women consume tranquillizers more frequently than men.

Results. There is a significant correlation ($p = < 0.05, > 0.01$) between sex and tranquillizer consumption as shown in Table 32.

Table 32. *Sex-specific distribution of tranquillizer consumption*

	NR (%)	Yes (%)	No (%)	%	n
Men	11.5	6.5	82	100	60
Women	2	18	80	100	60
Total	7	12	81	100	120
	$x^2 = 7.777$	$p = < 0.05, > 0.01$			

Of the probands indicating regular consumption, 11 are women.

Working Hypothesis IV. Women consume amphetamines more frequently than men.

Results. There is no significant correlation between sex and amphetamine consumption. A trend supports the working hypothesis. Of the 4 probands indicating amphetamine consumption, 3 were women.

The first working hypotheses are falsified by the findings; the latter two are supported.

11.4.4 Sex and Evaluation of One's Own Drug Consumption

Working Hypothesis. Women, more frequently than men, evaluate their drug consumption as normal.

Results. There is a highly significant correlation ($p = < 0.001$) between sex and the evaluation of one's own drug consumption. Although only 30% of the men describe their drug consumption as "normal," 71.5% of the women do. On the other hand, 3 women indicate that their drug consumption is pathological. This attitude did not appear at all among the men.

11.4.5 Work Time

Three working hypotheses concerned the correlation between the number of hours of daily work and the consumption of amphetamines, morphines, and barbiturates, but the number of probands is too small to permit any relevant statements. Only the working hypothesis concerning the consumption of tranquillizers can be elaborated.

Working Hypothesis. The consumption of tranquillizers increases in proportion to the increasing number of daily workhours.

Results. There are no significant correlations ($p = < 0.10, > 0.05$) between daily worktime and tranquillizer consumption. The working hypothesis is falsified.

11.4.6 Attitude Towards of Season

The three working hypotheses concerning the subjective experience of the season as a tolerable stressor cannot be elaborated because the number of probands per category is too small to permit relevant statements.

Working Hypothesis. Probands who experience the season as an intolerable stressor have a higher tranquillizer consumption than others.

Results. There are no significant correlations between the subjective experience of the season and the quantity of tranquillizer consumption.

11.4.7 Attitude Towards the Season and Self-Evaluation of the Probands' Drug Consumption

Working Hypothesis. Probands who experience the season as intolerable evaluate their drug consumption as nonnormal more frequently than those who experience it as a tolerable stressor.

Results. There is a significant correlation ($p = < 0.05, > 0.02$) between the subjective experience of the season and the self-evaluation of drug consumption. Probands who experience the seyson as an intolerable stressor indicate that their drug consumption is harmful (25%) or pathologic (6%) and also probands who experience the season as a tolerable stressor believe that their drug consumption is harmful (7%) or pathologic (1%). The working hypothesis is supported.

11.4.8 Marital Status

Working Hypothesis. The drug consumption of unmarried probands is higher than the drug consumption of married probands.

Results. There is no significant correlation between drug consumption and marital status.

11.4.9 Occupational Roles

Working Hypothesis. Housewives have the highest drug consumption. Probands working in the tourist facilities have the next highest. Mountain guides and ski instructors have the lowest drug consumption.

Results. There is no significant correlation ($p = > 0.10$) between the occupational roles and drug consumption. There is, however, a tendency which partly supports the working hypothesis – the proportion of nonconsumers to consumers is 3 to 1 for probands working in tourist facilities, 9 to 1 for mountain guides and ski instructors, 17 to 1 for artisans and workers, 4 to 1 for commercial and bureaucratic employees, and 5 to 1 for housewives.

11.4.10 Type of Constitution

Working Hypothesis. Leptosomes have a higher drug consumption than pycnics or athletic types of constitution.

Results. There is no significant correlation between type of physical constitution and drug consumption.

11.4.11 Family Environment

Working Hypothesis. There were several working hypotheses concerning the correlation between drug consumption and childhood environment, number of developmental problems, level of education, social mobility, and family problems.

Results. There are no significant correlations between all the above items and drug consumption.

11.4.12 Daily Work Hours

Working Hypothesis. Drug consumers more frequently indicate a maximal work time than nonconsumers.

Results. There are highly significant correlations ($p = < 0.01, > 0.001$) between the drug consumption and daily work time. While 29% of the drug consumers indicate a maximal work time of more than 15 hours daily, only 4% of the nonconsumers indicate maximal work time. The findings support the working hypothesis.

11.4.13 Psychosomatic Symptoms

Working Hypothesis. Drug consumers indicate psychosomatic symptoms more often than nonconsumers.

Results. There is no significant correlation between drug consumption and the indication of psychosomatic symptoms. There is a trend, however, favoring the working hypothesis – 95% of the drug consumers indicate psychosomatic symptoms as opposed to 79% of the nonconsumers.

11.4.14 Attitude Towards a Possible Economic Crisis

Working Hypothesis. Drug consumers indicate being afraid of a possible economic crisis more often than nonconsumers.

Results. There is no significant correlation between drug consumption and the attitude towards a possible economic crisis.

11.4.15 Self-Evaluation of Health

Working Hypothesis. Drug consumers indicate impaired health more often than nonconsumers.

Results. There is a highly significant correlation ($p = <0.01, >0.001$) between drug consumers and self-evaluation of health. While only 15% of the nonconsumers indicate feeling unhealthy at the time of the interview, 43% of the consumers do.

11.4.16 Correlations Between Smoking, Alcohol Consumption, and Drug Consumption

Working Hypothesis. There is a direct correlation between consumption of tobacco, alcohol, and drugs.

Results. There is no significant correlation between the consumption of tobacco and drugs or between the consumption of alcohol and drugs. There is a tendency for drug consumers to consume tobacco (44%), while nonconsumers are more frequently nonsmokers (29%).

11.5 Total Drug Consumption and Self-Evaluation of Drug Consumption

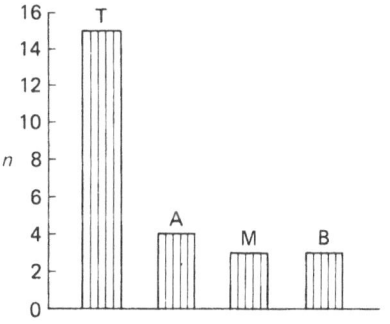
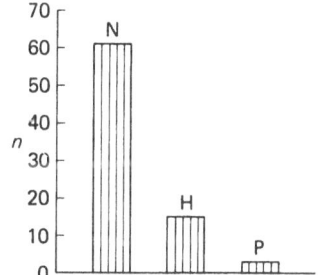

Fig. 40. Total distribution of the different types of drug consumption. T, tranquillizers; A, amphetamines, M, derivates of morphine; B, barbiturates

Fig. 41. The distribution of the different categories of self-evaluation of drug consumption. N, normal; H, harmful; P, pathological

11.6 Discussion of Results

A comparison of my results with the epidemiologic results of the international literature is difficult, if not impossible, for the following reasons:

- My results stem from a representative sample of the total population of a village, while the samples investigated in the international literature are samples of urban areas, students, total populations of a country, special social classes, special age groups, hospitalized patients, or chronic drug consumers.
- Given my operational definition (cf. p. 254) I can speak only of habitual or regular drug consumption, but not of excessive consumption, addiction, or physical dependence. It can be assumed, however, that habitual consumers who take a drug two or more times a week have at least a psychological drug dependence.

Given these limitations, a few of the results are discussed briefly.

11.6.1 Frequency of Habitual Drug Consumption

As it is generally known, the tendency for dissimulation by drug consumers, whether consciously or unconsciously motivated, is high. In the function of the village doctor, I used to warn people against drug abuse. An observer who intervenes actively in the field of investigation influences the results; therefore, we can assume that the actual drug consumption of the village is higher than indicated by the probands. In several cases, I could verify that my assumption was correct.

As expected, the consumption of tranquillizers is highest; 12% of the probands regularly consume tranquillizers, while the consumption of other drugs is rather low. Of the three probands who indicated taking drugs of the morphine-type, two consumed codeine containing drugs and 1 proband morphine containing drugs; 3% of the sample indicated regular consumption of amphetamine containing drugs and 3% consumed barbiturates regularly.

The tranquillizer consumption of the village in 1970, although such a comparison is questionable, corresponds to the tranquillizer consumption in the United States in 1960 (cf. p. 253). The tranquillizer consumption in Saas-Fee may be regarded as rather high.

Cannabis, cocaine, hallucinogens, and opiates, with the exception of the 3% mentioned above, are not indicated and, as far as the direct field observation was reliable, not yet consumed in 1970.

11.6.2 Polytoxicomania

According to the definition used in this study, I cannot strictly speak of polytoxicomania, but, rather, of habitual and simultaneous drug consumption of two or more drugs.

Only three indicated that they regularly consumed tranquillizers and barbiturates (2 probands) or tranquillizers and amphetamine containing drugs (1 proband).

There is no statistically significant correlation between drug consumption (cf. p. 259) and alcohol consumption, or between drug consumption and tobacco consumption. Thus, it can be assumed that the tendency towards polytoxicomania was low in 1970. This is probably linked to the fact that the value patterns governing drug consumption are strictly prohibitive, with the exception of the consumption of tranquillizers. By and large, the population assumes that tranquillizer consumption is harmless.

I expect that the situation in 1980 will be quite different and that the percentage of polytoxicomania will be increased.

11.6.3 Variables Influencing Drug Consumption

Most of the working hypotheses are not supported by the findings. In some cases, the number of probands is too small to permit relevant statements. In other cases, the findings of the questionnaire contradict the results of the direct field observation and of the interview with key persons.

11.6.3.1 Age

With the exception of the consumption of drugs of the morphine-type (cf. p. 255) the group of 45-55-years-olds indicates the highest percentage of consumption. These probands find themselves in a psychobiological and psychosocial crisis. They are at an age where role accumulation, responsibility, and overwork are highest; where family problems or economic problems are highest; and where the coping resources can be exhausted and the general psychic energy decreased. Since the achievement level remains, or should remain, and since the coping potential and energy resources decrease, drug consumption becomes a strategy for coping with stress. This is especially clear in the case of amphetamine containing drug consumption — all the probands consuming amphetamine containing drugs are of this age group.

The oldest and the youngest probands indicate the lowest drug consumption. This is probably related to the fact the role specific demands decrease or do not yet increase and that the value pattern of these two age groups are prohibitive, although for different reasons.

Corresponding to the highest drug consumption of the 45-55-years-olds, they are also the group (cf. p. 256) who most often declares its own drug consumption as harmful — more than one-third of this group, compared to 12.5% of the standard distribution, think that their drug consumption is harmful.

Compared to the indications given by Kielholz et al. (cf. p. 253), there are important differences in my sample. The group of the 15-25-years-olds does not consume drugs at all. This finding differs considerably from the comparable reports of Angst, Bättig, Battegay, and Gnirrs (cf. p. 253). The nonpermissive value pattern and the fact that, in 1970, the village was not yet within the network of the modern drug market are probably responsible for protecting the youth from drug experiences.

Unlike the sample of Kielholz (cf. p. 253), the group of the 35-45-years-olds is not especially at risk, while the age group of the 45-55-years-olds is most at risk.

11.6.3.2 Sex

With the exception of the consumption of the morphine-type drugs (cf. p. 256), the drug consumption of women is higher than that of men. The specific proportions are the following: morphine-type drugs, men to women = 3 to 2; barbiturates, men to women = 1.5 to 3; tranquillizer, men to women = 6.5 to 18; and amphetamine containing drugs, men to women = 1.5 to 5.

Compared to the findings of the international literature (cf. p. 253), there is a high correlation in the sex-specific distribution of drug consumption.

The sex-specific differences are less clear-out where the self-evaluation of drug consumption is concerned (cf. p. 256). While only 30% of the men assume that their drug consumption is normal, 71.5% of the women do. This interesting discrepancy is due probably to the fact that the consumption of tranquillizers is not considered harmful. On the other hand, corresponding to the sex-specific rates of consumption, 5% of the women declare that their drug consumption is harmful, while none of the men do.

11.6.3.3 Marital Status

In my sample, there are fewer single probands among the drug consumers than among the nonconsumers (cf. p. 258), but the differences are not significant. Since there were no separated or divorced probands in the sample, a comparison with the findings of other authors (cf. p. 253) cannot be made.

11.6.3.4 Personality, Sociocultural, and Socioeconomic Factors

While Kielholz (cf. p. 252) finds the leptosome-asthenic constitution more frequent in drug consumers, this is not the case in my sample (cf. p. 258). The difference might be due to the difference of the compared samples.

I did not find any support for the hypothesis that drug consumers come more often from a disturbed early environment (cf. p. 252) or that they more frequently indicate developmental problems (cf. p. 252) than nonconsumers. Although drug consumers more frequently indicate family problems (cf. p. 258) than nonconsumers, the differences are not statistically significant.

Drug consumers, more often than nonconsumers (cf. p. 257), experience the season as an intolerable stressor. They indicate psychosomatic symptoms (cf. p. 259), and are afraid of a possible economic crisis (cf. p. 259). Although these differences are not statistically significant, they suggest that these drug consumption have a primary response disposition in common − they more often interpret a situation as a stressor than non-consumers do.

Almost one-third (29%) of the drug consumers work more than 15 hours per day (cf. p. 257) while only 4% of the nonconsumers indicate maximal worktimes. Possibly, drug consumers belong to a more active personality type, but it is more probable that individuals who are overworked have a tendency to maintain their achievement level by means of drugs. This latter interpretation is supported by my findings (cf. p. 259) − while 43% of the drug consumers indicate not being "healthy" at the moment of the interview, only 15% of the nonconsumers do.

Drug consumers more frequently have a higher education (cf. p. 258) and more often indicate greater social mobility (cf. p. 258) than nonconsumers; however, the differences are not statistically significant.

There are some interesting, but insignificant, correlations between occupational roles and drug consumption (cf. p. 258). Innkeepers have the highest drug consumption (27%), followed by housewives (20%). Artisans and workers have the lowest drug consumption (6%). Innkeepers and probands working in the tourist facilities have a hectic work rhythm while housewives often have a role accumulation which makes them more vulnerable to stressors. They consume drugs to cope better with stress. This interpretation is substantiated by the already mentioned fact that probands with long workhours indicate greater drug consumption than those with shorter workhours — more than half of the probands who work 15 hours or more per day are habitual tranquillizer consumers. Although they have personality features of a perfectionist and obsessional type, my epidemiologic approach did not include any psychometric tests for direct interviews and, thus, any definite statements about the personality type would be mere speculation.

11.6.4 Final Remarks

The results illustrate that women, age 45-55, are the main consumers of tranquillizers. Their work situation with its long workhours, role accumulation at home and in the business, and heavy responsibilities seem to be the primary factors favoring drug consumption. Thus, drug consumption has mainly the utilitarian function of maintaining the performance and achievement level of a person.

Drug consumption in the village is essentially due to situational factors in the web of the social organization. Personality structure seems to play a minor role. Expectedly, drug consumption in 1980 will be higher because the social organization in the village will have the same patterns and because chronic stress is likely to push an increasing number of individuals to drug consumption. I assume that increasing consumption will make the value patterns more permissive and this permissiveness will increase drug consumption.

12. Consumption of Tobacco

12.1 Introduction

The second report of the Royal College of Physicians of London (331), issued in 1970, concludes that cigarette smoking today is a cause of death as important as were the epidemics of the last century and that from a standpoint of health policy, the consumption of tobacco is the same challenge for humanity today as typhoid fever, cholera, tuberculosis, and other epidemics were in the last century.

The idea that smoking is harmful and that it shortens life was first presented by Pearl (f. 331, p. 24) in 1938. For various reasons, especially commercial and hedonistic ones, this warning had no effect. In 1948, an editorial of the Journal of the American Medical Association (f. 331, p. 24) argued that moderate smoking does not diminish the life expectancy of persons who have no special counter indication.

However, as long ago as 1950, the study of Doll and Hill (cf. 309, p. 219) proved that there are significant statistical correlations between smoking and lung cancer. Only in 1962, when the first report of the Royal College of Physicians of London (cf. 309, p. 22) was published, physicians and the public were alarmed, since it offered a great number of facts supporting the harmful effects of smoking. In the following years, other studies proved that smoking is more harmful than had been assumed. The Hammond study (f. 338), for instance, investigated 36, 975 so-called statistical twins (i.e., smokers and nonsmokers whose life data correspond in at least 25 important factors). It showed that at the end of the investigation, 1,385 of the smokers and only 662 of the nonsmokers had died and death from lung cancer occurred in 12 of the nonsmokers as compared to 110 of the smokers.

In 1968 and 1970, a case of chronic bronchitis or of a vascular disease, which was directly related to chronic smoking, rarely appeared in the general practice. Pipe smoking in Saas-Fee, widerspread up to the beginning of our century and enjoyed by many of the older women, was out of fashion. Cigarette smoking was considered damaging to one's health. There was evidence, however, that it became more fashionable every year, even for women and adolescents. Cigar and pipe smoking were considered rare phenomena.

I included smoking in the questionnaire for three main reasons — it is a general health problem, according to the international literature; smoking seemed to increase in the village; and it was important for the comparison in 1980.

12.2 International Literature

Only a few aspects of smoking, relevant to my investigation, are discussed in this context.

12.2.1 Physiochemical and Pharmacodynamic Aspects

In tabacco smoke, there are over 1000 particles (331, 338) which are potentially harmful, especially if their diameter is small enough to pass through the bronchioli into the alveolar system of the lungs. The composition of these substances depends on the type of tobacco plant, the methods of production, and the type of smoking behavior, as pointed out by Ague (6). It is well-known that smokers who smoke a cigarette down to the butt have an increased intake of nocive substances.

There are four major groups of harmful substances (331, p. 37 ff) in tobacco:

- Cancerproducing substances (e.g., polycyclic aromatic hydrocarbons, polonium) and substances which inhibit the cancerinhibiting effect (e.g., phenoles, fatty acids)
- Irritating substances (e.g., acroleine), which increase the secretion of the bronchioli and/or have a ciliostatic effect
- Nicotine, which imitates the function of neurotransmitters with a stimulating and, later, inhibiting effect. As Ague (5, 6) stresses, nicotine influences the central nervous system, thus changing the psychological state and producing, dependent on the subjective effect, dependence or rejection of smoking. Nicotine influences the cardiovascular system (331, p. 421); Adrenaline and noradrenaline secretion increases and heart rhythm, volume per contraction, and blood pressure increase. Nicotine increases the coagulation time and produces a vasoconstriction. Nicotine produces (338) a stress reaction which is not triggered by the environment and, therefore, nonfunctional.
- Carbonmonoxide has a high affinity to hemoglobine, pushing away oxygen of its carrier and decreasing its transport by abour 10%.

12.2.2 Health Consequences of Smoking

The most important consequences of smoking (309, 331, 338, 354) are the following:

- Inflammatory-degenerative disorders of the pulmonal system (e.g., bronchitis, emphysema)
- Neoplasic transformations (e.g., carcinoma of the mouth, glottis, lungs, sometimes stomach, pancreas, and bladder)
- Inflammatory-degenerative transformations and disorders of the cardiovascular system (e.g., claudicatio intermittens, angina pectoris, infarctus of the myocarde)
- Inflammatory deseases of the gastrointestinal tract (e.g., stomach ulcer ulcus duodeni)
- Effects on the intrauterine life, probably due to a decrease of oxygen, producing smaller infants and even stillbirths, as mentioned by Russel et alia 309, p. 221)
- Such rare disorders as nicotine-amblyopia, liver cirrhosis, and inflammatory transformation of the palate and the gengiva

Health disorders due to smoking increase the general morbidity and influence the economy of a country to an astonishing extent. Godber (cf. 309, p. 21) estimates that the English industry loses 20 times more workers by smoking than by wage strikes and Ball (f. 309, p. 21) estimates that, in England, each year between 5.000 and 8.000 hospital beds are occupied by patients with health problems due to smoking.

Retrospective and prospective studies (331) prove that the life expectancy of smokers is significantly decreased. In 1964, the American Surgeon General's Report (354) came to the conclusion that cigarette smoking in men, and to a slightly lesser extent in women, leads to a 70% increase of the age-specific death rate. Probands who stopped smoking before they participated in this study still have a deathrate increased by 40%. Four major studies, made in the USA, Canada, and England (f. 331), came to similar conclusions.

According to another study made in Great Britain in 1968 (f. 331, p. 27) there were 31.000 more deaths among the 35-64-years old male smokers than are expected in non-smokers. Similarly, Lowe (cf. 309, p. 221) made a study in England and Wales showing that every year 38.000 male smokers and 4.000 female smokers die earlier than nonsmokers. The second report of the Royal College of Physicians of London (331), published in 1971, showed that in every year England 20.000 – 24.000 men between 35 and 64 die prematurely because they are smokers.

A ministerial report from West Germany (f. 338) came to the following conclusions: in 1972, 140.000 individuals died "because they smoked" and in 1970, 23, 706 individuals died due to lung cancer as compared to 18.753 individuals who died due to traffic accidents.

Almost all of these studies argue that the harmful effect of smoking is directly correlated to the number of cigarettes per day.

It is a controversial question whether or not cigars and pipes are less harmful than cigarettes. The authors of the four studies mentioned above (331 p. 24) came to the conclusion that cigar smokers have an only slightly shorter life expectancy than nonsmokers. A study by the American Health Department (354) came to similar conclusions. A study made in Canada (f. 331, p. 11) of 78.000 retired men and 14.000 retired women concludes that the life expectancy of pipe and cigar smokers is equal to that of nonsmokers.

There are studies which argue, however, that the opposite holds true. A followup study with 293,658 American veterans (354, p. 8) concludes that the death rate of pipe and cigar smokers is significantly increased if the smoker consumes more than four pipes or cigars daily. German and Swiss studies (331, p. 54) even argue that pipe and cigar smokers have a higher death rate than cigarette smokers.

The issue, then, is far from being completely elucidated.

12.2.3 Variables Influencing Smoking

12.2.3.1 Age

New Studies (337) indicate that an increasing number of young people smoke. McKennel and Thomas (245) report statistics illustrating that the daily cigarette smoking of adolescents and adults shows little differences – 21% of the adolescents and 15% of the adults smoke less than 5 cigarettes daily.

On the other hand, the daily cigarette smoking decreases rapidly after the age of 60, as Russel (309) reports.

Russel (309, p. 224) points out that the pressure of advertising, the influence of the peer group, the mass media, and the example of the adults and the value patterns they suggest induce adolescents to smoke increasingly. They associate maturity, success, luck, openmindedness, sensuality, and sexual potence with cigarettes.

Early onset of smoking (331, p. 51) is a factor of risk. Prospective studies (331, p. 84) prove that young smokers risk dieing from myocardium infarctus two to three times more often than nonsmokers. Older smokers have a death risk one and a half times higher.

12.2.3.2 Sex

Men smoke much more than women, but there is a new trend (338) for increased smoking in women. Russel (309) reports the following data: 9% of the men and 18% of the women smoke less than 5 cigarettes per day, 18% of the men and 34% of the women smoke 5-10 cigarettes per day, 41% of the men and 37% of the women smoke 11-20 cigarettes per day, 22% of the men and 11% of the women smoke 21-30 cigarettes per day and 10% of the men and no women smoke 30 or more cigarettes per day.

An English study (331) indicates that girls smoke more frequently than they used to. This tendency is new, but since women smoke less and inhale less (331, p. 33) their risk of diminished life expectancy is still less significant than in men. Today (i.e., autumn 1978), these findings are replaced by alarming American reports showing that the life expectancy of female smokers in America is drastically reduced.

12.2.3.3 Personality

Twin studies (331, p. 111) proved that monocygotic twins, even when reared in a different environment, have a higher concordance in their smoking behavior than could be expected. Thus, genetic factors seem to influence smoking.

Individuals of the behavioral type A (331) smoke much more frequently than others; they are impulsive, extroverted, seek fun and activity; love risks, and are aggressive against authority. They have a tendency to get divorced, change their occupational roles, and cause car accidents. These are, however, tendencies (331, p. 112) and not statistically significant comparisons with nonsmokers.

Little is known about the unconscious motivations for smoking. One study (331), p. 111) found that smoking cigarettes correlates with the age of weaning; persons able to give up smoking were weaned before the age of 8 months and probands unable to give up smoking were weaned at the age of 4.7 months. Another study (331) did not find correlations between early childhood "oral behavior" and smoking.

More is known about the conscious motivations for smoking. The motivations indicated most often (331, p. 110) are stimulation, fun, reduction of tensions, anger, anxiety, craving for nicotine and automatic fixated habituation without pleasure. Based on these conscious motivations leading to smoking and which make it impossible to quit smoking, different types of smokers have been postulated. Tomkins (cf. 234, p. 279) proposes the following typology:

- Positive-affectsmokers (i.e., smoking serves the gaining of pleasure)
- Negative-affect-snokers (i.e. smoking serves the reduction of tensions
- Habituation smokers (i.e. affectively neutral automatism)
- Addictive smokers (i.e., smoking serves the decrease of disagreeable and painful symptoms of deprivation)

An English study (331, p. 110) differentiates between two types:

– Smoking is motivated by inner needs (e.g., anxiety or pleasure)
– Smoking is motivated by social factors, (e.g., insecurity or group constraint).

These latter types are further differentiated into "consonant smokers" who accept smoking and do not want to quit it and "dissonant smokers" who do not accept their smoking and would like to stop. "Dissonant smokers" often smoke to satisfy inner needs, whereas "consonant smokers" often smoke for purely social reasons.

McKennel and Thomas (245) divide the group of individuals who smoke for the satisfaction of inner needs into two types: smokers who smoke because of nervous irritation and those who smoke for satisfaction.

According to Russel (309), smokers often are not only extremely nicotine dependent, they also have a great number of neurotic symptoms, are depressed, and have many social problems. Given the widespread consumption of tobacco, the reliability and specificity of such a statement is, in my view, questionable.

12.2.3.4 Habituation and Addiction

As Russel (309, p. 26) emphasizes, the permissive social climate induces certain learning processes which, combined with the pharmacodynamic effect of nicotine, are the main determinant factors for habituation, dependence, and addiction. The favorable climate is created by a general availability of tobacco, the prestige value of being "in", group constraints, and value centered advertising campaigns connecting smoking with youth, health, and happiness.

Half of the smokers would like to quit smoking, as McKennel and Thomas (245) stress. Other authors (331) report that one-fifth of the regular smokers, especially the young smokers, give up smoking, although often only temporarily. One-third of the older smokers give up smoking before the age of 70. According to Russel (309, p. 221), three out of four smokers try to quit smoking at least once, but only one out of four succeeds. "Consonant smokers" are more successful in quitting smoking than ,,dissonant smokers."

As the Royal College of Physicians of London (331) reports, in 1968, the industry in Great Britain spent about 12.2 million pounds for advertising. The same pattern is found in other countries, therefore, smoking cannot decrease as fast as it would be desirable from a health point of view. In 1970, the Swiss population consumed 3320 cigarettes per person, the United States 3850 East Germany 2500, and Austria 2340.

12.3. Methods of Data Collection

The methods of data collection correspond to those used throughout the study.

Fifteen items in the questionnaire deal with tobacco consumption. The questions are about the daily consumption of cigarettes, cigars, and pipes; the self-evaluation of smoking; the conscious motives for smoking; and the conscious motives for not quitting smoking. I formulated 19 working hypotheses.

50 probands indicated cigarette smoking. Since the number of cigar and pipe smokers (n = 13) was too small to permit separate elaboration, they were examined as a single category.

12.4 Working Hypotheses About Smoking and Results

12.4.1 Sex

Working Hypothesis I. Men smoke more frequently and smoke a greater number of cigarettes per day than women.

Results. There is a statistically significant correlation (p = <0.001) between sex and the number of cigarettes smoked daily (Table 33).

Table 33. Sex specific distribution of smoking

Cigarettes	Men	Women	%	n
0 - 5	29	52	100	81
5 - 10	3	10	100	13
15	11	2	100	13
20	3	3	100	6
>20	7	-	100	7
Total	60	60	100	120

$$x^2 = 21.46 \ p = <0.001$$

The findings support the working hypothesis.
Working Hypothesis II. Only men smoke cigars and pipes.
Results. There is a highly significant correlation (p = <0.001) between sex and cigar or pipe smoking; 13 men and none of the women smoke cigars and pipes.

12.4.2 Age

Working Hypothesis I The younger age groups smoke more cigarettes per day than the older ones.

Results. There is a highly significant correlation (p = <0.01, >0.001) between age and cigarette smoking. Nonsmokers and small quantity smokers are more frequent in the older age groups than in the younger. All other quantities are most frequently in the younger and middle age groups. There is, however, a relatively great number (n = 10) of the two youngest age groups who smoke only 5-10 cigarettes per day.
The findings support the working hypothesis.

Working Hypothesis II. The daily pipe and cigar consumption is smallest in the youngest groups and increases with increasing age.

Results. There is a highly significant correlation ($p = <0.001$) between age and pipe or cigar smoking. There is one proband between 15 and 35, two probands between 35 and 55, and 10 probands between 55 and 75 years old who smoke cigars or pipes.

The working hypothesis is supported.

12.4.3 Sex and Self-Evaluation

Working Hypothesis. Men have a higher tendency to declare their own smoking is harmless than women.

Results. There is a significant correlation ($p = <0.01, >0.001$) between sex and self evaluation of smoking 15 men indicate their smoking as not harmful 13 men and 9 women as slightly harmful, and 9 men and 2 women as harmful.

The working hypothesis is supported.

12.4.4 Age and Self-Evaluation

Working Hypothesis. Younger probands have a tendency to evaluate their smoking as harmful and older probands have a tendency to evaluate it as harmless.

Results. There is no significant correlation between age and self-evaluation of smoking.

The working hypothesis is falsified.

12.4.5 Self-Evaluation and Amount of Cigarette Smoking

Working Hypothesis. The tendency to evaluate smoking as harmful increases with an increasing amount of cigarette smoking.

Results. There is a highly significant correlation ($p = <0.001$) between the number of cigarettes smoked per day and self-evaluation of smoking. Probands who rarely smoke evaluate their smoking as harmless. Probands who smoke quantities indicate it as harmful.

The working hypothesis is supported.

12.4.6 Self-Evaluation and Amount of Pipe and Cigar Smoking

Working Hypothesis. Pipe and cigar smokers show a tendency to evaluate their smoking as harmless.

Results. There is a highly significant correlation ($p = <0.001$) between pipe and cigar smoking and self-evaluation. Probands who indicate "harmless" are more frequently pipe or cigar smokers than the standard distribution would have us expect.

The results support the working hypothesis.

12.4.7 Motivations

Working Hypothesis I. All motivations, with the exception of "insecurity," are more frequently indicated by men than women.

Results. There is a highly significant correlation ($p = <0.001$) between sex and the motivation "nervousness." For this motivation, however, the working hypothesis is falsified because it is indicated more frequently by women.

There is a highly significant correlation ($p = <0.01, >0.001$) between sex and the motivation "insecurity," which is indicated by only 1 women.

There is a highly significant correlation ($p = <0.01, >0.001$) between the motivation "wish to be adult" and sex; the motivation is indicated by 6 men and no women. The result supports the working hypothesis.

There is a significant correlation ($p = <0.001$) between sex and the motivation "imitation of others;" it is indicated by 11 men and no women. The result supports the working hypothesis.

Working Hypothesis II. The motivations for not quitting smoking "one must enjoy life after all" and "there is no need to quit smoking" is more frequently indicated by women; all the other motivations are more frequently dicated by men.

Results. There is a highly significant correlation ($p = <0.01, >0.001$) between sex and the categories "one must enjoy life after all" or "there is no need to quit smoking." Both motivations are indicated more frequently by men. This result falsified the first part of the working hypothesis.

There is a highly significant correlation ($p = <0.1, >0.001$) between sex and the categories "I don't have the will to do it," "I fear the symptoms of withdrawal," "I already tried several times without success." All these motivations are indicated more frequently by men. The results support the second part of the working hypothesis.

12.4.8 Developmental Problems

Working Hypothesis. Smokers indicate developmental problems more frequently than nonsmokers.

Results. There is a highly significant correlation ($p = <0.001$) between developmental problems of smokers and nonsmokers. 66% of the smokers and only 35% of the nonsmokers indicate one or several developmental problems.

There is a highly significant, but puzzling, correlation ($p = <0.001$) between the number of cigarettes smoked daily and developmental problems. Probands who smoke little or excessively (i.e., fewer than 10 or more than 20 cigarettes per day) indicate in 75-80% developmental problems, while probands who smoke average quantities (i.e., 10-20 cigarettes per day) indicate in only 41% developmental problems. This finding is somewhat contradictory and will be discussed below (see Chap. 4.).

There is a significant correlation ($p = <0.02, >0.01$) between the developmental problem "pavor nocturnus" and smokers or nonsmokers. Smokers indicate the symptom four times more than nonsmokers.

There is a significant correlation ($p = <0.2, >0.01$) between the developmental problem "onychophagia" and smokers or nonsmokers. Smokers indicate the symptom two times more than nonsmokers.

Generally, the findings support the working hypothesis.

12.4.9 Work Hours

Working Hypothesis. Smokers indicate more workhours than nonsmokers.

Results. There is no significant correlation between number of cigarettes and workhours, although there is a tendency in favor of the hypothesis. Of the 17 probands indicating 10-20 cigarettes per day, 9 work over 12 hours and, of the 13 probands indicating more than 20 cigarettes per day, 8 work more than 12 hours per day.

However, the hypothesis is essentially falsified.

12.4.10 Subjective Experience of the Season

Working Hypothesis. Smokers experience the season as an intolerable stressor more often than nonsmokers.

Results. There is no significant correlation between smokers or nonsmokers and the way the season is experienced.

The hypothesis is falsified.

12.4.11 Educational Background

Working Hypothesis. Smokers indicate an insufficient education more often than nonsmokers.

Results. There is no significant correlation between education and smokers or nonsmokers.

The hypothesis is falsified.

12.4.12 Attitude Toward a Possible Economic Crisis

Working Hypothesis. Smokers indicate being afraid of a possible economic crisis more often than nonsmokers.

Results. There is no significant correlation between smokers or nonsmokers and the attitude towards a possible economic crisis.

The hypothesis is falsified.

12.4.13 Self-Evaluation of Health

Working Hypothesis. Smokers indicate feeling ill more often than nonsmokers.

Results. There is no significant correlation between the self-evaluation of the proband's health and smokers or nonsmokers.

The hypothesis is falsfied.

12.4.14 Self-Evaluation of Drug Consumption

Working Hypothesis. Smokers assume that their drug consumption is harmful more often than nonsmokers.

Results. There is a highly significant correlation ($p = <0.001$) between the self-evaluation of drug consumption and smokers or nonsmokers. Only 28% of the smokers, but 67% of the nonsmokers, indicate their drug consumption as normal and 20% of the smokers, but only 12% of the nonsmokers, indicate their smoking as harmful.

The working hypothesis is supported.

12.4.15 Physical Constitution

Working Hypothesis. Smokers are athletes more often than leptosomes and leptosomes more often than pycnics.

Results. There is no significant correlation between the type of physical constitution and smoking, although there is a tendency in favor of the working hypothesis.

12.4.16 Basic Data Concerning the Amount of Smoking

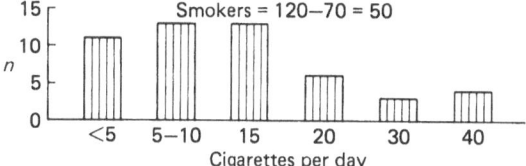

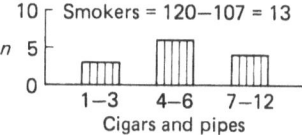

Fig. 42. Distribution of the quantities of daily cigarette smoking

Fig. 43. The distribution of the quantities, of daily cigar or pipe smoking

12.5 Discussion of Results

12.5.1 Consumption of Tobacco

Smoking in Saas-Fee in 1970 was not yet a severe health problem. Only 42% of the probands are smokers; 11% (13 probands) smoke more than 20 cigarettes daily (cf. Fig. 42) and, of the 13% who smoke pipes or cigars, only 4 probands smoke more than 7 pipes or cigars per day.

Even if probands often indicate smaller quantities of smoking, the dissimulation tendency is low because it is not shameful or guilt producing to be a smoker. The daily consumption of all probands is 675 cigarettes. The yearly consumption of one smoker 2005 cigarettes. Considering the fact that the sample did not include individuals under 15 or over 75 years old and these two groups are approximately one-quarter of the population of Saas-Fee, the yearly amount of cigarettes per capita is about 1640. Compared to the Swiss average (cf. p. 266) of 3.320 cigarattes per year per capita, the consumption in the village is only half as high.

12.5.2 Age

Age has a determinant influence on smoking and nonsmoking. Nonsmokers and probands smoking less than five cigarettes per day (cf. p. 269) belong mainly to the two oldest age groups (55-75). This corresponds indirectly to the observation of Russel (cf. p. 266) that smoking decreases after the age of 60, a fact related to their nonpermissive value patterns concerning cigarette smoking. In the older generations in the village, the nonpermissive value pattern still prevails; however, it changes in the younger generations (cf. p. 270). Probands smoking maximal quantities of cigarettes belong to the younger and middle age groups. 77% of the pipe or cigar smokers, however, belong to the two oldest groups (cf. p. 270).

The extent to which the nonpermissive attitude still plays a role, even in the younger generations, can be indirectly deduced from the finding (cf. p. 270) that smokers of the younger and middle age groups tend to evaluate their smoking as harmful.

12.5.3. Sex

Women do not smoke cigars or pipes, although pipe smoking was common among older women up to 1951. The finding that cigarette smoking in the village is increasing among younger women corresponds with reports in the international literature (cf. p. 266).

In order to permit a comparison with the findings of Russel (cf. p. 267), the percentage of the sex-specific consumption of cigarettes is — less than 5 cigarettes per day, man to women = 0 10%; 5-10 cigarettes per day; men to women = 13-27%; 11-20 cigarettes per day; men to women = 58-33%; and more than 20 cigarettes per day, men to women = 19 – 0%. These results correspond essentially to the findings by Russel (f.p. 267). There are, however, no women smoking maximal quantities and no men smoking fewer than 5 cigarettes per day.

The sex-specific differences in the self-evaluation of smoking are important (cf. p 270). Men usually indicate that their own smoking is harmful; women that it is harmless.

There are major sex-specific differences in the motivation for smoking and the reasons which make it impossible to quit smoking (cf. p. 271). The motivations "nervousness" and "insecurity" are indicated more often by women while the motivations "wish to be adult" and "imitation of others" are indicated more often by men. All the reasons which make it impossible to stop smoking are indicated more often by men.

12.5.4 Conscious Motivations for Smoking

The motivations for smoking in the questionnaire were "nervousness," "insecurity," "wish to be adult," and "imitation of environment." The further motivations, added by probands, were "addiction," "fun," "boredom," "habituation," and "change." The number of added motivations was too low to permit statistical elaboration.

The motivation "insecurity" is indicated by one woman only (cf. p. 271). "nervousness" is most frequently indicated and has an equal sex distribution (cf. p. 271). "Wish to be adult" and "imitation of behavior of the environment" is indicated by men only. This might be due to the fact that the advertising industry sells cigarettes as symbols of virility, adventure, and erotic success.

"Nervousness" can be interpreted as a motivation for smoking or a result of smoking. It is indicated most frequently. Since Wiener (367, 368) introduced the cybernetic model of explanation, the monolinear cause-effect thinking is devaluated. From a behavioral perspective, cause or effect is defined arbitrarily because it depends on the viewpoint of the observer. Thus, "nervousness" can be both cause and effect.

Comparing my results with the categories of Tomkin (cf. p. 267), it seems that the number of "negative-effect smokers" in the village prevails. Comparing my results to the categories of McKennel and Thomas (cf. p. 268), the smokers of the village can be subsumed mainly in the group of "nervous irritation smokers."

12.5.5 Habituation and Dependence

The main reasons indicated which make it impossible to quit smoking are "lack of will" ($n = 19$), "no need to stop" ($n = 18$), "repetitive unsuccessful efforts at quitting" ($n = 10$), "fear of known withdrawal symptoms" ($n = 8$), and "it is important to have fun in life" ($n = 5$).

These reasons are more frequently indicated by men than women. More than one-third (38%) "do not have the will to quit." These smokers can be considered "dissonant smokers;" they wich to stop but are unable to do so. More than one-third (36%) are "consonant smokers:" they find it unnessecary to quit. One-sixth (16%) are addicted smokers, according to the terminology of Tomkins (cf. p. 267); they are afraid of withdrawal symptoms and, therefore, unable to stop.

12.5.6 Personality

Smokers, more frequently than nonsmokers, indicate developmental problems (cf. p. 271). There are significant correlations between onychophagia or pavor nocturnus and smoking.

Probands who smoke little or exceedingly (i.e., less than 10 or more than 20 cigarettes per day) indicate developmental problems more often than probands with an average cigarette consumption (i.e., between 10 and 20 per day) (cf. p. 270). A possible explanation for this finding is that the former probands have control problems. The alternative strategy for coping with their control problems is either to smoke very little or to smoke too much.

There are statistically significant differences between the drug consumption of smokers and nonsmokers. Smokers, more often than nonsmokers, do not indicate drug consumption (cf. p. 273); however, smokers, more often than nonsmokers, evaluate their drug consumption as harmful. Since 52% of the smokers do not evaluate their drug consumption at all, it can be assumed that they have a dissimulation tendency, probably connected with their self-image. Given these findings, which indirectly support the findings of Russel (cf. p. 267), we can assume that smokers, more often than nonsmokers, had a neurotic development.

It is questionable as to whether or not our smokers are really more active than non-smokers and whether or not they do belong to the behavioral type A (cf. p. 267). My data (cf. p. 272) indicate that 38% of the smokers, but only 27% of the non-smokers, work less than 10 hours per day. On the other hand, individuals smoking between 10 and 20 or more cigarettes per day (i.e., 53-61%) work 12 hours or more daily (cf. p. 272). The second half of the results indirectly supports the hypothesis that smokers belong to the behavioral type A.

Smokers and nonsmokers do not show major differences in relation to workhours, differences in the way they experience the season, nor how they evaluate their educational background. Many of the working hypotheses about these differences between smokers and nonsmokers were falsified by the findings.

Smokers do not have a higher anxiety level than nonsmokers (cf. p. 272); 41% of the nonsmokers and only 36% of the smokers indicate being afraid of a possible economic crisis and 5% of the nonsmokers and 20% of the smokers are indifferent towards a possible economic crisis. The question is, whether or not the conscious attitudes are congruent with the unconscious ones. The modern times create idols and the *Leitbild* of the courageous maverick who is afraid of nothing. Identification with such idols wards off anxiety. This fact may be indirectly corroborated by the following result, although it is not statistically significant — 24% of the nonsmokers and only 16% of the smokers felt that they were not in good health at the moment of the interview.

My field observations suggested that most of the smokers had an athletic constitution, while the pycnic constitution was rather rare among smokers. The results correspond with this observation (cf. p.   ). The question is, however, whether or not the type of constitution, in itself, and the corresponding structure of temperament and affectivity play a determinant role or to what extent the official image, which is specific for a certain type of constitution, is the determinant. It is possible, for instance, that pycnics have a more syntonic reaction to the environment and, therefore, need fewer "crutches" in interactions, while leptosomes need smoking in order to diminish the anxiety before or during human interactions. It is also possible that men with an athletic constitution identify more easily with the rugged cowboy or the tough mile runner image projected by advertise ments, thus, smoking would be a partial behavior of a more global behavior pattern.

13. Psychiatric Disorders

13.1 Introduction

Does stress influence the prevalence and incidence of neurotic and psychotic decompensations? As yet, this question has not been answered definitively. It is, indeed, difficult to answer. As an overview of the psychiatric literature shows, the fact that it is rarely asked in this form may be a basic reason why it has not been answered.

The brief review of the literature which follows is based on the assumption that investigators are, in fact, implicitly referring to stress and stressors when they speak of life events, social determinants, and environmental or ecological factors.

The review of the literature has been limited to findings and concepts relevant to my approach. It should be understood that the data collected in the village (cf. p. 283) are fragmentary and, thus, cannot directly test the hypothesis of an interconnection between social change, stress, and psychiatric disorders sensu strictu.

13.2 Methods of Case Finding

Before discussing the interconnection between stress and psychiatric disorders, a "psychiatric case" has to be defined.

Problems of definition often start in the epidemiologic area, exactly at the point where they seem to be resolved in clinical psychiatry. This fact may be exemplified by two definitions of neurosis proposed in clinical psychiatry. Schwidder (322, p. 353) defines a neurosis as "a pathological disturbance in the elaboration of experience with symptoms of abnormal experience, behavior, and/or disturbed somatic functional processes." Ernst (cf. 322) defines a neurosis as "a psychological disturbance which, in a descriptive manner, excludes such disorders as psychopathia, endogenous psychoses, psychosomatic disorders, somatic disorders, and ubiquitous norm variants." Ernst (cf. 322) stresses that it is difficult to operate with such definitions in the epidemiologic area.

Reid (293, p. 20) insists that we need more operational definitions for epidemiologic purposes. An operational definition, for instance, would describe a psychiatric disorder as a disturbance of emotionality or adaptation which leads to hospitalization or the incapacity to work. However, as Mechanic (249, p. 7) points out, such a definition runs the risk of confusing treatment in a hospital, with treated prevalence, or, even, with the so-called true prevalence. The criterion of "need to be treated" or of treatment itself is helpful for the operational definition of a "case," as Dohrenwend et al. (76, p. 160) mention, but at the same time, such a definition is of limited operational range, especially when the influence of social factors needs to be evaluated.

The observer plays a major part in the case finding. As Kleiner (188, p. 208) observes, the psychiatrist often has to rely on diagnostics made by persons who judge and evaluate a "case" differently. Shepherd (326, p. 281) successfully avoids this obstacle by defining a "case" as a patient whose subjective and/or objective state induces him to consult a qualified doctor who makes a psychiatric diagnosis. This criterion operates in terms of a population who consults therapeutic facilities *(Inanspruchnahme-Population).* Such a definition was used in epidemiologic studies by Faris and Dunham (97) in Chicago, Hollingshead and Redlich (153) in New Haven, and Häfner (135, p. 203) in Mannheim.

Nevertheless, even such an apparently clear and unambiguous definition is based upon a complex labeling process. A labeling process is a social process which depends upon many factors and ultimately decides whether or not when, and where a person consults a treatment facility and, thus, becomes an official patient. According to Svendsen (cf. 293, p. 19 ff), labeling depends mainly on three factors — a population factor, a hospital factor, and a threshold factor. The threshold factor depends on the seriousness of the disorder which, in turn, depends on the medical evaluation and general attitude of the public. Moreover, the threshold factor depends on the tolerance of bizarre behavior and the status of the hospital or the treatment facility as an effective therapeutic institution.

All these factors influencing the labeling process have a special impact in rural areas. Wilken (Zur Epidemiologie und Ökologie psychiatrischer Erkrankungen, unpublished manuscript) stresses that the differences between rural and urban rates of incidence appear in a new light as soon as we consider hospitalization as an act of social control. A similar stands is taken by Kleiner (188, p. 208).

13.3 Investigators and Techniques of Investigation

As Strotzka (346) points out, the reliability and the validity of many epidemiologic studies are insufficient. Even those made by qualified investigators with an important technical investment are often criticised for their methodological insufficiency. Dohrenwend et al. (76, p. 160) question the validity of the measurement techniques of the renowned Manhattan Midtown Study and the Stirling Country Study.

The intensity of a study influences the reported prevalence of clinically serious, but not previously diagnosed or treated, disorders, as Zola (cf. Wilken: op. cit.) emphasizes. A similar view is held by Mechanic (249, p. 4) who states that it is one of the basic principles of epidemiology that investigations are as good as the techniques used for case identification. What is viewed as a "case" depends on the training and skill of the individual investigators, as Essen-Moeller (93, p. 23) states.

Given this state of affairs, there are increasing efforts to improve the methods of investigation. A general consensus seems to be developing around the technical know-how of such improvements. Katz (183, p. 150) postulates that a standardized interviewing technique is of essential importance. The epidemiologic research of psychological or somatic disorders can be based on the direct clinical examination, questionnaires, or information offered by health care administrations, as Richman (295, p. 257) proposes. Even when the case finding methods are extensive, only a portion of the "cases" are included because only a portion of them end up in the case register, a point rightly stressed by Richman (295, p; 259).

A more detailed strategy for investigation is indicated by Goldberg (117). He suggests an overall plan with basic data (e.g., name, marital status). He, then, proposes making a nonstructured anamnesis, a semistructured interview which is directed toward the presence of symptoms and a supplementary nonstructured interview which is concerned with the exact family anamnesis. Finally, the plan should include a rating scale so that the entire investigation leads to an exact diagnosis.

13.4 Problems of Transcultural Diagnosis

As Wilken (op. cit.) points out, notions of health and illness gleaned in the investigation of a hospitalized population and used in the so-called true-prevalence studies lead to exaggregated incidence and prevalence rates. In an average population, there are many states, identical with certain states found in hospitalized patients, which need no treatment. Schwidder (322, p. 357) reports that this is one of the reasons why some studies (e.g., Manhattan Midtown Study) claim that only 17% of the population are free from psychiatric disorders. Wilken (op. cit.) points out that these astronomic prevalence rates of nonnormal individuals are due to a circular conclusion based on wrong premises.

Keupp (cf. Wilken op. cit.) reviewing different types of definitions, comes to the conclusion that the usual definitions of psychic health and illness do indicate very little about the congruence with the object they claim to define; the definitions indicate much more about the value patterns of the person who makes the definitions. Therefore, the labeling discussed by Wilken (op. cit.) focuse on the way in which norms are constructed, how they are controlled, and how deviant behavior is sanctioned in a given subculture.

The subcultural differences are also stressed by Dohrenwend et al. (76, p. 160) and Mechanic (249, p. 9). The latter emphasizes that case interviews are often of a limited value since individuals in certain subcultures do not or cannot indicate their symptoms. According to Dohrenwend et al. (76, p. 160), it is the way in which distress is expressed in a given subculture which becomes the main problem in measuring psychiatric disorders in a general population. They outline that the relation between objective psychological disturbance and the inability to play certain roles introduces problems which can be resolved only by a psychiatric interview.

13.5 Incidence and Prevalence of Mental Disorders

13.5.1 Problems of Definition

Incidence and prevalence of mental disorders need an exact definition in order to avoid major errors. Especially, the so-called true-prevalence studies do not reach the high aspiration level proclaimed by their authors, as Wilken (op. cit) makes clear.

According to Reid (293, p. 17), the incidence can be expressed in three ways – as the number of days of illness of a person during a certain time span within an exposed population, as the total number of days of illness of a person, and as the total number of days of illness of a person per period of illness. However, Dunham (83) questions whether or not the duration of neurotic and psychotic disorders can really be measured since it is arbitrary to define beginning or end of an illness.

As Reid (293, p. 17) states, prevalence is defined as the number of illnesses multiplied with the average duration of illness.

13.5.2 Rates of Morbidity·

The definition of the rate of morbidity differs from author to author and from country to country. In a study made in 1929, Brugger (cf. 293, p. 25) found that the rate of morbidity of all psychiatric disorders in a district was 1.31%. On the other hand, Häfner and Reimann (136) found a rate of incidence of 10.74% in a study made in Mannheim in 1955.

The differences are even more important in international studies. Dohrenwend and Dohrenwend (79) compared 25 studies (i.e., 12 from the USA, 15 from Europe, 6 from Asia, and 2 from Africa) and found that the rates of incidence of psychiatric disorders varied from 1.7% to 64% for the USA, 1% to 33% in Europe, 0.8% to 3% in Asia, and 40% to 50% in Africa. The overall results varied between 0.8% and 64%, and there seems to be little doubt that these variations are due more to the investigative techniques than to the real differences in the rates of distribution.

The rates of incidence differ more or less, depending on whether or not the studies report incidence rates of neurotic or psychotic disorders. As Mechanic (249, p. 6) points out, the rates of incidence of psychotic disorders (e.g., schizophrenia) oscillate only between 0.25% and 1% when the investigators use the same definition for schizophrenia. The frequency of neuroses and personality disorders however, oscillate much more, as Schwidder (322), Strotzka (346), Leighton et al. (208), and Shepherd (325) outline. Ernst (cf. 322, p. 356) explains these differences by the fact that ideas about normality and neuroses differ greatly from observer to observer.

Given these discrepancies in the incidence rates, a few studies shall be briefly discussed. In the so-called Stirling County Study, Leighton et al. (208) found the following morbidity rates: psychosomatic disorders (59.5%), psychoneuroses (51.9%), personality disorders (6.0%), sociopathias (i.e., alcoholism, dissociality) (5.8%), mental retardation (4.8%), organic brain syndromes (2.5%), and psychoses (0.9%).

Srole et al. (339), using a rather broad definition of "disorders," found in the Manhattan Midtown Study that more than 80% of the population suffered from mental disorders. Hagnell (139, p. 213), using a more restrictive definition to investigate the Swedish village of Lundby, found an incidence rate of mental disorders of 15.6%.

Cooper et al. (63, p. 299), using a well defined investigative technique, studied the patients of 46 general practices in Greater London and found a 1-year prevalence rate for all mental disorders of 140% among the adults at risk. Three years later, 44% of the diagnosed cases were without symptoms, whereas 14% showed more or less serious states. Shepherd et al. (326) found a prevalence rate of 15.4%, while Strotzka (346) found a prevalence rate of 18.9% in his study of the rural area Kleinburg.

Häfner and Reimann (136, p. 341) investigated the correlations between the incidence of mental disorders and ecological factors found by Faris and Dunham (97) and others. Their study included those inhabitants of Mannheim who, in 1956, had consulted specialized medical facilities for their mental disorders or mental retardation for the first time. According to these criteria, the incidence rate found was 10.74%, a figure which includes the incidence rate of 1.53% for mental retardation.

Finally, Häfner (135, p. 208) examined seven international studies and found that the incidence rate of mental disorders oscillated between 11.9% and 5.8%, while the prevalence rate oscillated between 20.51% and 15.2%.

13.6 Influencing Socioecological Factors

Today, it is generally acknowledged that incidence and prevalence rates of mental disorders are influenced by socioecological factors. The studies of Faris and Dunham (97), Häfner and Reimann (136), Hollingshead and Redlich (153), Leighton et al. (208), Srole et al. (339), and others postulated such influence and found fairly important statistical correlations supporting this hypothesis.

As Reid (293, p. 20) points out, Vermeylen demonstrated that during the military occupations of World War II, the rates of hospitalization decreased in many countries. This happened even when the hospital system was intact, suggesting that increased national and social integration were responsible for this fact.

However, this conclusion is questioned by Häfner (135, p. 204) who points out that the ecological distribution of neuroses and mental crises cannot be studied on the basis of the hospitalized population alone.

Different ecological variables are discussed in the international literature.

13.6.1 Family

According to Wilken (op. cit.), the breakdown of the social organization of a family provokes public social control and leads to an increase of the morbidity rate or, rather, the hospitalization rate. This statement is widely supported by the experiences of family therapists – by Bowen (37), Haley (140, 141), Minuchin (253-255), Wynne (374, and many others.

13.6.2 Society

Rural and urban areas have different degress of tolerance for bizarre behavior, which influence their rates of incidence and vary the prevalence. Studying a rural district in Michigan, Lemert cf. Wilken: op. cit.) found an astonishing tolerance for psychotic behavior. Roth and Luton (cf. Wilken: op. cit.), studying a rural area in Tennessee, report that only half of the psychotic population was hospitalized. A comparable study, made in the urban area of Baltimore, showed that three-quarters of the psychotic population was hospitalized.

13.6.3 Sex

According to Rutter (310, p. 82), there is no doubt that men are less resistent to stress than women. It seems that men are more vulnerable when exposed to psychosocial stressors; however, as we have seen in the chapter on psychosomatics, this hypothesis is questionable.

13.6.4 Coexistence of Psychosomatic Disorders

Eastwood (85, p. 91) reports that Leighton et al. (208) and Shepherd et al. (326) found a positive correlation between psychic and somatic disorders. Eastwood (85, p. 91) assumes that neurotic patients consult doctors more frequently and are ill more often than nonneurotics. Schwidder (322), reviewing the international literature, comes to a similar conclusion.

13.6.5 Stress

The question as to whether or not life events and/or psychosocial stressors influence the incidence and prevalence of mental disorders is still in dispute; however, it becomes increasingly apparent that positive correlations exist and that methodological improvements in the techniques of investigation are yielding more significant results than were previously thought possible.

Brown and Birley (42, p. 321) stress that the influence of psychosocial stressors, life changes, or life events is still controversial. They stress that in reviewing the international literature they found only "common sense" judgments, speaking pro or con for such an influence. They also point out that the frequently mentioned "stressful event" might already be a sign of the onset of an illness. Discussing the international literature, Brown et al. (43, p. 74) found that some authors assume a causal connection between stress and life events and that psychiatric morbidity cannot be proven. Other authors claim that life events have a partial or a determining influence. Brown et al. (43, p. 74) demonstrate that methodological errors increase the chance of a positive correlation between life events and mental disorders. Based on two studies made in London, they assume that this correlation exists between life events and depressive disorders. They conclude that three main reasons are responsible for the fact that most investigations find only negative correlations between life events and schizophrenic or depressive disorders – the selection of an adequate sample of comparison, the definition of the timespan between event and onset of disorder, and the criteria used for the description of the qualitative or quantitative nature of life events.

Brown et al. (44) described a method which makes it possible to differentiate between formative effects and triggering effects. Formative effects are present when the disorder would probably not, or not yet, have started without the life events; this is the case in depression. Triggering effects are present when the factors involved gave the last push for the onset of the disorder which would have started anyway; such a triggering effect is found in schizophrenia. The hypothesis of the formative effect is supported by Stein and Susser (343) who described it in the case of psychological loss, especially widowhood.

Dohrenwend (80, p. 13) claims that short term stressors increase the rate of psychic morbidity and that they correlate positively with schizophrenia decompensation. Such a view is questioned by Mechanic (249, p. 17) who claims that psychotic decompensations do not increase significantly during bombing attacks or other acute events. Nor is it proven, according to Mechanic (249, p. 17), that urbanism and hectic life style increase the rate of psychotic decompensations. There is evidence, however, that long lasting stress results in mental disorders and these vanish as soon as the stress vanishes.

In my opinion, such contradictory views are founded mainly on terminological uncertainties. Several authors do not differentiate between stressors and stress, or an event, per se, and the way in which such an event is experienced. My findings (cf. p. 216) that the frequency of psychosomatic stress reactions is positively correlated to the way in which the season is experienced, but not to the amount of worktime, suggests that such differentiations are crucial.

13.6.6 Suicidality

Ever since the famous suicide study of Durkheim, suicide is viewed as an indicator of stress. Many authors assume that the rate of suicide is a direct indicator of the social disintegration which creates an important field of stressors and can lead as far as total anomie.

Kreitman (203, p. 355) views suicide as a form of symbolic communication and, therefore, suicide should be studied as a social, and not individual, phenomenon. This social dimension is stressed by Häfner (135, p. 11) who points out that the pressure of confirmity and imitation play a determinant role. It is well-known that suicide can reach epidemic proportions in certain countries, at certain times, and under certain conditions. For instance, Goethe's publication of Die Leiden des jungen Werthers seems to have triggered a suicidal wave throughout Europe.

Interestingly enough, the suicide rate decreases whenever the population moves into an important crisis. As Häfner (135, p. 213) reports, the suicide rate of men decreased in Germany during the war, while it increased during the economic crisis; however, it is difficult to know how many of the war casualties were actually masked suicides.

13.7 Methods of Data Collection

In 1970, my lack of specialized psychiatric training did not permit adequate field interviews and reliable diagnoses of the incidence and prevalence of psychiatric disorders. Furthermore, the case register of the general practice was useless for the purpose of this study.

Given this situation, I applied a method of casefinding which seemed to be as reliable as possible under the circumstances. It corresponded to the method used by Häfner and Reimann (136).

I wrote to every psychiatric inpatient and outpatient hospital in Switzerland, provided a name register, and asked if they had treated patients from the village in the previous 50 years. I also asked for the exact diagnosis and the number and duration of treatments.

The replies proved, and this is rather interesting to note, that the psychiatric patients of the village had been treated all over the country. Some patients had consulted remote clinics, probably for the purpose of anonymity and because there were no satisfactory treatment facilities in the nearby area.

A case, according to my definition, is a patient treated in a psychiatric inpatient or outpatient facility in Switzerland. The advantage of such an operational definition is that the reliability of the diagnosis is high. The disadvantage is that patients treated by private practitioners or in nonpsychiatric treatment facilities are not included. Because I knew that the probands would not answer questions dealing with mental disorders, just as they did not answer questions concerning sexual behavior, I did not include these questions in the questionnaire.

Given this specific casefinding method, we can assume that the following prevalence and incidence of mental disorders is lower than in reality; however, my operational definition is adequate for the purpose of the followup study because the same method of case finding will be used in 1980.

13.8 Results

13.8.1 Distribution of First Diagnoses

The number of patients treated, primarily in inpatient facilities is so small that only the overall distribution is indicated. Finer analysis of the data, according to socioecological factors (e.g., sex, age, social class), would not yield significant results. In order to permit an overview of the change in the incidence rates of the last 50 years, all the first diagnoses are included in Table 34.

Table 34. *Overall distribution of the first diagnoses between 1921 and 1970*

	1921-30		1931-40		1941-50		1951-60		1961-70	
	M	F	M	F	M	F	M	F	M	F
Schizophrenia	2	1	1	1	3	1	2	1	3	2
Endogenous depression									1	
Alcoholism					1				4	
Organic brain disorders									2	1
Reactive depressions								1		2
Neuroses		1				1	1		2	
Homosexuality									1	
Psychosomatic disorders										1
Mental retardation						1				
Epilepsy										2
Psychopathia										
Involutive depression										1
Total	2	2	1	1	4	3	3	2	13	9

There are several interesting observations:

— A general, although irregular, increase in the frequency of diagnoses and, with it, of patients during the 50-year period.
— The morbidity of men is higher than that of women. This is true for the distribution within the decades and within the different nosological categories.
— "Schizophrenia" is mentioned often, while "endogenous depression" is mentioned only once. This distribution does not correspond to general epidemiological data of these nosological entities.
— In the first decade after 1951, not a single man is treated for alcoholism while, in the following decade, four are. This corresponds to the findings discussed earlier (cf. p. 219) which suggest that high alcohol consumption is related to the increasing number of stressors after 1951which took some time to produce official alcoholics.

13.8.2 Development of Rates of Incidence

Calculating the incidence rates per decade (i.e., the number of first diagnoses per decade), we find the following results shown in Fig. 44.

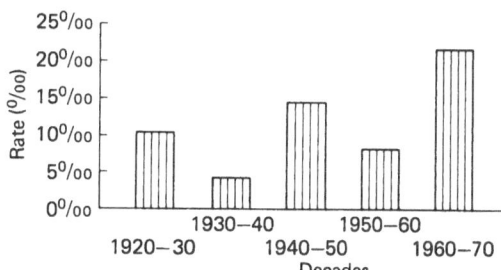

Fig. 44. Rates of incidence of first diagnoses in the 5 decades

The incidence rate is — 4 : 378 x 1000 = 0.58% for the 1st decade; 2 : 457 x 1000 = 4.37% for the 2nd decade; 7 : 489 x 1000 = 14.31 % for the 3rd decade; 5 : 621 x 1000 = 8.05% for the 4th decade; and 16 : 756 x 1000 = 21.16% for the 5th decade. The overall tendency is one of a linear increase, although the rate oscillates — it decreases in the 1930s and 1950s. These results will be discussed later.

13.8.3 Prevalence Rate in 1970

The prevalence rate of psychiatric disorders in 1970 can be calculated:

$$\text{Prevalence rate} = \frac{5}{800} \times 100 = 6.25\%$$

13.8.4 Duration of Hospitalization

The duration of hospitalization increases over the decades. This means that more patients stay longer in treatment facilities. There are sex-specific differences. With the exception of the first decade, men have a longer duration of hospitalization. This coincides with the higher incidence of first diagnoses of men (Fig. 45).

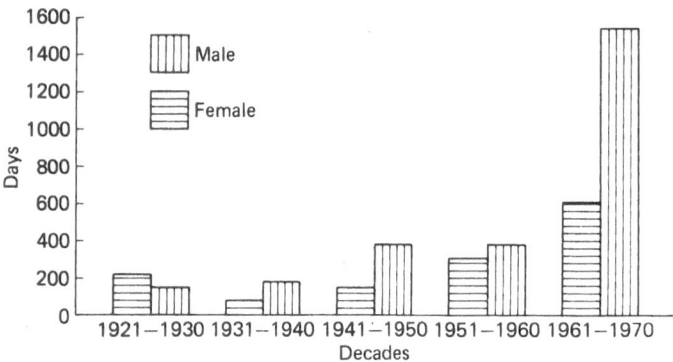

Fig. 45. Development of the duration of hospitalization from 1921 to 1970

13.9 Discussion of Results

13.9.1 Representativeness of My Results

The results of this study are insufficient for the following reasons:

- My lack of specialized psychiatric training in 1970.
- The case register of the general practice in the village was unreliable.
- The diagnoses of village patients, provided by different psychiatric treatment facilities, were essentially reliable. The reliability of diagnoses provided by psychiatrists is, however, questioned by a group of authors (i.e., 79, 143, 183, Wilken: (Zur Epidemiologie und Ökologie psychiatrischer Erkrankungen, unpublished manuscript), 249, 370).
- There was no network of private psychiatrists in the nearby area, therefore, there were no data available.
- The psychiatric inpatient treatment facility in the nearby area was not frequently consulted by the villagers for mainly sociocultural and political reasons.
- There had been changes in the diagnostic trends over the years.

Although the basic data for a comparison in the next cross-sectional study, in 1980, will have to be collected in the same way, we will need supplementary data to better understand the mental health situation in Saas-Fee. They should fulfill the general criteria postulated by Goldberg (117), Katz (183), and Richman (295, p. 257).

13.9.2 Case Finding

My operational definition of a case is a patient treated in a psychiatric inpatient or out-patient facility in Switzerland. This definition is similar to that used by Faris and Dunham (97), Häfner and Reimann (136), Hollingshead and Redlich (153), Reid (293), and Shepherd (325). It is clear and easy to handle and control; however, it it too narrow to provide sufficient information about the psychiatric morbidity of a population, as postulated by Dohrenwend et al. (76). Consequently, my results are below the actual morbidity rates.

The morbidity rates are influenced by different factors (293, p. 19 ff; Wilken: op. cit.). There is a tolerance for bizarre behavior in the village, an observation confirmed in other rural areas by Lemert (cf. Wilken: op. cit.) and Roth and Luton (cf. Wilken: op. cit.). In 1970, there were three schizophrenic men and one schizophrenic woman with quite obvious psychotic behavior in the village. They were looked upon as being "funny" or "somewhat strange," but this fact did not lead to a further labeling process or hospitalization. According to key informants, before 1951, the tolerance towards strange behavior (i.e., mainly hallucinatory, maniform, or paranoid behavior) was even greater.

13.9.3 Distribution of First Diagnoses

There is a general increase in the number of first diagnoses (cf. p. 284), a phenomenon which lends itself to several interpretations:

- An increase in population increased the absolute number of morbidity.
- Increasing social change introduced new value patterns and new sanctions for deviant behavior. In earlier periods, for instance, a schizophrenic could function well as a shepherd or fieldworker, but tourism and the new distribution of work provided fewer ecological niches in which such a person could function without disturbing others or being disturbed themselves. Today, bizarre behavior is scapegoated more quickly and a social ostracism leads to hospitalization.
- In 1970, the supreme law governing life in tourist facilities was to guarantee the peace and satisfaction of the guests. Although the labeling attitude towards bizarre behavior was more quickly defined as needing treatment, conspicuously deviant behavior was still tolerated more readily than in the cities.

13.9.4 Sex and Mental Health Disorders

Men have a higher morbidity rate than women, especially as far as alcoholism and psychosis are concerned. The increased rate of alcoholism is easily explained (cf. p. 284), but the male-specific increase of other first diagnoses is difficult to interpret. On the one hand, it might be due to higher vulnerability of men exposed to psychosocial stressors, as assumed by Rutter (310, p. 82). Brown (41) and Brown et al. (44), however, point out that such stressors would only have a triggering effect upon schizophrenia, and the overrepresentation of male psychotics would still not been explained. On the other hand, a given society might tolerate bizarre behavior from women more easily because women can be physically controlled or psychotic women can function adequately in ecological niches, for instance, at home away from social interactions which could decompensate them.

13.9.5 Prevalence Rate

The prevalence rate (cf. p. 285) was 6.25% in 1970. Again, this rate is probably lower than the actual prevalence rate. Since my case definition is restrictive, the results cannot be compared to the international literature.

13.9.6 Development of Incidence Rates

The incidence rates (cf. p. 285) show an overall tendency to increase, despite a decrease in the 1930s and 1950s. How can this decrease be explained?

According to all available information, the economic crisis of the 1930s produced a stagnation in the tourist development, but it increased the coherence and social integration of families and the village as a whole. A similar process occurred in the 1950s. All the social forces were focused upon building up the tourist resort, a situation which produced an increased coherence and integration of the families. Whenever social integration increases, the labeling process changes; there is less scapegoating of marginal individuals and less excluding them from the social context.

In the 1960s, the decade before my investigation, the incidence rate was 21.16%. Again, the actual incidence rate was probably higher. Comparison with the data of Strotzka (346) or Shepherd et al. (326) is not possible. These authors indicate an incidence rate per year while I indicate it per decade. Reducing my incidence rate per 10 years to an incidence rate per one year, mine is far below those reported by several authors. It is possible that the different casefinding methods are responsible for this fact.

In my data there are two officially diagnosed cases of only neurosis (cf. p. 284).

As Eastwood (85), Leighton et al. (208), Schwidder (322), and Shepherd et al. (326) point out, there are many neuroses, personality disorders, and alcoholic syndromes concealed among psychosomatic disorders. Alcoholism can be viewed, according to my field observations, as a strategy to cope with neurotic and psychotic anxieties.

13.9.7 Duration of Hospitalization

Figure 45 (cf. p. 286) indicates that the duration of hospitalization for men is higher than women. This correlation is due primarily to the higher prevalence and incidence rate of men.

13.9.8 Suicide

The only known suicide within the 5 decades before my investigation was committed by a man hospitalized for endogenous depression; the only psychotic depression ever diagnosed in the village. I have no other indications of suicide attempts in the decade before my investigation or prior to that time. There are several protective factors which might be responsible for that fact:

- The prohibitive attitude of the Roman Catholic Church still had an important impact on the villagers (cf. p. 148). A religious system creates order and meaningfulness in the stream of random life events and, thus, protects against anomie and existential desperation.

- Possibly some of the hunting or mountain accidents were masked suicides. They were further camouflaged by the family to avoid the sanction of the Church. Suicide was a mortal sind and, thus, for centuries, the Roman Catholic Church forbid that these sinners would be buried in the consecrated earth.
- The high social integration of families and the village as a whole had a protective function as observed in other contexts by Häfner (135) and Kreitman (203).

13.9.9 Stress and Psychiatric Morbidity

My method used does not permit valuable statements about the quantitative correlations between stress and psychiatric morbidity.

The direct field observation, however, suggests that, in 1970, there were neuroses and personality disorders influenced by the problems produced by the cultural lag during the process of socialization. The syngenetic program, built up during the phase of the cultural lag, is contradictory in many of its elements, a fact producing stressors which influence individuals and their coping potentials.

14. Crime

14.1 Introduction

The direct field observation showed that delinquent behavior in the village was nonsignificant in 1970. Therefore, this chapter is added only for the sake of completeness.

Delinquent behavior is one of the stress indicators of a population and a means of communicating a threatened homeostasis of a human system.

14.2 International Literature

Given the qualitative and quantitative insignificance of delinquent behavior in the village, only a gew points of view, relevant for this study, will be discussed.

14.2.1 Definition of Delinquent Behavior

What is labeled "delinquent behavior" depends mainly upon the social value patterns and the efficiency of social control. In this sense, Sack (311, p. 979) defines delinquent behavior as "an offense against a norm which is controlled by a certain sanction." A similar definition is given by Wheeles (cf. 311, p. 997), who defines it as a behavior which objectively offends a norm and which, moreover, is perceived by the social environment as deviant from the norm.

It seems to me that these definitions – though generally accepted and unequivocal in the context of criminality studies – are too broad. After all, drunkenness may be a norm deviance sanctioned by social ostracism, but it is not necessarily viewed as delinquent behavior. A more satisfactory definition should include a description of the type of behavior and the type of sanction.

14.2.2 The Delinquent

It is generally assumed that individuals of the lowest social class are more likely to become delinquent because social control, personal motivations, and a specific milieu push the individual in this direction.

Glueck and Glueck (cf. 301, p. 141) showed that individuals of those groups who have no satisfying emotional bonds and no internalization of the prevalent value patterns of their society are especially at risk. This is often the case in the lower social classes which may have a dysfunctional family structure, as Minuchin et al. (254) pointed out in his structural study of the families of slums.

This view is shared by Rosenmayr (301, p. 142), who emphasizes the "deferred gratification pattern" in which members of the middle classes are trained during the socialization process. Such a gratification pattern makes possible the renouncing of the immediate gratification for the sake of future gratification. The lower classes, with their more restricted life goals and realization possibilities, seem to prefer immediate gratification in a life that promises no satisfying future. Once trained in this pattern, an individual has reduced capacities of enduring frustration, and acting out becomes the appropriate strategy for coping with stress. Contemporary observations suggest that emotionally deprived middle and upper class children go through similar frustrations and, therefore, become prone to delinquent behavior. Thus, it seems that the social organization of a family is a more important determinant for delinquent behavior than the economic situation.

Fromm (110, p. 120) views a deficient "superego formation" as a central personality deficit leading to delinquent behavior. He emphasizes (110, p. 128) the following sociopsychological mechanism which disposes an individual to delinquent behavior: low sublimation possibility, social reinforcement of individual aggressive impulses directed towards the upper classes, the satisfaction of narcissistic needs in the delinquent act, and the possibility of interpreting the delinquent behavior as an attempt to redistribute the wealth more evenly. Rosenmayr (301, p. 143 ff) writes that such an attempt does not seem inappropriate for lower class individuals with limited economic possibilities.

Hacker (134, p. 21 ff), stressing the social and individual effects of control of aggression and aggressiveness in adolescents, comes to similar conclusions. The mechanism of acting out, punishment, and building up of new aggressions, along with the inability to endure frustration, degenerates into a self-steering vicious circle since acting out does not have a cathartic function. Hacker (134, p. 34) writes that it can lead to a paradoxical increase of aggression. Plack (283, p. 340) claims that criminality is "the neurosis of the little man" who lacks the social setup of the middle and upper classes for becoming neurotic in a socially accepted form.

14.2.3 Social Environment

All the hypotheses and concepts outlined before stress the importance of the social environment. Haley (140, p. 2 ff), however, emphasizes that it is impossible to separate the individual from its social context if we want to understand deviant or symptomatic behavior. Social environment and individual delinquent behavior are interdependent. As Plack (283, p. 303) states, the criminal has a social function because he expresses the repressed intensions of those who are more successful in controlling them. This lack of control is a general feature of the dysfunctional family structures. As Minuchin et al. (254) demonstrated, disorganized lower class families with a poor parental executive favor acting out anger and aggressions.

Fromm (110, p. 130) argues that it is impossible to decide whether or not delinquent behavior is due to "drives" or the socioeconomic structure of a society — both the organization of "drives" and society shape and determine each other. The interconnection between economic situation and delinquency is statistically proven according to Fromm

(110, p. 115) – corn prices and criminality (i.e., thefts) are directly proportional to each other. It is held by Oswald (266, p. 45) and Plack (283, p. 22) that prescribed values and delinquency are interdependent, although this correlation is difficult to prove. The same holds true for the correlation between delinquency and the socioeconomic situation, as Levi and Anderson (218, p. 75) outline in their discussion of the problems of urbanization.

Sack (311, p. 976 ff) argues that Lacasagne's dictum, *les sociétés ont les criminels qu'elles méritent* (societies have the criminals they deserve), is more the expression of a moralistic attitude than a critical evaluation of the object of investigation. Sack (311, p. 976 ff) views that the delinquent behavior as the final product in a complex chain of interactions whose elements influence each other in multiple ways. According to Sack (311, p. 983), formal control (e.g., criminal law) and informal social control (e.g., influence of friends, peer group) reinforce or inhibit delinquent behavior.

What Habermas (133, p. 177) analyzed in another context can be applied to delinquency – the crime appears as a socially determined norm deviance which is heaped upon the helpless individual as his private problem and which can be secondarily controlled by formal control. The primary problem now appears as a problem which can be resolved by purely administrative-bureaucratic procedures. In other words, the dysfunctional homeostasis of a society is, first, projected into the individual and, second, treated by bureaucratic-legalistic means.

14.2.4 Statistics of Crime

Statements about delinquent behavior are primarily based on statistics of criminality. This method of casefinding is operational, but restrictive. As Levi and Anderson (218, p. 75) point out, statistics of criminality have a low degree of reliability and, therefore, are difficult to interpret. Sack (311, p. 998 ff) emphasizes that especially the question of the unreported cases *(Dunkelziffer)* is far from being resolved theoretically.

14.3 Methods of Data Collection

In 1970, the village gave the impression that criminality was not an important stress indicator. Felonies were unknown or had not been reported, at least not over the last century. The aggressive interactions (e.g., verbal and/or physical fights during carnival or election periods) and the rare thefts committed mainly by adolescents were viewed by the population as a slight norm deviance, not as a criminal act. Although such behaviors were rejected, they did not lead to major formal sanctions.

For obvious reasons, the questionnaire could not be used for the elucidation of criminal behavior. I decided to rely on the statistics of criminality. Since the village was in the process of building up a bureaucracy adapted to the modern era, there were no statistics available before 1968. Statements of the development of criminal behavior before and after the construction of the road are therefore missing. The data presented are from 1968, 1969, and 1970.

14.4 Results

As Table 35 indicates, only thefts were reported. Mainly, objects in easily accessible locations were stolen. All thefts are not important from a quantitative standpoint.

Table 35. *Quality and quantity of the delicts committed from 1968 to 1970*

Quantity	Quality of delicts	
6	Thefts	in public enterprises
1	Thefts	of mail
1	Thefts	in a military institution
1	Thefts	in a shop
4	Thefts	in warehouses
1	Thefts	on a construction plot
26	Thefts	in public places and hotels
1	Thefts	in a campground
1	Thefts	in a public swimming pool
5	Thefts	in the street
1	Thefts	in an apartment
1	Thefts	in a cellar
1	Thefts	in a mountain cabin
5	Thefts	in cars
4	Thefts	of car equipment
46	Thefts	of skis
2	Thefts	of copper objects
21	Nondelivery	of found objects
Total 128	Thefts	

Only a few of these thefts were adjudicated (see Table 36).

Table 36. *Quality and quantity of committed and adjudicated delicts*

Year	Origin of offender	Profession	Sex	Delicts
1968	Village	Worker	M	Thefts in cars
1968	Foreign country	Artist	M	Embezzlement
1968	Foreign country	Employee	F	Fraud
1969	Foreign country	Employee	F	Burglary in hotel
1969	Canton Wallis	Mechanic	M	Burglary
1969	Canton Wallis	Handyman	M	Burglary
1969	Foreign country	Employee	F	Theft on construction site
1969/ 1970	Foreign country	Employee	F	Nondelivery of found objects
1970	Canton Wallis	Mechanic	M	Burglaries in hotel
1970	Switzerland	Employee	M	Suspicion of drug consumption

Total: 10 delinquents, 9 thefts, 1 suspicion of drug consumption

The annual rate of reported and adjudicated crimes varies between three and four incidents. There was only one villager convicted for theft. The professional categories suggest that all the convicted delinquents, possibly with the exception of the artist, belong to the lower social class. The sex distribution is six males and four females.

14.5 Discussion of Results

According to my case definition, cases reported in the statistics of criminality only are taken into consideration, though Levi and Anderson (218, p. 75) and Sack (311, p. 998 ff) emphasize that these data have to be interpreted cautiously.

The number of reported delicts is probably lower than the actual number of delicts. Given the numerous tourists (i.e., approximately 800,000 per year), the number of delicts is low. The quota of adjudicated delicts is only 9.25%, a fact due mainly to the migration intensity of a tourist resort.

All the delicts, with the exception of "suspicion of drug consumption," are thefts or burglaries. All the delinquents, with the possible exception of the artist, are from the lower social classes, an indicator of the unequal distribution of property, a higher incidence of social disintegration, or the fact that lower class members are caught more easily.

Fromm (110, p. 120 ff) points out that the lower classes are especially motivated to delinquent behavior. The great number of employees and workers who are among the delinquents corroborate Fromm's statement. Moreover, these individuals, with one exception, do not belong to the native population and, thus, are not subject to the same social control as the villagers, a fact which favors delinquency, as stressed by Rosenmayr (301, p. 141) and Sack (311, p. 983). Social contradictions (i.e., the unequal distribution of property and surplus profit produced with common effort) become the personal problem of the individual, as described by Habermas (133, p. 171). The deviance is bureaucratically resolved via formal social control (i.e., by convicting the person) and a report in the official statistics of criminality.

Since there seem to be no delinquent villagers, with one exception, it can be assumed that the prohibitive value and deferred gratification patterns are still existing. The villagers express stress by drinking, smoking, psychosomatic symptoms, or drug consumption. The ritualized control of aggression within the social organization and the motoric release of aggression in sports and hard work seems to function as escape valves. Moreover, the economic situation allows the villagers to own most of the objects which might otherwise be stolen.

Finally, the main protective agent seems to be the family. It is still structurally intact and essentially fulfills its basic functions (i.e., it offers a good economic base and an effective socialization process). Thus, the syngenetic program contains the prohibitive value patterns needed to inhibit delinquent acts.

15. Epilogue

At the beginning of the 19th century, Zurbriggen (cf. 308) closed his chronicle with the following sentences, cast in an old-fashioned language, and giving the impression that he almost had to justify his lifelong work, "Some people will say that I valued this valley too highly. Perhaps. But then I ask these critics to tell me which other mountain valley has so early won its freedom? Which valley has produced so many scholars of an ecclesiastic or worldly type? Which one has produced so many important persons who have given so many founds *(Pfrumbden)* and prebends *(Gotteshäuser),* although being poor, and which one has produced such a great number of wise men for the Church and of intelligent men for the high political positions and so many warm patriots and industrious people?"

More than 150 years later, the present diachronic study, aimed at the description of this same valley and of one of its villagers, Saas-Fee, is published. There is no need for justification; however, if I gave one, it would be different from that of the old chronicler.

I attempted to describe the village process of Saas-Fee with a holistic-syngenetic concept. I tried to show that the structural and functional organization of such a microcosm is of a very complex nature. A village is a human system, composed of many subsystems, and interrelated in multiple interactions on different levels of hierarchy. The village, an open human system, has tried to maintain its homeostasis over the centuries by multiple transformations and a continuous exchange of matter-energy and information with its environment.

There were times when the village process underwent transformations at a high rate of speed and recalibration (i.e., the overall adjustment to social change was very difficult). There were other times when the village process slowed down and when each year, each decade, or each century brought the same reality the past had had to offer. There were times when the village seemed to sleep and, like the Alps, was petrified in the condition of a never changing, tradition directed rural society. There also were times when the village was not only awake, but alarmed by the rapidly advancing social process.

Tourism, introduced in Saas-Fee in the middle of the last century and accelerated in its qualitative and quantitative impact in the middle of this century, opened a new chapter in the village history. The turning of the pages produced stress and the villagers coped with it by choosing all the strategies human beings had invented since they left the mythical paradise. They worked hard, prayed to their Lord, cunned, fought, gave in, adapted, emigrated, drank, smoked, consumed drugs, and developed psychosomatic symptoms, depressions, and "craziness." Not all these coping strategies had the same value and many, while helpful in the immediate situation, created more stress and disorders in the longrun. Life is a constant battle against the increasing entropy, and this battle had its victories and its defeats. For a contemporary observer, it is difficult, it not impossible, to decide what were the victories and what the defeats.

It has been a fascinating endeavor to study the village and describe how it changed its form of social organization over the centuries. The old organizations never completely vanished and the new organizations were never completely new. One form of organization slipped into the other, as one sand dune moves into the other. Social organizations were transformed in the same way in which wind and erosion transform the faces of valleys and mountains into new faces which are the old ones in different positions within the space-time continuum. Change refers to what is redundant, what is stable in the continuous turmoil of transformations, and what remains of itself behind the mask of a turbulent cosmic dance. What is redundant is that human beings are extremely flexible in their struggle for survival and in their quest for what they consider to be a decent life.

The old unit, man-environment, still exists in the village, although the villagers have changed their relationship towards the environment. Their former isolation in the wild mountains has turned into an unexpected opportunity to build up an attractive tourist resort. Again, this opportunity has two faces. The old fears of a wild nature have been replaced by the new fears to depend upon the international economic and political situation with its unpredictable changes. The former existential anxiety has only changed its face. Something might happen which would stop people from visiting the village. This possibility constitutes a permanent threat.

What would be the consequences if this threat became true? The mountains and glaciers of The Pearl of the Alps would again become the walls imprisoning the village in isolation and socioeconomic deprivation. For the time being, there is no evidence that such a thing might happen in the near future. The number of tourists is still increasing, debts are being repaid, and new investments made. The villagers seem to live better today than ever before.

The villagers march to the rhythm of an invisible drummer, and this rhythm is pretty fast. Rapid social change has created a torrent in which fragments of old structures swim towards the sea of entropy. It also carries new structures, islands of life which work against entropy and build up new structures. Creativity is fighting entropy.

The village process is full of contradictions. It exemplifies the time-honored teachings symbolized in the ancient Chinese T'ai-chi T'u, The Diagram of the Supreme Ultimate — life is composed of Yin and Yang, of dark and light, good and bad, positive and negative, male and female, giving and taking. The more a process veers towards one extreme of the complementarity of Yin and Yang, the more it bears in itself the potential for its opposite. In 1970, Saas-Fee was in the vortex of rapid social change. The drummer might change his rhythm one day and slow down again.

The village changed and is still changing. This author changed and is still changing. As Levi-Strauss (221, p. 43) proclaimed, "The field of research with which every anthropological career begins, is the mother and wetnurse of doubt, the philosophical attitude par excellence." The Saas-Fee study offered me both, it nourished me with doubt, but it also gave me understanding; understanding of the world, the village, and last, but not least, of myself.

References

1. Ackoff, R.L., Emery, F.E.: On purposeful systems. Chicago, New York: Aldine. Atherton 1972
2. Adler, A.: Menschenkenntnis. Frankfurt, Hamburg: Fischer 1966
3. Adorno, T.W.: Eingriffe, neun kritische Modelle. Frankfurt: Suhrkamp 1963
4. Ague, C.: Nicotine content of cigarettes and the smoking habits: their relevance to subjective ratings of preferences in smokers. Psychopharmacologia *24*, 326-330 (1972)
5. Ague, C.: Nicotine and smoking: effects upon subjective changes in mood. Psychopharmacologia *30*, 323-328 (1973)
6. Ague, C.: Smoking patterns, nicotine intake at different times of day and changes into cardiovascular variables while smoking cigarettes. Psychopharmacologia *30*, 135-144 (1973)
7. Arensberg, K.M.: Die Gemeinde als Objekt und als Paradigma. In: Handbuch der empirischen Sozialforschung, Koenig, R. (ed.), Vol. 1, pp. 498-521. Stuttgart: Enke 1962
8. Aitken, R.C.B.: Methodology of research in psychosomatic medicine. Brit. Med. J. *4*, 285-287 (1972)
9. Almond, G.A.: Politische Systeme und politischer Wandel. In: Theorien des sozialen Wandels. Zapf, W. (ed.), pp. 211-227. Cologne, Berlin: Kiepenheuer & Witsch 1971
10. Amsler, R.: L'alcoolisme en milieu rural. VIIIe Congrès de l'association de médecine rurale, Luchon, Juin 1958. Concours Méd. *41/42* (1958)
11. Angst, J., Baumann, U., Mueller, U., Ruppen, R.: Epidemiologie des Drogenkonsums im Kanton Zürich. Arch. Psychiatr. Nervenkr. *217*, 11-24 (1973)
12. Antonelli, F., Ancona, L.: Metodologia nella ricerca psico-somatica. Med. Psicoanal. (Roma) *17*, 103-111 (1972)
13. Bacon, S.D.: Alcohol and complex society. In: Society, culture and drinking. Pittman, D.J., Snyder, C.R. (eds.), pp. 78-93. New York; Wiley 1962
14. Bales, R.F.: Attitudes toward drinking in the Irish culture. In: Society, culture and drinking. Pittman, D.J., Snyder, C.R. (eds.), pp. 157-187. New York: Wiley 1962
15. Barry III, H., Blane, K.T.: Birth order as a method of studying environmental influences in alcoholism. Ann. N.Y. Acad. Med. *197*, 172-178 (1972)
16. Bateson, G.: Naven. San Francisco: Stanford University Press 1958
17. Bateson, G.: Steps to an ecology of mind. New York: Ballantine Books 1972
18. Bateson, G., Jackson, D.D., Haley, J., Weakland, J.A.: Toward a theory of the double-bind. In: Communication, family and marriage. Human communication. Jackson, D.D. (ed.) Vol. 1, pp. 31-54. Palo Alto: Science and Behavior Books 1968
19. Battegay, R., Muehlemann, R.: Pilotstudie in einer Rekrutenschule betreffend Alkoholkonsum, Drogenerfahrung und Rauchergewohnheiten. Schweiz. Arch. Neurol. Neurochir. Psychiatr. *113*, 109-135 (1973)
20. Becker, W.: Frauen-Alkoholismus. Ther. Ggw. *110*, 400-410 (1971)
21. Bellmann, D., Hein, W., Trapp, W., Zang, G.: Ansatz zu einer Theorie der Provinz. Ungleiche regionale Entwicklung im Kapitalismus. In: Kursbuch 39, Enzensberger, H.M., Michel, K.M., Wieser, H. (eds.), pp. 108-127, Berlin: Rotbuch 1975
22. Bellwald, A., Jaeger, E.: Touristische Planung Alpendorf, Dorf- und Regionalplanung im Auftrag der Gemeinde Saas-Fee, 1973.
23. Bendix, R.: Die vergleichende Analyse historischer Wandlungen. In: Theorien des sozialen Wandels. Zapf, W. (ed.), pp. 177-187. Cologne, Berlin: Kiepenheuer & Witsch 1971
24. Bendix, R.: Modernisierung in internationaler Perspektive. In: Theorien des sozialen Wandels. Zapf, W. (ed.), pp. 505-512. Cologne, Berlin: Kiepenheuer & Witsch 1971

25. Benedict, R.: The Chrysanthemum and the sword. Pattern of Japanese culture. New York: World Publishing 1967
26. Bernard, J.: Community disorganization. Int. Encycl. Soc. Sci. *3*, 163 (1968)
27. Berner, P.: Der Alkoholismus im ländlichen Milieu. In: Arbeitstagung über Alkoholismus. Kryspin-Exner, K. (ed.), pp. 236-254. Vienna: Romayor 1962
28. Von Bertalanffy, L.: Robots, men and minds. New York: Braziller 1967
29. Von Bertalanffy, L.: General systems theory. New York: Braziller 1968
30. Blaser, P., Poeldinger, W.: Spzialpsychiatrische Erhebungen. Bern, Stuttgart: Huber 1968
31. Bloch, E.: Gespräch über Ungleichzeitigkeit. In: Kursbuch 39. Enzenberger, H.M., Michel, K.M., Wieser, H. (eds.), pp. 1-9. Berlin: Rotbuch 1975
32. Blumer, H.: Symbolic interaction: An approach to human communication. In: Approaches to human communication. Dudd, R.W., Ruben, B.D. (eds.), pp. 401-419. Rochelle Park, New Jersey: Hayden 1972
33. Bodenmueller, L.: Geschichtliches über Lawinen und Waldbrände beim Gletscherdorf Sass-Fee. Wir Walser *2*, 27-34 (1973)
34. Bolte, K.M.: Vertikale Mobilität. In: Handbuch der empirischen Sozialforschung. Koenig, R. (ed.), pp. 1-42. Stuttgart: Enke 1969
35. Boulding, K.E.: Economics and general systems. In: The relevance of general systems theory. Laszlo, E. (ed.), pp. 77-92. New York: Braziller 1972
36. Bowen, M.: Alcoholics as viewed through family systems theory and family psychotherapy. Ann. N.Y. Acad. Sci. *233*, 115-122 (1974)
37. Bowen, M.: Theory in the practice of psychotherapy. In: Family Therapy: Theory and practice. Guerin, P.J. (ed.), pp. 42-90. New York: Gardner Press Inc. 1976
38. Brady, J.V.: Toward a behavioral biology of emotion. In: Emotions, their parameters and measurement. Levi, L. (ed.), pp. 17-46. New York: Raven Press 1975
39. Braeutigam, W.: Pathogenetische Theorien und Wege der Behandlung in der Psychosomatik (mit Beschreibung einer Form stationärer und ambulanter Therapie). Nervenarzt *44*, 354-363 (1974)
40. Brede, K.: Die Pseudo-Logik psychosomatischer Störungen; Überlegungen zu einem soziologischen Organisumuskonzept. In: Psychoanalyse als Sozialwissenschaft. Lorenzer, A., Dahmer, H., Horn, K., Brede, K., Schwanenberg, E. (eds.), pp. 152-198. Frankfurt: Suhrkamp 1971
41. Brown, G.W.: Life events and psychiatric illness: Some thoughts on methology and causality. J. Psychosom. Res. *16*, 311-320 (1972)
42. Brown, G.W., Birely, J.L.T.: Social percipitants of severe psychiatric disorders. In: Psychiatric epidemiology. Proceedings of the international symposium held at Aberdeen University, 1969. Hare, E.H., Wing, J.K. (rds.), pp. 321-325). London, New York, Toronto: 1970
43. Brown, G.W., Sklair, F., Harris, T.O., Birely, J.L.T.: Life events and psychiatric disorders; part 1: some methodological issues. Psychol. Med. *3*, 74-87 (1973)
44. Brown, G.W., Harris, T.O., Peto, J.: Life events and psychiatric disorders. Part II: Nature of casual link. Psychol. Med. *3*, 159-176 (1973)
45. Bruner, J.S.: On knowing. Essays for the left hand. New York: Atheneum 1976
46. Bruun, K.: The significance of roles and norms in the small group for individual behavioral changes while drinking. In: Society, culture and drinking. Pittman, D.J., Snyder, C.R. (eds.), pp. 293-303. New York: Wiley 1962
47. Buck, C., Hobbs, G.E.: The problems of specifity in psychosomatic illness. J. Psychosom. Res. *3*, 227-233 (1959)
48. Bunzel, R.: The role of alcoholism in two Central American cultures. Psychiatry *3*, 361-387 (1940)
49. Cadwallader, M.L.: Die kybernetische Analyse des sozialen Wandels. In: Theorien des sozialen Wandels. Zapf, E. (ed.), pp. 141-146. Cologne, Berlin: Kiepenheuer & Witsch 1971
50. Campbell, A.A., Katona, G.: L'enquete échantillon: techniques de recherches socio-psychologiques. In: Les méthodes de recherche dans les sciences sociales. Festinger, L., Katz, D. (eds.), Vol. 1, pp. 23-68. Paris: Presses universitaires de France 1963
51. Cannel, C., Kahn, R.L.: L'interview comme méthode de collecte. In: Les méthodes de recherche dans les sciences sociales. Festinger, L., Katz, D. (eds.), Vol. 2, pp. 385-437. Paris: Presses universitaires de France 1963

52. Cassirer, E.: The philosophy of symbolic forms. Vol. 1: Language. New Haven, London: Yale University Press 1955
53. Cassirer, E.: The philosophy of symbolic forms. Vol. 2: Mythical thought. New Haven, London: Yale University Press 1955
54. Chafetz, M.E.: Alcoholism and alcoholic psychosis. In: Comprehensive Textbook of Psychiatry II. Friedman, A.M., Kaplan, H.I., Sadock, B.J. (eds.). Baltimore: Williams & Wilkins 1975
55. Chotjewitz, P.O.: Neuland-Leben in der Provinz. In: Kursbuch 39. Enzenberger, H.M., Michel, K.M., Wieser, H. (eds.), pp. 10-32. Berlin: Rotbuch 1975
56. Christian, P., Hahn, P.: Der Herzinfarkt in psychosomatischer und anthropologischer Sicht. Internist *13*, 421-424 (1972)
57. Ciompi, L.: Katamnestische Untersuchungen zur Entwicklung des Alkoholismus im Alter. In: Gerontology. Steinmann, B. (ed.), pp. 279-284. Bern, Stuttgart, Wien: Huber 1973
58. Clinard, M.B.: The public drinking house and society. In: Society, culture and drinking. Pittman, D.J., Snyder, C.R. (eds.), pp. 270-292. New York: Wiley 1962
59. Coddington, R.D.: The significance of life events as etiologic factors in the diseases of children. A study of normal population. J. Psychosom. Res. *16*, 205-213 (1972)
60. Coddington, R.D.: The significance of life events as etiologic factors in the diseases of children. A study of professional workers. J. Psychosom. Res. *16*, 7-18 (1972)
61. Connor, R.G.: The self-concepts of alcoholics. In: Society, culture and drinking. Pittman, D.J., Snyder, D.R. (eds.), pp. 455-467. New York: Wiley 1962
62. Cooper, B., Sylph, J.: Life events and the onset of neurotic illness: An investigation in general practice. Psychol. Med. *3*, 421-435 (1973)
63. Cooper, B., Eastwood, M.R., Sylph, J.: Psychiatric morbidity and social adjustment in a general practice population. In: Psychiatric epidemiology. Proceedings of the international symposium held at Aberdeen University, 1969. Hare, E.H., Wing, J.K. (eds.), pp. 299-309. London, New York, Toronto: 1970
64. Cremerius, J.: Is the Psychosomatic disease a nosological entity? In: Program Abstracts, 4th Congress of the International College of Psychosomatic Medicine, pp. 20-21, Kyoto 1977
65. Cronholm, B.: Ethology, psychiatry and psychosomatic medicine. Reports from the Laboratory for Clinical Stress Research, Karolinska Institut, Stockholm, No. 39, Sept. 1974
66. Daheim, H.: Soziologie der Berufe. In: Handbuch der empirischen Sozialforschung. Koenig, R. (ed.), Vol. II, pp. 358-407. Stuttgart: Enke 1969
67. Dahmer, H.: Psychoanalyse und historischer Materialismus. In: Psychoanalyse als Sozialwissenschaft. Lorenzer, A., Dahmer, H., Horn, K., Brede, K., Schwanenberg, E. (eds.), pp. 60-92. Frankfurt: Suhrkamp 1971
68. Dahrendorf, R.: Sozialer Wandel. In: Wörterbuch der Soziologie. Bernsdorf, W. (ed.), p. 102. Stuttgart: Enke 1969
69. Dahrendorf, R.: Zu einer Theorie des sozialen Konflikts. In: Theorien des sozialen Wandels. Zapf, W. (ed.), pp. 108-123. Cologne, Berlin: Kiepenheuer & Witsch 1971
70. Davies, J.C.: Eine Theorie der Revolution. In: Theorien des sozialen Wandels. Zapf, W. (ed.), pp. 399-417. Cologne, Berlin: Kiepenheuer & Witsch 1971
71. Davis, K.: Sozialer Wandel und internationale Beziehungen. In: Theorien des sozialen Wandels. Zapf, W. (ed.), pp. 484-499. Cologne, Berlin: Kiepenheuer & Witsch 1971
72. Deutsch, K.W.: Soziale Mobilisierung und politische Entwicklung. In: Theorien des sozialen Wandels. Zapf, W. (ed.), pp. 329-350. Cologne, Berlin: Kiepenheuer & Witsch 1971
73. Deutsch, K.W.: Neue Forschungsmethoden, Modelle, Theorien. In: Theorien des sozialen Wandels. Zapf, W. (ed.), pp. 188-210. Cologne, Berlin: Kiepenheuer & Witsch 1971
74. Deutsch, K.W.: Macht und Kommunikation in der internationalen Gesellschaft. In: Theorien des sozialen Wandels. Zapf, W. (ed.), pp. 471-483. Cologne, Berlin: Kiepenheuer & Witsch 1971
75. Dobzhansky, T.: Evolution at work. In: Ideas from human evolution. Selected essays, 1949-1961. Howells, B. (ed.), pp. 19-35. New York: Atheneum 1967
76. Dohrenwend, B.P., Chin-Shong, E.T., Egri, G., Mendelsohn, F.S., Stoker, J.: Mesures of psychiatric disorder in contrasting class and ethnic groups; a preliminary report of on-going research. In: Psychiatric epidemiology. Proceedings of the international symposium held at Aberdeen University, 1969. Hare, E.H., Wing, J.K. (eds.), pp. 159-202. London, New York, Toronto: 1970

77. Dohrenwend, B.S.: Social class and stressful events. In: Psychiatric epidemiology. Proceedings of the international symposium held at Aberdeen University, 1969. Hare, E.H., Wing, J.K. (ed.), pp. 313-319. London, New York, Toronto: 1970

78. Dohrenwend, B.S.: Life events as stressors: A methodological inquiry. J. Health Soc. Behav. *14*, 167-175 (1973)

79. Dohrenwend, B.S., Dohrenwend, B.P.: The problems of validity in field studies of psychological disorders. J. Abnorm. Psychol. *70*, 52-69 (1965)

80. Dollard, J.: Drinking mores and the social class. J. Stud. Alcohol (1945)

81. Du Bois, R.: Santé et société, une hypothèse sur la sociogénèse des troubles fonctionnels. Psychosom. Med. *3/4*, 218-222 (1972/73)

82. Duebi, H.: Saas-Fee und Umgebung; ein Führer durch Geschichte, Volk und Landschaft des Saas-Thales. Bern: Franke 1946

83. Dunham, H.W.: Discussion. In: Psychiatric epidemiology. Proceedings of the international Symposium held at Aberdeen University, 1969. Hare, E.H., Wing, J.K. (eds.), pp. 225-227. London, New York, Toronto: 1970

84. Durant, W.: Kulturgeschichte der Menschheit, das Zeitalter der Reformation. Vol. 18. Zurich: Ex Libris

85. Eastwood, M.R.: Psychiatric morbidity and physical state in a general practice population. In: Psychiatric epidemiology. Proceedings of the international symposium held at Aberdeen University, 1969. Hare, E.H., Wing, J.K. (eds.), pp. 291-298. London, New York, Toronto: 1970

86. Eastwood, M.R., Trevelyan, M.H.: Stress and coronary heart disease. J. Psychosom. Res. *15*, 289-292 (1971)

87. Eastwood, M.R., Trevelyan, M.H.: Psychosomatic disorders in the community. J. Psychosom. Res. *16*, 381-386 (1972)

88. Eibl-Eibesfeldt, I.: Grundriß der vergleichenden Verhaltensforschung. Munich, Zurich: Piper 1974

89. Einstein, A., Infeld, L.: The Evolution of Physics. New York: Simon & Schuster 1938

90. Eisenstadt, S.N.: Sozialer Wandel, Differenzierung und Evolution. In: Theorien des sozialen Wandels. Zapf, W. (ed.), pp. 75-94. Cologne, Berlin: Kiepenheuer & Witsch 1971

91. Erickson, J.M., Pugh, W.M., Gunderson, E.K.E.: Status congruency as a predictor of job satisfaction and life stress. Appl. Psychol. *56*, 523-525 (1972)

92. Erikson, E.H.: Identität und Lebenszyklus. Frankfurt: Suhrkmap 1971

93. Essen-Moeller, E.: Discussion. In: Psychiatric epidemiology. Proceedings of the international symposium held at Aberdeen University, 1969. Hare, E.H., Wing, J.K. (eds.), pp. 23-26. London, New York, Toronto: 1970

94. Etzioni, A.: Elemente einer Makrosoziologie. In: Theorien des sozialen Wandels. Zapf, E. (ed.), pp. 147-176. Cologne, Berlin: Kiepenheuer & Witsch 1971

95. Evreux, R.: Consommation d'alcool et jeunesse rurale. Rev. Alcool. *11*, 10-14 (1965)

96. Falk, G.: The contribution of the alcohol culture to alcoholism in America. Br. J. Addict. *65*, 9-17 (1970)

97. Faris, R.E.L., Dunham, H.W.: Mental disorders in urban areas: An ecological study of schizophrenia and other psychosis. Chicago: University of Chicago Press 1939

98. Field, P.B.: A new cross-cultural study of drunkenness. In: Society, culture and drinking. Pittman, D.J., Snyder, C.R. (eds.), pp. 48-74. New York: Wiley 1962

99. Fouquet, P.: Alcohol and religions. In: Alkohol und Alkoholismus. 27th International Congress, Frankfurt 1964. Hamm/Westf., Hamburg: Neuland 1965

100. Frankl, V.: The doctor and the soul; from psychotherapy to logotherapy. New York: Vintage Books 1973

101. Freud, S.: Gesammelte Werke, Vol. VIII. Frankfurt: Fischer 1940

102. Freud, S.: Gesammelte Werke, Vol. IX. Frankfurt: Fischer 1940

103. Freud, S.: Gesammelte Werke, Vol. X. Frankfurt: Fischer 1940

104. Freud, S.: Gesammelte Werke, Vol. XIII. Frankfurt: Fischer 1940

105. Freud, S.: Das Unbehagen der Kultur. Gesammelte Werke, Vol. XIV, Frankfurt: Fischer 1940

106. Freud, S.: Die Zukunft einer Illusion. Gesammelte Werke, Vol. VIV. Frankfurt: Fischer 1940

107. Freud, S.: Gesammelte Werke, Vol. XV. Frankfurt: Fischer 1940

108. Freud, S.: Gesammelte Werke, Vol. XVI. Frankfurt: Fischer 1940
109. Freud, S.: Gesammelte Werke, Vol. XVII. Frankfurt: Fischer 1940
110. Fromm, E.: Analytische Sozialpsychologie und Gesellschaftstheorie. Frankfurt: Suhrkamp 1970
111. Fromm, E.: Das Menschenbild bei Marx. Mit den wichtigsten Teilen der Frühschriften von Karl Marx. Frankfurt: Europäische Verlagsanstalt 1972
112. Fuerstenberg, F.: Religionssoziologie. In: Handbuch der empirischen Sozialforschung. Koenig, R. (ed.), pp. 1102-1122. Stuttgart: Enke 1969
113. Gabriel, E.: Über die soziale Bedingtheit des Alkoholismus. In: Arbeitstagung über Alkoholismus. Kryspin-Exner, K. (ed.), pp. 259-261. Vienna: Romayor 1962
114. Gehlen, A.: Die Seele im technischen Zeitalter; Sozialpsychologische Probleme in der industriellen Gesellschaft. Hamburg: Rowohlt 1957
115. Gibbins, R.J., Walters, R.H.: Three preliminary studies of psychoanalytic theory of alcohol addiction. Quart. J. Stud. Alcohol 21, 618-641 (1960)
116. Globetti, G., Pomery, G.: Characteristics of community residents who are favorable toward alcohol education. Ment. Hyg. 54, 411-415 (1970)
117. Goldberg, D.P.: The reliability of a standardised psychiatric interview suitable for use in communites surveys. In: Psychiatric epidemiology. Proceedings of the international symposium held at Aberdeen University, 1969. Hare, E.H., Wing, J.K. (eds.), pp. 283-290. London, New York, Toronto: 1970
118. Grace, W.I., Graham, D.T.: Relationship of specific attitudes and emotions to certain bodily diseases. In: Psychosomatics classics. Gottschalk, L.A., Knapp, P.H., Reiser, M.F., Sapira, J.D., Shapiro, A.P. (eds.), pp. 225-242. Basel, Munich, Paris, London, New York, Sydney: Karger 1958
119. Grassi, E.: Kunst und Mythos. Hamburg: Rowohlt 1957
120. Grinker, R.R.: Psychiatry in broad perspective. New York: Behavioral Publications 1975
121. Groen, J.J.: Influence of social and cultural patterns on psychosomatic diseases. Psychother. Psychom. 18, 189-215 (1970)
122. Groen, J.J.: The measurement of emotion and arousal in the clinical physiological laboratory and in medical practice. In: Emotions, their parameters and measurements. Levi, L. (ed.), pp. 727-746. New York: Raven Press 1975
123. Guntern, G.: Alcoolisme et environment, Schweiz. Rundschau Med. (Praxis) 63, 1149-1155 (1974)
124. Guntern, G.: Sozialer Wandel und seelische Gesundheit. Der Wandel eines Bergdorfes vor der Agrikultur zum Gastgewerbe. Psychiatr. Clin. 7, 287-313 (1974)
125. Guntern, G.: Changement social et consommation d'alcool dans un village de montagne. Schweiz. Arch. Neurol. Neurochir. Psychiatr. 116, 353-411 (1975)
126. Guntern, G.: Die Langzeitstudie Alpendorf: Ein Paradigma für das Studium langfristig wirkender, psychosozialer Stressoren. Schweiz. Arch. Neurol. Neurochir. Psychiatr. 121, 97-113 (1977)
127. Guntern, G.: Alpendorf: tourisme, changement social, stress et problemes psychiatriques. Soc. Psychiatr. 13, 41-51 (1978)
128. Guntern, G.: Alpendorf: Transactional processes in a human system. Reports from the Laboratory for Clinical Stress Research. Karolinka Institute, Stockholm, No. 76, March 1978
129. Guntern, G.: Transactional topology: a meta-theoretical model of human communication. In: Ethology and communication in mental health. Corson, S.A. (ed.). New York: Pergamon Press to be published
130. Guntern, G.: Die kopernikanische Revolution in der Psychotherapie: der Wandel vom psychoanalytischen zum systemischen Paradigma. Familiendynamik, interdisziplinäre Zeitschrift für Praxis und Forschung, Zurich, 1980.
131. Guntern, G.: Epistemology and basic concepts of structural family therapy. to be published
132. Guntern, G.: Psychosomatic symptoms, indicators of a disturbed transactional field. 4th Congress of the International College of Psychosomatic Medicine, Kyoto 1977, to be published
133. Habermas, J.: Legitimationsprobleme im Spätkapitalismus. Frankfurt: Suhrkamp 1973

134. Hacker, F.: Materialien zum Thema Aggression; Gespräche mit Adalbert Reif und mit Bettina Schattat. Vienna, Munich, Zurich: Molden 1972

135. Häfner, H.: Der Einfluß von Umweltfaktoren auf die seelische Gesundheit; Ergebnisse, Möglichkeiten und Grenzen der Forschung. Psychiatr. Clin. 7, 199-225 (1974)

136. Häfner, H., Reimann, H.: Spartial distribution of mental disorders in Mannheim, 1965. In: Psychiatric epidemiology. Proceedings of the international symposium held at Aberdeen University, 1969. Hare, E.H., Wing, J.K. (eds.). pp. 341-354. London, New York, Toronto: 1970

137. Haes, J.L.: Drinking patterns and the influence of friends and family. Quart. J. Stud. Acohol 16, 178-185 (1955)

138. Hagen, E.E.: Traditionalismus, Statusverlust, Innovation. In: Theorien des sozialen Wandels. Zapf, E. (ed.), pp. 351-361. Cologne, Berlin: Kiepenheuer & Witsch 1971

139. Hagnell, O.: The incidence and duration of episodes of mental illness in a total population. In: Psychiatric epidemiology. Proceedings of the international symposium held at Aberdeen University, 1969. Hare, E.H., Wing, J.K. (eds.), pp. 213-224. London, New York, Toronto: 1970

140. Haley, J.: Strategies of psychotherapy. New York: Grune & Stratton 1963

141. Haley, J.: Problem solving therapy. San Francisco, Washington, London: Jossey-Bass 1976

142. Hardyck, C.D., Moos, R.M.: Sampling problems in studies of psychosomatic disorders: Difficulties in determining personality correlates. J. Psychosom. Res. 10, 171-182 (1966)

143. Hare, E.H.: Discussion. In: Psychiatric epidemiology. Proceedings of the international symposium held at Aberdeen University, 1969. Hare, E.H., Wing, J.K. (eds.), pp. 228-232. London, New York, Toronto: 1970

144. Harmon, D.K., Maruda, M., Holmes, T.H.: The social readjustment rating scale: a cross-cultural study of Western Europeans and Americans. J. Psychosom. Res. 14, 391-400 (1970)

145. Hartmann, H.: Ego psychology and the problem of adaptation. New York: International Universities Press 1958

146. Hartmann, H.: Die Grundlagen der Psychoanalyse. Stuttgart: Klett 1972

147. Haynal, A.: Freud und Piaget. Psyche 3, 242-272 (1975)

148. Heath, D.B.: Drinking patterns of the Bolivian Camba. In: Society, culture and drinking. Pittman, D.J., Snyder, D.R. (eds.), pp. 22-36. New York: Wiley 1962

149. Heintz, P.: Sozialer Wandel. In: Fischer Lexikon, Vol. 10: Soziologie, p. 268. Frankfurt: Fischer 1958

150. Heisenberg, W.: The physical principles of quantum theory. In: Physical thought from the presocratics to the Quantum physicists. Sambursky, S. (ed.), pp. 517-519. New York: Pica Press 1975

151. Hes, J.P.: Drinking in a Yemenite rural settlement in Israel. Br. J. Addict. 65, 293-296 (1970)

152. Hinkle, L.E., Christenson, W.N., Kane, R.D., Ostfeld, A., Theteford, W.N., Wolff, H.G.: An investigation of the relationship between life experience, personality characteristics and general susceptibility. In: Psychosomatics classics. Gottschalk, L.A., Knapp, P.H., Reiser, M.F., Sapira, J.D., Shapiro, A.P. (eds.), pp. 225-242. Basel, Munich, Paris, London, New York, Sydney: Karger 1958

153. Hollingshead, A.B., Redlich, F.C.: Social class and mental illness. New York: Wiley 1958

154. Holmes, T.H., Rahe, R.H.: The social readjustment rating scale. J. Psychosom. Res. 11, 213 (1967)

155. Holmes, T.S., Holmes, T.H.: Short-term intrusions into the life style routine. J. Psychosom. Res. 14, 121-132 (1970)

156. Homans, G.C.: The nature of social science. New York: Harcourt, Braze & World 1967

157. Homans, G.C.: Funktionalismus, Verhaltenstheorie und sozialer Wandel. In: Theorien des sozialen Wandels. Zapf, W. (ed.), pp. 95-107. Cologne, Berlin: Kiepenheuer & Witsch 1971

158. Hordern, A.: Tranquillity denied. In: Psychopharmacology, sexual disorders and drug abuse. Ban et al. (eds.). Amsterdam, London: North-Holland Publishing 1973

159. Horkheimer, M.: Gesellschaft im Übergang. Frankfurt: Fischer Athenäum 1972

160. Horn, K.: Insgeheime kulturalistische Tendenzen der modernen psychoanalytischen Orthodoxie. Zum Verhältnis von Subjektivem und Gesellschaftlichem in der Ich-Psychologie. In: Psychoanalyse als Sozialwissenschaft. Lorenzer, A., Dahmer, H., Horn, K., Brede, K., Schwanenberg, E. (eds.), pp. 93-151. Frankfurt: Suhrkamp 1971

161. Horney, K.: Neue Wege der Psychoanalyse. München: Kindler
162. Horstmann, K.: Horizontale Mobilität. In: Handbuch der empirischen Sozialforschung. Koenig, R. (ed.), Vol. II, pp. 43-64. Stuttgart: Enke 1969
163. Horton, D.: The functions of alcohol in primitiv societies: a cross cultural study. Quart. J. Stud. Alcohol 4, 199-320 (1943)
164. Hoselitz, D.F., Merrill, R.S.: Sozialer Wandel in unterentwickelten Ländern. In: Handbuch der empirischen Sozialforschung. Koenig, R. (ed), Vol. II, pp. 567-603. Stuttgart: Enke 1969
165. Hummel, H.J.: Psychologische Ansätze zu einer Theorie des sozialen Verhaltens. In: Handbuch der empirischen Sozialforschung. Koenig, R. (ed.), Vol. II, pp. 1157-1277. Stuttgart: Enke 1969
166. Imseng, G.: Die Chronik des Saas-Tales und die Entwicklung der Fremdenindustrie von 1851-1952.
167. Imseng, K.: Saas-Thal; Querschnitt durch die Ur-, Früh- und Siedlungsgeschichte mit besonderer Berücksichtigung des Saas-Thales. Privatverlag 1973
168. Imseng, W.: Der Sommer in Saas-Fee. Saas-Fee: Verlag des Verkehrsvereins 1967
169. Imseng, W.: Der Winter in Saas-Fee. Saas-Fee: Verlag des Verkehrsvereins 1970
170. Irgens-Jensen, O.: The use of alcohol in an isolated area of Northern Norway. Br. J. Addict. 65, 181-185 (1970)
171. Jackson, D.D. (ed.): Communication, family and marriage; Human communication, Vol. 1. Palo Alto: Science and Behavior Books1967
172. Jackson, D.D. (ed.): Therapy, communication and change; Human communication, Vol. 2. Palo Alto: Science and Behavior Books 1967
173. Jackson, J.K.: Alcoholism and the family. In: Society, culture and drinking. Pittman, D.J., Snyder, D.R. (eds.), pp. 472-492. New York: Wiley 1962
174. Jacobs, M.A., Spilken, A.Z., Norman, M.M., Anderson, L.S.: Patterns of maladaptation and respiratory illness. J. Psychosom. Res. 15, 63-72 (1971)
175. Jaeggi, U.: Berggemeinden im Wandel. Eine empirisch-soziologische Untersuchung in vier Gemeinden des Berner Oberlandes. Bern: Haupt 1965
176. Jantke, C.: Vorindustrielle Gesellschaft. In: Soziologie. Ein Lehr- und Handbuch zur modernen Gesellschaftskunde. Gehlen, A., Schelsky, H. (eds.), pp. 93-120. Düsseldorf, Cologne: Diederichs 1955
177. Jaynes, J.: The origin of consciousness in the breakdown of the bicameral mind. Boston: Houghton, Mifflin 1976
178. Jellinek, E.M.: Cultural differences in the meaning of alcoholism. In: Society, culture and drinking. Pittman, D.J., Snyder, D.R. (eds.), pp. 356-368. New York: Wiley 1962
179. Jellinek, E.M.: Phases of alcohol addiction. In: Society, culture and drinking. Pittman, D.J., Snyder, C.R. (eds.), New York: Wiley 1962
180. Jessor, R., Collins, M.I., Jessor, S.L.: On becoming a drinker; social-psychological aspects of an adolescent transition. Ann. N.Y. Acad. Sci. 197, 199-213 (1972)
181. Kaplan, M.A.: Transformationsregeln internationaler Systeme. In: Theorien des sozialen Wandels. Zapf, W. (ed.), pp. 500-504. Cologne, Berlin: Kiepenheuer & Witsch 1971
182. Katz, D.: Les études sur terrain. In: Les méthodes de recherche dans les sciences sociales. Festinger, L., Katz, D. (eds.), Vol. 1, pp. 68-119. Paris: Presses universitaires de France 1963
183. Katz, M.M.: Discussion of the previous three papers. In: Psychiatric epidemiology. Proceedings of the international symposium held at Aberdeen University, 1969, Hare, F. H., Wing, J.K. (eds.), pp. 149-155. London, New York, Toronto: 1970
184. Kaufmann, L.: Familie, Kommunikation, Psychose. Stuttgart, Vienna: Huber 1972
185. Keller, M.: The definition of alcoholism and the estimation of its prevalence. In: Society, culture and drinking. Pittman, D.J., Snyder, C.R. (eds.), pp. 310-329. New York: Wiley 1962
186. Kielholz, P., Ladewig, D.: Die Drogenabhängigkeit des modernen Menschen. München: Lehmanns 1972
187. Kielholz, P., Battegay, R., Ladewig, D.: Drogenabhängigkeit. In: Psychiatrie der Gegenwart, Kistzer, K.P., Meyer, S.E., Müller, M., Strömgren, E. (eds.), Vol. II/2, pp. 497-564. Berlin, Heidelberg, New York: Springer 1972

304

188. Kleiner, R.J.: Discussion. In: Psychiatric epidemiology. Proceedings of the international symposium held at Aberdeen University, 1969. Hare, E.H., Wing, J.K. (eds.), pp. 205-209. London, New York, Toronto: 1970
189. Knoetig, H.: Energiefluß und Informationsfluß als komplimentäre Anteile jeder Wechselwirkung zwischen Organismus und Umwelt. Helgoländer wiss. Meeresuntersuchungen *14*, 279-290 (1966)
190. Knoetig, H.: Bemerkungen zum Begriff Humanökologie. Humanökologische Blätter *2/3*, 3-140 (1972)
191. Koenig, R.: Soziologie der Familie. In: Soziologie. Ein Lehr- und Handbuch zur modernen Gesellschaftskunde. Gehlen, A., Schlesky, H. (eds.), pp. 121-158. Düsseldorf, Cologne: Diederichs 1955
192. Koenig, R.: Gemeinde. In: Fischer Lexikon, Vol. 10: Soziologie, p. 74. Frankfurt: Fischer 1958
193. Koenig, R.: Die Beobachtung. In: Handbuch der empirischen Sozialforschung. Koenig, R. (ed.), Vol. 1, pp. 107-135. Stuttgart: Enke 1962
194. Koenig, R.: Soziologie. Fischer Lexikon, Vol. 10: Soziologie, pp. 280-288. Frankfurt: Fischer 1967
195. Koenig, R.: Gemeinde. In: Wörterbuch der Soziologie. Bernsdorf, W. (ed.), p. 334. Stuttgart: Enke 1969
196. Koenig, R.: Soziologie der Familie. In: Handbuch der empirischen Sozialforschung. Koenig, R. (ed.), Vol. II, pp. 172-305. Stuttgart: Enke 1969
197. Koenig, R.: Einige Bemerkungen über die Bedeutung der empirischen Forschung in der Soziologie. In: Handbuch der empirischen Sozialforschung. Koenig, R. (ed.), Vol. II, pp. 1278-1291. Stuttgart: Enke 1969
198. Koetter, H.: Agrarsoziologie. In: Soziologie. Ein Lehr- und Handbuch zur modernen Gesellschaftskunde. Gehlen, A., Schlesky, H. (eds.), pp. 204-237. Düsseldorf, Cologne: Diederichs 1955
199. Koetter, H.: Landbevölkerung im sozialen Wandel. Ein Beitrag zur ländlichen Soziologie. Düsseldorf, Cologne: Diederichs 1958
200. Koetter, H.: Stadt-, Land-Soziologie. In: Handbuch der empirischen Sozialforschung. Koenig, R. (ed.), Vol. II, pp. 604-621. Stuttgart: Enke 1969
201. Kohut, K.: Narzißmus, eine Theorie der psychoanalytischen Behandlung narzißtischer Persönlichkeitsstörungen. Frankfurt: Suhrkamp 1976
202. Korzybski, A.: Science and Sanity. Lancaster, Pennsylvania: International Non-Aristotelian Library 1933
203. Kreitman, N.: Subcultural aspects of attempted suicide. In: Psychiatric epidemiology. Proceedings of the international symposium held at Aberdeen University, 1969. Hare, E.H., Wing, J.K. (eds.), pp. 355-359. London, New York, Toronto: 1970
204. Kur-Verkehrsverein Saas-Fee. Jahresbericht für das Geschäftsjahr 1970
205. Kutter, M.: Abschied von der Werbung. Niederteufen/Appenzell: Niggli 1976
206. Lawrence, J.J., Maxwell, M.A.: Drinking and socio-economic status. In: Society, culture and drinking. Pittman, D.J., Snyder, C.R. (eds.), pp. 141-145. New York: Wiley 1962
207. Lazarus, R.S.: Psychological stress and the coping process. New York: McGraw-Hill 1966
208. Leighton, D.C., Harding, I.S., MacKlin, D.B., MacMillan, A.M., Leighton, A.H.: The character of danger, the Stirling County Study of psychiatric disorder and socio-cultural environment, Vol. 3. New York: Basic Books 1963
209. Lemert, E.M.: Alcoholism and the socio-cultural situation. Quart. J. Stud. Alcohol *17*, 306-317 (1956)
210. Lemert, E.M.: The occurrence in sequence of events in the adjustment of families to alcoholism. Quart. J. Stud. Alcohol *21*, 679-697 (1960)
211. Lemert, E.M.: Alcohol, values and social control. In: Society, culture and drinking. Pittman, D.J., Snyder, C.R. (eds.), pp. 553-571. New York: Wiley 1962
212. Lerner, D.: Die Modernisierung des Lebensstils: Eine Theorie. In: Theorien des sozialen Wandels. Zapf, W. (ed.), pp. 362-381. Cologne, Berlin: Kiepenheuer & Witsch 1971
213. Levi, L.: Psychological stress and disease: A conceptual model. In: Life stress and illness. Gunderson, E.K.E., Rahe, R.H. (eds.), pp. 8-33. Springfield, Illinois: Thomas 1974

214. Levi, L.: Stress, Distress and psychosocial stimuli. In: Occupational stress. McLean, A. (ed.), pp. 31-46. Springfield, Illinois: Thomas 1974

215. Levi, L.: Situation stressante, réactions de stress et maladies. In: Symposium medical international "Stress, maladies de la civilisation et vieillissement", Paris 28-29 avril 1975, pp. 26-38. Laboratoires Robert et Carrière 1975

216. Levi, L. (ed.): Emotions, their parameters and measurement. New York: Raven Press 1975

217. Levi, L.: Parameters of emotions: an evolutionary and ecological approach. In: Emotions, their parameters and measurement. Levi, L. (ed.), pp. 705-712. New York: Raven Press 1975

218. Levi, L., Anderson, L.: Population, environment and quality of life: A contribution to the United Nations world population conference. Royal Ministry for Foreign Affaires, Stockholm 1974

219. Levi-Strauss, C.: Tristes tropiques. Paris: Plon 1955

220. Levi-Strauss, C.: La pensée sauvage. Paris: Plon 1962

221. Levi-Strauss, C.: Cultural anthropology. New York: Basic Books 1963

222. Levi-Strauss, C.: Das Ende des Totemismus. Frankfurt: Suhrkamp 1965

223. Levi-Strauss, C.: The elementary structures of kinship. Boston: Beacon Press 1969

224. Levi-Strauss, C.: The raw and the cooked. Introduction to a science of mythology. New York: Harper & Row 1969

225. Lienert, G.A.: Die Konfigurationsfrequenzanalyse: Ein neuer Weg zu Typen und Syndromen. Klin. Psychol. Psychother. *19*, 99-115 (1971)

226. Lockwood, D.: Soziale Integration und Systemintegration. In: Theorien des sozialen Wandels. Zapf, W. (ed.), pp. 124-140. Cologne, Berlin: Kiepenheuer & Witsch 1971

227. Lorenzer, F.: Symbol, Interaktion und Praxis. In: Psychoanalyse als Sozialwissenschaft. Lorenzer, A., Dahmer, H., Horn, K., Brede, K., Schwanenberg, E. (eds.), pp. 9-59. Frankfurt: Suhrkamp 1971

228. Luban-Plozza, B.: Soziodynamik der Familie als medizinisches Problem. Präventivmed. *17*, 319-329 (1972)

229. Luborsky, L.L., Docherty, I.P., Penick, S.: Onset conditions for psychosomatic symptoms: a comparative review of immediat observation with retrospective research. Psychosom. Med. *35/3*, 187-204 (1973)

230. Lucisano, B.: Il valore stressante degli eventi. Med. psicoanal. (Roma) *17*, 125-133 (1972)

231. Luftseilbahnen Saas-Fee AG: Geschäftsrechnung 1973

232. Lundquist, G.A.R.: Klinische und sozio-kulturelle Aspekte des Alkoholismus. In: Psychiatrie der Gegenwart, 2nd ed., Vol. II/2. pp. 363-388. Berlin, Heidelberg, New York: Springer 1972

232a. Mackenroth, G.: Bevölkerungslehre. In: Soziologie; ein Lehr- und Handbuch zur modernen Gesellschaftskunde. Gehlen, A., Schelsky, H (eds.), pp. 46-92. Düsseldorf, Köln: Diederichs 1955

233. Maddox, G.L.: Teenage drinking in the United States. In: Society, culture and drinking. Pittman, D.J., Snyder, C.R. (eds.), pp. 230-245. New York: Wiley 1962

234. Mair, J.M.M.: Psychological problems and cigarette smoking. J. Psychosom. Res. *14*, 277-283, 1970

235. Malinowski, B.: Magic, science and religion. New York: Doubleday 1964

236. Malinowski, B.: La sexualité et sa répression dans les societés primitives. Paris: Paillot 1967

237. Marcuse, H.: Kultur und Gesellschaft, Vol. 2. Frankfurt: Suhrkamp 1965

238. Marcuse, H.: Der eindimensionale Mensch, Soziologische Texte. Studien zur Ideologie der fortgeschrittenen Industriegesellschaft. Neuwied: Luchterhand 1967

239. Martindale, D.: Introduction. In: Exploration in social changes. Zollschau, G.K., Hirsch, W. (eds.). Boston: Houghton Mifflin 1964

240. Marx, K.: Zur Kritik der politischen Ökonomie. Berlin: Dietz 1972

241. Matussek, P., Egenter, R.: Ideologie, Glaube und Gewissen. Diskussion an der Grenze zwischen Moraltheologie und Psychotherapie. Munich, Zurich: Droemer-Knaur 1965

242. Mayntz, R., Ziegler, R.: Soziologie der Organisation. In: Handbuch der empirischen Sozialforschung. Koenig, R. (ed.), Vol. II, pp. 444-513. Stuttgart: Enke 1969

243. Mc Clelland, D.C.: The achieving society. Toronto: Collier-MacMillan 1961

244. Mc Cord, W., Mc Cord, J.: A longitudinal study of the personality of alcoholics. In: Society, culture and drinking. Pittman, D.J., Snyder, C.R. (eds.), pp. 413-430. New York: Wiley 1962

245. Mc Kennel, A.C., Thomas, R.K.: Adults and adolescent smoking habits and attitudes. A report on a survey carried out for the Ministry of Health. S.S. 353/B, October 1967

246. Mead, M.: Cultural patterns and technical change. New York: New American Library 1955

247. Mead. M.: Geschlecht und Temperament in primitiven Gesellschaften. Hamburg: Rowohlt 1959

248. Mead, M.: Mann und Weib. Das Verhältnis der Geschlechter in einer sich wandelnden Welt. Hamburg: Rowohlt 1960

250. Mendel, G.: Generationskrise. Eine soziopsychoanalytische Studie. In: Literatur der Psychoanalyse. Mitscherlich, A. (ed.), Frankfurt: Suhrkamp 1972

251. Miller, J.G.: Living Systems: Basic concepts. Behav. Sci. *10*, 193-237 (1965)

252. Miller, J.G.: Living systems: Structure and process. Behav. Sci. *10*, 337-379 (1965)

253. Minuchin, S.: Families and family therapy. Cambridge, Massachusets: Harvard University Press 1974

254. Minuchin, S., Montalvo, B., Guerney, B.G., Rosman, B.L., Schumer, F.: Families of the slums. New York: Basic Books 1967

255. Minuchin, S., Rosman, B.L., Baker, L.: Psychosomatic families. Anorexia nervosa in context. Cambridge: Harvard University Press 1978

256. Mitscherlich, A.: Die Unwirklichkeit unserer Städte. Anstiftung zum Unfrieden. Frankfurt: Suhrkamp 1966

257. Moldenhauer, P.: Beziehungen zwischen psychosomatischem Syndrom, Verhalten in der Gruppe und Selbst. Eine Fallstudie. Dyn. Psychiatr. *6/18*, 33-56 (1973)

258. Moore, W.E.: Social change. In: Int. Encycl. Soc. Sci. *14*, 366 (1968)

259. Morgenthaler, F., Parin, P., Parin-Matthey, G.: Die Weißen denken zuviel. Psychoanalytische Untersuchungen bei den Dogon in Westafrika. Zürich: Atlantis; Munich: Kindler 1963

260. Morgenthaler, F., Parin, P., Parin-Matthey, G.: Fürchte deinen Nächsten wie dich selbst. Psychoanalyse und Gesellschaft. Am Modell der Agni in Westafrika. Frankfurt: Suhrkamp 1971

261. Musaph, H.: Introduction of the discussion: the influence of social and cultural patterns on psychosomatic disorders. Psychother. Psychosom. *18*, 239-242 (1970)

262. Myrdal, J.: Report from a Chinese village. London: Pilador Pan Books 1975

263. Navratil, L.: On etiology of alcoholism. Quart. J. Stud. Alcohol *20*, 236-244 (1959)

264. Nelson, P., Mensh, I.N., Hecht, E., Schwartz, A.N.: Variables in the reporting of recent life changes. J. Psychosom. Res. *16*, 465-471 (1972)

265. Nitsch, J.R.: Industrielle Beanspruchung als psychologisches Problem. Rehabilitation *12*, 68-77 (1973)

266. Oswald, H.: Die überschätzte Stadt. In: Texte und Dokumente zur Soziologie. Popitz, H. (ed.), Olten, Freiburg: Walter 1966

267. Palola, E.G., Dorpat, T.L., Larson, W.R.: Alcoholism and suicidal behavior. In: Society, culture and drinking. Pittman, D.J., Snyder, C.R. (eds.), pp. 511-534. New York: Wiley 1962

268. Park, P.: Problem drinking and role deviation study in incipient alcoholism. In: Society, culture and drinking. Pittman, D.F., Snyder, C.R. (eds.), pp. 431-454. New York: Wiley 1962

269. Parin, P.: Das Mikroskop der vergleichenden Psychoanalyse und die Makrosozietät. Psyche *1*, 1-25 (1976)

270. Parsons, T.: The social system. Glencoe, Illinois: Free Press 1951

271 Parsons, T.: An outline of the social system. In: Theories of society. Parsons, T. (ed.), Vol. 2, pp. Glencoe, Ill.: Free Press 1961

272. Parsons, T.: Evolutionäre Universalien der Gesellschaft. In: Theorien des sozialen Wandels. Zapf, W. (ed.), pp. 55-74. Cologne, Berlin: Kiepenheuer & Witsch 1971

273. Parsons, T.: Das Problem des Strukturwandels: Eine theoretische Skizze. In: Theorien des sozialen Wandels. Zapf, W. (ed.), pp. 35-54. Cologne, Berlin: Kiepenheuer & Witsch 1971

274. Pflanz, M.: Sozialer Wandel und Krankheit: Ergebnisse der medizinischen Soziologie. Stuttgart: Enke 1962

275. Piaget, J.: Psychologie der Intelligenz. Olten, Freiburg: Walter 1972

276. Piaget, J.: The language and thought of the child. New York: New American Library 1974

277. Piaget, J.: L'équilibration des structures cognitives. Paris: Presses universitaires de France 1975

278. Piaget, J., Imhelder, B.: The gaps in empiricism. In: Beyond Reductionism. Koestler, A., Smythies, J.R. (eds.), pp. 118-148. New York: Hutchinson 1969

279. Pichler, E.: Wertmaßstäbe und sozio-kulturelle Wirkungsbedingungen beim Alkoholismus. In: Arbeitstagung über Alkoholismus. Kryspin-Exner, K. (ed.), pp. 255-258. Wien: Romayor 1962

280. Pittman, D.J.: International overview: social and cultural factors in drinking patterns, pathological and nonßpathological. In: Alkohol und Alkoholismus. 27th International Congress, Frankfurt 1964. Hamm/Westf., Hamburg: Neuland 1965

281. Pittman, D.J., Snyder, C.R. (eds.): Society, culture and drinking. New York: Wiley 1962

282. Pittman, D.J., Wayne, G.: Criminal careers of the chronic drunkenness offender. In: Society, culture and drinking. Pittman, D.J., Snyder, C.R. (eds.), pp. 535-546. New York: Wiley 1962

283. Plack, A.: Die Gesellschaft und das Böse. Eine Kritik der herrschenden Moral. München: List 1967

284. Popper, K.R., Eccles, J.C.: The self and its brain. An Argument for Interactionism. Berlin, Heidelberg, New York: Springer 1977

285. Portmann, A.: Biologische Fragmente zu einer Lehre vom Menschen. Basel: Schwabe 1944

286. Pschyrembel, W.: Praktische Gynäkologie. Berlin: De Gruyter 1968

287. Rahe, R.H., Lind, E.: Psychosocial factors and sudden cardiac death: a pilot study. J. Psychosom. Res. *15*, 19-24 (1971)

288. Rahe, R.H., Kean, J.D., Arthur, R.J.: A longitudinal study of life change and illness patterns. J. Psychosom. Res. *10*, 355-366 (1967)

289. Rahe, R.H., Romo, M., Bennett, L., Siltanen, P.: Recent life changes, myocardial infarction and abrupt coroanry death. Studies in Helsinki. Arch. Intern. Med. *33*, 221-228 (1971)

290. Rapaport, A.: The search for simplicity. In: The relevance of general systems theory. Laszlo, E. (ed.), pp. 13-30. New York: Braziller 1972

291. Redfield, R.: The little community. Viewpoints for the study of a human whole. Stockholm: Almquist & Wiksells 1955

292. Reich, W.: Charakteranalyse. Cologne, Berlin: Kiepenheuer & Witsch 1970

293. Reid, D.D.: Epidemiologische Methoden in der psychiatrischen Feldforschung. Stuttgart: Thieme 1966

294. Ribeiro, D.: Der zivilisatorische Prozess. Frankfurt: Suhrkamp 1971

295. Richman, A.: The use of case-registers of psychiatric care in epidemiological research of mental disorders. In: Psychiatric epidemiology. Proceedings of the international symposium held at Aberdeen University, 1969. Hare, E.H., Wing, J.K. (eds.), pp. 257-272. London, New York, Toronto: 1970

296. Richter, H.E.: Eltern, Kind und Neurose. Die Rolle des Kindes in der Familie. Hamburg: Rowohlt 1970

297. Riesman, D.: Die einsame Masse. Eine Untersuchung der Wandlungen des amerikanischen Charakters. Hamburg: Rowohlt 1966

298. Robins, L.N., Bales, W.M., O'Neal, P.: Adult drinking patterns of former problem children. In: Society, culture and drinking. Pittman, D.J., Snyder, C.R. (eds.), pp. 395-412. New York: Wiley 1962

299. Rocher, G.: Le changement social, Vol. 3. Paris: Point 1968

300. Roghman, K.J., Haggerty, R.J.: Family stress and the use of healts services. Int. J. Epidemiol. *1*, 279-286 (1972)

301. Rosenmayr, L.: Hauptgebiete der Jugendsoziologie. In: Handbuch der empirischen Sozialforschung. Koenig, R. (ed.), Vol. II, pp. 65-171. Stuttgart: Enke 1969

302. Rosenmayr, L.: Soziologie des Alters. In: Hanbuch der empirischen Sozialforschung. Koenig, R. (ed.), Vol. II, pp. 306-357. Stuttgart: Enke 1969

303. Rostow, W.W.: Die Phase des Take-off. In: Theorien des sozialen Wandels. Zapf, W. (ed.), pp. 286-311. Cologne, Berlin: Kiepenheuer & Witsch 1971

304. Rubington, E.: "Failure" as a heavy drinker: the case of the chronic drunkenness offender of Skid Row. In: Society, culture and drinking. Pittman, D.J., Snyder, C.R. (eds.), pp. 146-153. New York: Wiley 1962

305. Ruch, L.O., Holmes, T.H.: Scaling of life change: Comparison of direct and indirect methods. J. Psychosom. *15*, 221-227 (1971)

306. Ruesch, J., Bateson, G.: Communication, the social matrix of psychiatry. New York: Norton 1951

307. Rueschenmeyer, D.: Partielle Modernisierung. In: Theorien des sozialen Wandels. Zapf, W. (ed.), pp. 382-398. Cologne, Berlin: Kiepenheuer & Witsch 1971
308. Ruppen, P.J.: Die Chronik des Saas-Thales von 1200 bis 1851.
309. Russel, H.M.A.: Tabacco and the nations health. In: Drugs, alcohol and tabacco in Britain. Zacune, J., Hensman, C., Heinemann, W. (eds.), pp. 209-229. London: Medical Books 1971
310. Rutter, M.C.: Discussion. In: Psychiatric epidemiology. Proceedings of the international symposium held at Aberdeen University, 1969. Hare, E.H., Wing, J.K. (eds.), pp. 69-86. London, New York, Toronto: 1970
311. Sack, F.: Probleme der Kriminalsoziologie. In: Handbuch der empirischen Sozialforschung. Koenig, R. (ed.), Vol. II, pp. 961-1049. Stuttgart: Enke 1969
312. Sangree, W.H.: The social functions of beer drinking in Bantu Tiriki. In: Society, culture and drinking. Pittman, D.J., Snyder, C.R. (eds.), pp. 6-21. New York: Wiley 1962
313. Satin, D.G.: Life stresses and psychosocial problems in the hospial emergency unit. Soc. Psychiatry 7, 119-126 (1972)
314. Schelsky, H.: Industrie- und Betriebssoziologie. In: Soziologie. Ein Lehr- und Handbuch zur modernen Gesellschaftskunde. Gehlen, A., Schelsky, H. (eds.), pp. 159-203. Düsseldorf, Cologne: Diederichs 1955
315. Scherhorn, G.: Soziologie des Konsums. In: Handbuch der empirischen Sozialkunde. Koenig, R. (ed.), Vol. II, pp. 834-862. Stuttgart: Enke 1969
316. Scheuch, E.K.: Soziologie der Freizeit. In: Handbuch der empirischen Sozialforschung. Koenig, R. (ed.), Vol. II, pp. 735-833. Stuttgart: Enke 1969
317. Schmidbauer, W., Vom Scheidt, J.: Handbuch der Rauschdrogen. München: Nymphenburger 1971
318. Schneider, P.B.: Zum Verhältnis von Psychoanalyse und psychosomatischer Medizin. Psyche 1, 21-49 (1973)
319. Schnidrig, A.L.: Das Walser Haus. Wir Walser 11/2, 2-3 (1973)
320. Schuckit, M.A.: Family history and half-sibling research in alcoholism. Ann. N.Y. Acad. Sci. 197, 121-125 (1972)
321. Schwanenberg, E.: Psychoanalyse versus Sozioanalyse oder die Aggression als kritisches Problem im Vergleich von Freud und Parsons. In: Psychoanalyse als Sozialwissenschaft. Lorenzer, A., Dahmer, H., Horn, K., Brede, K., Schwanenberg, E. (eds.), pp. 199-236. Frankfurt: Suhrkamp 1971
322. Schwidder, W.: Klinik der Neurosen. In: Psychiatrie der Gegenwart, 2nd ed., Kisker, K.P., Meyer, S.E., Müller, M., Strömgren, E. (eds.), Vol. II/1, pp. 351-476. Berlin, Heidelberg, New York: Springer 1972
323. Selye, H.: The stress of life. New York: McGraw-Hill 1956
324. Shannon, C.A., Weaver, W.: The mathematical theory of communication. Chicago: Urbana University of Illinois Press 1949
325. Shepherd, M.: Psychiatric epidemiology and general practice. Introduction. In: Psychiatric epidemiology. Proceedings of the international symposium held at Aberdeen University, 1969. Hare, E.H., Wing, J.K. (eds.), pp. 281-282. London, New York, Toronto: 1970
326. Shepherd, M., Cooper, B., Brown, A.C., Kalton, G.W.: Psychiatric illness in general practice. London: Oxford University Press 1966
327. Silbermann, A., Luthe, H.O.: Massenkommunikation. In: Handbuch der empirischen Sozialforschung. Koenig, R. (ed.), Vol. II, pp. 675-734. Stuttgart: Enke 1969
328. Simmons, O.G.: Ambivalence and the learning of drinking behavior in a Peruvian community. In: Society, culture and drinking. Pittman, D.J., Snyder, C.R. (eds.), pp. 37-47. New York: Wiley 1962
329. Skinner, B.F.: Beyond freedom and dignity. Toronto, New York, London: Bantam & Vintage 1972
330. Skolnick, J.H.: Religious affiliation and the drinking behavior. Quart. J. Stud. Acohol 19, 452-470 (1958)
331. Smoking and health now. A report of the Royal College of Physicians of London. London: Pitman 1971
332. Snyder, C.R.: Culture and Jewish sobriety: the ingroup-outgroup factor. In: Society, culture and drinking. Pittman, D.J., Snyder, C.R. (eds.), pp. 188-225. New York: Wiley 1962

333. Solms, H.: Notwendige Abwandlungen der Behandlungsmethoden des chronischen Alkoholismus infolge regionaler Verschiedenheit der Trinksitten und der Alkoholkrankheiten. In: Arbeitstagung über Alkoholismus. Kryspin-Exner, K. (ed.), pp. 142-157. Wien: Romayor 1962
334. Solms, H.: Süchtigkeit als individual-pathologisches Schicksal und allgemein-menschliches Problem. In: Rauschmittel und Süchtigkeit. Probleme im Gespräch, Vol. 3, pp. 35-44. Bern, Frankfurt: Lang 1971
335. Solms, H.: Psychodynamik des Alkoholismus. In: Psychiatrie der Gegenwart. 2nd ed., Kisker, K.P., Meyer, S.E., Müller, M., Strömgren, E. (eds.), Vol. II/2, pp. 389-406. Berlin, Heidelberg, New York: Springer 1972
336. Somerhausen, C.: Warum wird von einem Drogenproblem gesprochen? In: Rauschmittel und Süchtigkeit. Probleme im Gespräch, Vol. 3. pp. 25-34. Bern, Frankfurt: Lang 1971
337. Spiegel, J.: Transactions, the interplay between individual, family and society. New York: Science House 1971
338. Spiegel-Magazin, 28/38, Sept. 16, 1974
339. Srole, L., Langner, T.S., Michael, S.T., Opler, M.K., Rennie, T.A.C.: Mental health in the metropolis: The Midtown Manhattan Study. New York: McGraw-Hill 1962
340. Stacey, R., Davies, J.: Drinking behavior in childhood and adolescence, an evaluative review. Br. J. Addict. 65, 203-212 (1970)
341. Stanway, R.G., Mullin, R.P.: The relationship of exercise response to personality. Psychol. Med. 3, 343-349 (1973)
342. Statistisches Jahrbuch des Kantons Wallis: Sitten 1970
343. Stein, Z., Susser, M.W.: Bereavement as precipitating event in mental illness. In: Psychiatric epidemiology. Proceedings of the international symposium held at Aberdeen University, 1969. Hare, E.H., Wing, J.K. (eds.), pp. 327-333. London, New York, Toronto: 1970
344. Stone, G.P.: Drinking styles and status arrangements. In: Society, culture and drinking. Pittman, D.J., Snyder, C.R. (eds.), pp. 121-140. New York: Wiley 1962
345. Strotzka, H.: Einführung in die Sozialpsychiatrie. Reinbek: Rowohl 1965
346. Strotzka, H.: Kleinburg, eine sozialpsychiatrische Feldstudie. Wien: Österreichischer Bundesverlag 1969
347. Strotzka, H., Grumiller, I.: Krankheit als soziales Phänomen. Internist 13, 403-408 (1973)
348. Supersaxo, P.: Fremdenverkehr in Saas-Fee von 1880-1960. Saas-Fee: Verlag des Verkehrsvereins Saas-Fee 1960
349. Taeschner, K.L.: Zur Epidemiologie und Äthiologie des Drogenkonsums Jugendlicher. Münch. Med. Wochenschr. 115, 2275-2279 (1973)
350. Tanter, R., Midlarsky, M.: Revolutionen. Eine Quantitative Analyse. In: Theorien des sozialen Wandels. Zypf, W. (ed.), pp. 418-440. Cologne, Berlin: Kiepenheuer & Witsch 1971
351. Thayer, L.: Communication-systems. In: The relevance of general systems theory. Laszlo, E. (ed.), pp. 93-122. New York: Braziller 1972
352. Theorell, T., Rahe, R.H.: Psychosocial factors and myocardial infarction: an in-patient study in Sweden. J. Psychosom. Res. 15, 25-31 (1971)
353. Theorell, T., Rahe, R.H.: Psychosocial factors and myocardial infarction: an out-patient study in Sweden. J. Psychosom. Res. 15, 33-39 (1971)
354. The health consequences of smoking. A Public Health Service review. US Department of Health, Education and Welfare. Public Health Service publication, Vol. 1696, 1967
355. Thomas, K.: Die künstlich gesteuerte Seele. Stuttgart: Enke 1970
356. Tjaden, K.H.: Soziales System und sozialer Wandel. Stuttgart: Enke 1972
357. Touraine, A.: Industriesoziologie. In: Handbuch der empirischen Sozialforschung. Koenig, R. (ed.), Vol. II. pp. 408-443. Stuttgart: Enke 1969
358. Trice, H.M.: The job behavior of problem drinkers. In: Society, culture and drinking. Pittman, D.J., Snyder, C.R. (eds.), pp. 493-510. New York: Wiley 1962
359. Trice, H.M., Wahl, R.J.: A rank order analysis of the symptoms of alcoholism. In: Society, culture and drinking. Pittman, D.J., Snyder, C.R. (eds.), pp. 369-381. New York: Wiley 1962
360. Uhlenhuth, E.H., Paykel, E.S.: Symptom configuration and life events. Arch. Gen. Psychiatry 28, 744-748 (1973)

361. Walton, H.S.: Personality as determinant of the form of alcoholism. Br. J. Psychiatry *114*, 761-766 (1968)
362. Warder, J., Ross, C.J.: Age and alcoholism. Br. J. Addict. *66*, 45-51 (1971)
363. Watzlawick, P., Beavin, J.H., Jackson, D.D.: Menschliche Kommunikation. Formen, Störungen, Paradoxien. Wien: Huber 1974
364. Watzlawick, P., Weakland, J., Fisch, R.: Changements, paradoxes et psychothérapie. Paris: Seuil 1975
365. Wein, H.: Zur Integration der neuen Wissenschaft vom Menschen. Psyche *4*, 721-741 (1959)
366. Weingarten, G.: Mental performance during physical exertion, the benefit of beeing physically fut. Int. J. Sport Psychol. *1*, 16-26 (1973)
367. Wiener, N.: Cybernetics. New York: Wiley and Sons 1948
368. Wiener, N.: The human use of human beings. Cybernetics and society. New York: Avon 1954
369. Wieser, S., Kunad, E.: Katamnestische Studien beim chronischen Alkoholismus und zur Frage von Sozialprozessen bei Alkoholikern. Nervenarzt *36*, 477-483 (1965)
370. Wing, J.K.: A standard form of psychiatric present state examination and a method for standardizing the classification of symptoms. In: Psychiatric epidemiology. Proceedings of the international symposium held at Aberdeen University, 1969. Hare, E.H., Wing, J.K. (eds.), pp. 93-108. London, New York, Toronto: 1970
371. Wittkower, E.D., Dubreuil, G.: Psychocultural stress in relation to mental illness. Soc. Sci. Med. *7*, 691-704 (1973)
372. Wolf, S.: Regulatory mechanisms and tissue pathology. In: Emotions, their parameters and measurement. Levi, L. (ed.), pp. 619-626. New York: Raven Press 1975
373. Wylie, L.: Dorf in der Vaucluse. Der Alltag einer französischen Gemeinde. Frankfurt: Fischer 1969
374. Wynne, L.C., Singer, M.T., Bartko, J.J., Tochey, M.L.: Schizophrenics and their families: Recent Research on parental communication. In: Developments in psychiatric research. Tanner, J.E. (ed.), pp. 1-75. Sevenoaks, Kent: Hodder and Stoughton 1977
375. Wyss, D.: Marx und Freud. Ihr Verhältnis zur modernen Anthropologie. Göttingen: Vandenhoeck & Wuprecht 1969
376. Wurzbacher, G., Pflaum, R.: Das Dorf im Spannungsfeld der industriellen Entwicklung. Stuttgart: Enke 1954
377. Zacune, J., Hensman, C., Heinemann, W.: Drugs, alcohol and tobacco in Britain. London: Medical Books 1971
378. Zapf, E. (ed.): Theorien des sozialen Wandels. Cologne, Berlin: Kiepenheuer & Witsch 1970
379. Zohman, B.L.: Emotional factors and coronary disease. Geriatrics *2*, 110-119 (1973)
380. Zucchi, '.: Ricerche sui rapporti fra l'alcoolismo dell' adulto e la tendenza all' alcool nelle prime eta della vita. Neuropsychiatria *12*, 389-425 (1956)
381. Zuckmayer, C.: Als wär's ein Stück von mir. Frankfurt: Fischer 1966
382. Zwaga, H.J.G.: Psychophysiological reactions to mental tasks: effort or stress? Ergonomics *1*, 61-67 (1973)

Subject Index

acculturation 4, 22, 31, 52, 101 ff., 113,
    158 ff., 173
agriculture 2, 65 ff., 140 ff.
achievement motivation 24, 60, 95
alcohol consumption and alcoholism 219 ff.
    age 220 f., 233, 234, 236, 243
    birth order 222, 241
    causes 228, 243 ff.
    consequences 230
    definition 219
    economic factors 226, 237, 242
    family 224, 235, 236, 241 f.
    function 227, 245
    genetic factors 222
    group 225
    marital status 221
    occupational roles 221 f., 237, 243 f.
    personality structure 223 ff., 235, 238 f.
    quantitative aspects 246 f.
    religion 222
    rural areas 230 f.
    sex 221, 236
    social mobility 222
    socialization 225, 235
    sociocultural factors 225, 231 f., 240 f.
    types 229, 247
Alemans 48
anthropology 6
architecture 8, 9, 62 ff., 132 f.

Burgunds 47

catastrophes 57 f., 78 ff.
Celtics 47 f.
character formation 31, 60 ff., 88 ff., 153 ff.
climate 44 f.
clubs and associations 53, 99 ff., 157 f.
communication
    means 45, 48, 58 ff., 130 f.
    mechanisms 92 ff.
    theories 4, 34
community
    budget 70
    Burgher 74, 99 f.
    municipal 49, 74, 97, 99 f., 134 f.

conspicuous consumption 2 f.
costumes 104 ff., 160 ff.
criminality 290 ff.
    definitions 290
    delinquent 290 f.
    social environment 291 f.
    statistics 292 f.
    types 292 f.
crisis
    personal 12, 147, 159, 245
    social 11, 147
    systemic 16, 147, 245
cross-sectional study 39
cultural lag 8, 18, 121, 146, 172
customs 81 f., 107 ff., 160 ff.
cybernetics 4, 18 ff., 33 f., 91 ff.

demographic subsystem 53 ff.
determinants and metadeterminants 87 ff.
diachronic perspective 45 ff.
drug consumption 249 ff.
    age 253, 255 f., 261
    causes 250 f.
    consequences 252
    definitions 250
    marital status 253, 258, 262
    occupational roles 254, 257, 258
    personality 252, 258, 262
    sex 253, 256 f., 261 f.
    social class 254
    socioeconomic factors 250 f., 258, 259, 262 f.
    types 250, 252, 254, 260 f.

ecological approach 12, 33 f.
ecological system 3, 42, 45 f., 53
economic base 4 f., 11, 33, 68 f., 89
economic development 10, 56 ff., 118, 119,
    129 f.
economic infrastructure 2, 11, 52, 62 f., 70
economy of subsistence 4 f., 89
elites 23
emigrations 5, 102
environment 3, 12, 42
ethnic blend 46 ff.
expiation behavior 78 ff.

Schriften-reihe Neurologie

Neurology Series

Herausgeber:
H. J. Bauer, G. Baumgartner,
A. N. Davison, H. Hänshirt,
P. Vogel

Die Bezieher des Archiv für Psychiatrie und Nervenkrankheiten, der Zeitschrift für Neurologie/Journal of Neurology und des Zentralblatt für die gesamte Neurologie und Psychiatrie erhalten die Schriftenreihe zu einem um 10 % ermäßigten Vorzugspreis.

Band 1: W. Kahle
Die Entwicklung der menschlichen Großhirnhemisphäre
1969. Antiquarisch
ISBN 3-540-04703-4

Band 2: A. Prill
Die neurologische Symptomatologie der akuten und chronischen Niereninsuffizienz
Befunde zur pathogenetischen Wertigkeit von Stoffwechsel-, Elektrolyt- und Wasserhaushaltsstörungen sowie zur Pathologie der Blut/Hirn-Schrankenfunktion. 1969. Antiquarisch
ISBN 3-540-04704-2

Band 3: K. Kunze
Das Sauerstoffdruckfeld im normalen und pathologisch veränderten Muskel.
Untersuchungen mit einer neuen Methode zur quantitativen Erfassung der Hypoxie in situ. 1969. Antiquarisch
ISBN 3-540-04705-0

Band 4: H. Pilz
Die Lipide des normalen und pathologischen Liquor cerebrospinalis. 1970. Antiquarisch
ISBN 3-540-05007-8

Band 5: F. Rabe
Die Kombination hysterischer und epileptischer Anfälle.
Das Problem der "Hysteroepilepsie" in neuer Sicht. Mit einem Geleitwort von E. Bay. 1970
ISBN 3-540-05008-6

Band 6: J. Ulrich
Die cerebralen Entmarkungserkrankungen im Kindesalter
Diffuse Hirnsklerosen. Mit einem Geleitwort von F. Lüthy. 1971
ISBN 3-540-05244-5

Band 7: K. H. Puff
Die klinische Elektromyographie in der Differentialdiagnose von Neuro- und Myopathien
Eine Bilanz. 1971
ISBN 3-540-05527-4

Band 8: K. Piscol
Die Blutversorgung des Rückenmarkes und ihre klinische Relevanz
1972. Antiquarisch
ISBN 3-540-05740-4

Band 9: M. Wiesendanger
Pathopysiology of Muscle Tone
1972
ISBN 3-540-05761-7

Band 10: H. Spiess
Schädigungen am peripheren Nervensystem durch ionisierende Strahlen
Mit ausführlicher englischer Zusammenfassung. 1972
ISBN 3-540-05763-3

Band 11: B. Neundörfer
Differentialtypologie der Polyneuritiden und Polyneuropathien.
1973
ISBN 3-540-06062-6

Band 12: H. Lange-Cosack; G. Tepfer
Das Hirntrauma im Kindes- und Jugendalter
Klinische und hirnelektrische Längsschnittuntersuchungen an 240 Kindern und Jugendlichen mit frischen Schädelhirntraumen. Unter Mitarbeit von H.-J. Schlesener. Mit einem Geleitwort von W. Tönnis. 1973
ISBN 3-540-06262-9

Band 13: S. Kunze
Die zentrale Ventrikulographie mit wasserlöslichen, resorbierbaren Kontrastmitteln
1974. Antiquarisch
ISBN 3-540-06782-5

Band 14: E. Sluga
Polyneuropathien
Typen und Differenzierung. Ergebnisse bioptischer Untersuchungen. 1974
ISBN 3-540-06945-3

Band 15: H. F. Herrschaft
Die regionale Gehirndurchblutung
Meßmethoden, Regulation, Veränderungen bei den cerebralen Durchblutungsstörungen und pharmakologische Beeinflußbarkeit. 1975
ISBN 3-540-07363-9

Band 16: R. Heene
Experimental Myopathies and Muscular Dystrophy
Studies in the Formal Pathogenesis of the Myopathy of 2,4-Dichlorophenoxyacetate. 1975
ISBN 3-540-07376-0

Band 17: T. Tsuboi; W. Christian
Epilepsy
A Clinical, Electroencephalographic and Statistical Study of 466 Patients. 1976
ISBN 3-540-07735-9

Band 18: E. Esslen
The Acute Facial Palsies
Investigations on the Localization and Pathogenesis of Meato-Labyrinthine Facial Palsies. With a foreword by U. Fisch. 1977
ISBN 3-540-08018-X

Band 19: J. Jörg
Die elektrosensible Diagnostik in der Neurologie
Mit einem Geleitwort von E. Bay. 1977
ISBN 3-540-08236-0

Band 20: S. Poser
Multiple Sclerosis
An Analysis of 812 Cases by Means of Electronic Data Processing. 1978
ISBN 3-540-08644-7

Band 21: M. Oehmichen
Mononuclear Phagocytes in the Central Nervous System
Origin, Mode of Distribution, and Function of Progressive Microglia, Parivascular Cells of Intracerebral Vessels, Free Subarachnoidal Cells, and Epiplexus Cells. Translated from the German by M. M. Clarkson. 1978
ISBN 3-540-08958-6

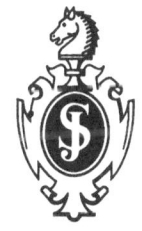

Springer-Verlag
Berlin
Heidelberg
New York

Monographien aus dem Gesamtgebiete der Psychiatrie Psychiatry Series

Herausgeber: H. Hippius, W. Janzarick, C. Müller

1. Band: K. Hartmann
Theoretische und empirische Beiträge zur Verwahrlosungsforschung
2., neubearbeitete und erweiterte Auflage. 1977. 16 Abbildungen, 34 Tabellen XII, 180 Seiten
ISBN 3-540-07925-4

2. Band: P. Matussek
Die Konzentrationslagerhaft und ihre Folgen
Mit R. Grigat, H. Haiböck, G. Halbach, R. Kemmler, D. Manteil, A. Triebel, M. Vardy, G. Wedel. 1971. 19 Abbildungen, 73 Tabellen. X, 272 Seiten
ISBN 3-540-05214-3

3. Band: A. E. Adams
Informationstheorie und Psychopathologie des Gedächtnisses
Methodische Beiträge zur experimentellen und klinischen Beurteilung mnestischer Leistungen. 1971. 12 Abbildungen. IX, 124 Seiten. ISBN 3-540-05215-1

4. Band: G. Nissen
Depressive Syndrome im Kindes- und Jugendalter
Beitrag zur Symptomatologie, Genese und Prognose
1971. 11 Abbildungen, 51 Tabellen. IX, 174 Seiten
ISBN 3-540-05493-6

5. Band: A. Moser
Die langfristige Entwicklung Oligophrener
Mit einem Vorwort von Chr. Müller. 1971. 4 Abbildungen, 30 Tabellen. X, 102 Seiten
ISBN 3-540-05599-1

6. Band: H. Feldmann
Hypochondrie
Leibbezogenheit. Risikoverhalten. Entwicklungsdynamik
1972. 36 Abbildungen, 5 Tabellen. VI, 118 Seiten
ISBN 3-540-05753-6

7. Band, S. Meyer-Osterkamp, R. Cohen
Zur Größenkonstanz bei Schizophrenen
Eine experimentalpsychologische Untersuchung. Mit einem einführenden Geleitwort von H. Heimann. 1973. 5 Abbildungen VII, 91 Seiten
ISBN 3-540-06147-9

8. Band: K. Diebold
Die erblichen myoklonisch-epileptisch-dementiellen Kernsyndrome
Progressive Myoklonusepilepsien – Dyssynergia cerebellaris myoclonica – myoklonische Varianten der drei nachinfantilen Formen der amaurotischen Idiotie 1973. 31 Abbildungen. IX, 254 Seiten. ISBN 3-540-06117-7

9. Band: C. Eggers
Verlaufsweisen kindlicher und präpuberalen Schizophrenien
1973. 3 Abbildungen. IX, 250 Seiten. ISBN 3-540-06163-0

10. Band: M. Schrenk
Über den Umgang mit Geisteskranken
Die Entwicklung der psychiatrischen Therapie vom „moralischen Regime" in England und Frankreich zu den „psychischen Curmethoden" in Deutschland 1973. 20 Abbildungen. IX, 194 Seiten. ISBN 3-540-06267-X

11. Band: Heinz Schepank
Erb- und Umweltfaktoren bei Neurosen
Tiefenpsychologische Untersuchungen an 50 Zwillingspaaren Unter Mitarbeit von P. E. Becker, A. Heigl-Evers, C. O. Köhler, Helga Schepank, G. Wagner 1974. 1 Abbildung, 82 Tabellen. VIII, 227 Seiten
ISBN 3-540-06647-0

12. Band: L. Ciompi, C. Müller
Lebensweg und Alter der Schizophrenen
Eine katamnestische Langzeitstudie bis ins Senium. 1976. 27 Fallbeispiele, 23 Abbildungen, 48 Tabellen. IX, 242 Seiten
ISBN 3-540-07567-4

13. Band: L. Süllwold
Symptome schizophrener Erkrankungen
Uncharakteristische Basisstörungen. 1977. 15 Tabellen. VIII, 112 Seiten. ISBN 3-540-08203-4

14. Band:
The Apallic Snydrome
Editors: G. Dalle Ore, F. Gerstenbrand, C. H. Lücking, G. Peters, U. H. Peters. With the editorial assistance of E. Rothemund 1977. 67 figures, 17 tables. XV, 259 pages (5 pages in German) ISBN 3-540-08301-4

15. Band: O. Benkert
Sexuelle Impotenz
Neuroendokrinologische und pharmakotherapeutische Untersuchungen. 1977. 33 Abbildungen, 20 Tabellen. VIII, 139 Seiten. ISBN 3-540-08427-4

16. Band: R. Avenarius
Der Größenwahn
Erscheinungsbilder und Entstehungsweise. 1978. VI, 98 Seiten. ISBN 3-540-08547-5

17. Band:
Psychiatrische Epidemiologie
Geschichte, Einführung und ausgewählte Forschungsergebnisse Herausgeber: H. Häfner Mit Beiträgen zahlreicher Fachwissenschaftler. 1978. 20 Abbildungen, 91 Tabellen. XII, 252 Seiten. ISBN 3-540-08629-3

18. Band:
Transmethylations and the Central Nervous System
Editors: V. M. Andreoli, A. Agnoli C. Fazio. 1978. 45 figures, 44 tables. VI, 185 pages ISBN 3-540-08693-5

19. Band:
Psychiatrische Therapie-Forschung
Ethische und juristische Probleme Herausgeber: H. Helmchen, B. Müller-Oerlinghausen Mit Beiträgen zahlreicher Fachwissenschaftler. 1978. XII, 180 Seiten. ISBN 3-540-08732-X

20. Band: R. M. Torack
The Pathologic Physiology of Dementia
With Indications for Diagnosis and Treatment 1978. 11 figures, 24 tables. VIII, 155 pages ISBN 3-540-08904-7

21. Band: G. Huber, G. Gross, R. Schüttler
Schizophrenie
Verlaufs- und sozialpsychiatrische Langzeituntersuchungen an den 1945-1959 in Bonn hospitalisierten schizophrenen Kranken 1979. 2 Abbildungen, 112 Tabellen. XIII, 399 Seiten
ISBN 3-540-09014-2

Springer-Verlag Berlin Heidelberg New York